Mundei.
2006.

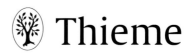

Peripheral Regional Anesthesia

An Atlas of Anatomy and Techniques

Gisela Meier, M.D.

Head of the Department of Anesthesia
and Interventional Pain Therapy
Oberammergau Center for Rheumatology
Oberammergau, Germany

Johannes Buettner, M.D.

Head of the Department of Anesthesia
Trauma Center
Murnau, Germany

422 illustrations

Thieme
Stuttgart · New York

Library of Congress Cataloging-in-Publication Data

Meier, Gisela, 1954 -
  [Atlas der peripheren Regionalanästhesie. English]
  Atlas of peripheral anesthesia techniques : anatomy, anesthesia, pain therapy / Gisela Meier, Johannes Buettner.
      p. ; cm.
  Includes bibliographical references and index.
  ISBN 3-13-139791-8 (alk. paper)—
  ISBN 1-58890-429-6 (alk. paper)
1. Conduction anesthesia—Atlases.
[DNLM: 1. Anesthesia, Conduction—Atlases. 2. Nerve Block—methods—Atlases. 3. Pain—prevention & control—Atlases. WO 300 M511a 2005a] I. Büttner, Johannes, 1650- II. Title.
  RD84.M45 2005
  617.9'64—dc22
          2005019630

This book is an authorized and revised translation of the German edition published and copyrighted 2004 by Georg Thieme Verlag, Stuttgart, Germany. Title of the German edition: Atlas der peripheren Regional-anästhesie. Anatomie - Anästhesie - Schmerztherapie

Translator: mt-g medical translation gmbh, Neu Ulm
Illustrators: Nikolaus Lechenbauer and Gerhard Schlich for Astra Zeneca; Peter Haller, Stuttgart

Important note: Medicine is an ever-changing science undergoing continual development. Research and clinical experience are continually expanding our knowledge, in particular our knowledge of proper treatment and drug therapy. Insofar as this book mentions any dosage or application, readers may rest assured that the authors, editors, and publishers have made every effort to ensure that such references are in accordance with **the state of knowledge at the time of production of the book.**
Nevertheless, this does not involve, imply, or express any guarantee or responsibility on the part of the publishers in respect to any dosage instructions and forms of applications stated in the book. **Every user is requested to examine carefully** the manufacturers' leaflets accompanying each drug and to check, if necessary in consultation with a physician or specialist, whether the dosage schedules mentioned therein or the contraindications stated by the manufacturers differ from the statements made in the present book. Such examination is particularly important with drugs that are either rarely used or have been newly released on the market. Every dosage schedule or every form of application used is entirely at the user's own risk and responsibility. The authors and publishers request every user to report to the publishers any discrepancies or inaccuracies noticed. If errors in this work are found after publication, errata will be posted at www.thieme.com on the product description page.

© 2006 Georg Thieme Verlag,
Rüdigerstrasse 14, 70469 Stuttgart, Germany
http://www.thieme.de
Thieme New York, 333 Seventh Avenue,
New York, NY 10001 USA
http://www.thieme.com

Typesetting by primustype Hurler GmbH, Notzingen
Printed in Germany by Grammlich, Pliezhausen
ISBN 3-13-139791-8 (GTV)
ISBN 1-58890-429-6 (TNY)   1 2 3 4 5

Foreword

Compared to general anesthesia, regional anesthesia can provide anatomically selective anesthesia with less interference with the patient's vital functions and a reduced need for opiates. Using a continuous catheter technique, the regional block can be transformed into a likewise selective analgesia with similar advantages for postoperative and other pain management.

Regional anesthesia is sometimes considered an art; this art can, however, be learnt by any interested anesthesiologist who has access to professional instructions and a good training program. The most exclusive form of regional anesthesia is peripheral nerve blockade, and for colleagues interested in practicing peripheral nerve and plexus blocks, this Atlas is an excellent source of clear and instructive descriptions of most clinically relevant extremity blocks. The art of peripheral nerve blockade is based on good anatomical understanding, careful handling of needles, catheters and patients, and good knowledge of pharmacology of local anesthetics. All these components are well presented in this Atlas.

Today's technology offers advanced assistance in localizing the target nerve; however, the use of electrostimulation or ultrasonography, for example, does not reduce the importance of anatomical knowledge. In my opinion, a competent anesthetist should also be able to find most peripheral nerves without this special equipment. And those readers who have carefully studied this Atlas will certainly be able to do that!

Nösund, Orust, Sweden   Dag E. Selander

Acknowledgements

The authors of this book consider themselves lucky to have had the continued support for many years of trusted colleagues and numerous friends. In the last decade we have been actively involved, both as speakers and tutors, in courses on anatomy for regional anesthesia and pain management at Innsbruck University, Austria. Thanks to Drs. Christoph Huber, Gottfried Mitterschiffthaler, and Asst. Prof. Herbert Maurer and their courses, the field of anatomy has been opened up for special clinical and anesthesiological questions. During this time we were able to discuss various questions pertaining to peripheral blocking techniques. Together we carried out scientific research at the Department of Anatomy in order to clarify specific problems. Our special thanks go to all our colleagues and friends at Innsbruck University.

Other colleagues in Germany and Austria, both in Anesthesia and in Anatomy, have kindly cooperated with the authors over years. There has been a long-standing exchange of experience among them. Asst. Prof. C. Dorn and Prof. Anderhuber (Graz University, Austria), Profs. J. Jage and Stofft (Mainz University, Germany), Profs. Kessler and H.-W. Korf (Frankfurt University, Germany), Profs. T. Standl and Z. Halata (Hamburg University, Germany), Dr. M. Gründling and Prof. Fanghänel (Greifswald University, Germany), and Prof. B. Freitag and Dr. S. Rudolph (Klinikum Südstadt Rostock, Germany) were very collegial and helpful and their cooperation lead to many new findings. In these institutes the authors also had the chance to regulary clarify anatomical details relevant to peripheral blocking. We received support from numerous colleagues and apologize that we are unable to mention all of them here. We thank all the members of the institutes.

We are especially grateful that the anatomists allowed us to take photographs of their specimens. Colleagues selflessly supplied photographic material. Dr. H. Kaiser (Rechberg Hospital Bretten, Germany) provided pictures showing complications of psoas compartment block. Profs. S. Kapral and P. Marhofer (Vienna University, Austria) have conducted scientific research on ultrasound techniques in guiding regional blockages and introduced them into clinical practice. They were kind enough to support us by providing ultrasound pictures. Many of the anatomical drawings for this book were produced by Mr. N. Lechenbauer. This was only possible with the support of B. Schmalz and R. Ploenes (AstraZeneca Co.). We also received active support in our own hospitals. In cooperation with the Department of Radiology at the Trauma Center Murnau, Germany (Director Dr. U. Esch), MRI pictures were taken using test persons in order to receive insight into deeper structures. Surgeons patiently waited for clinical pictures to be taken and members of staff made themselves available as test persons. Special thanks go to our staff. Dr. M. Neuburger (Trauma Center, Murnau) has been kind enough to let us have research results and took additional photographs and performed extra examinations. Drs. D. Lang (Trauma Center, Murnau) and C. Bauereis (Oberammergau Center for Rheumatology, Germany) have supported us in taking clinical pictures. Support from our own and other departments of our hospitals was so great that it is impossible to name everybody. We received a great deal of encouragement and many useful tips. This book is the result of many years of cooperation between anatomy and anesthesia. We would like to express our thanks to all those who have supported us along the way.

The *Atlas of Peripheral Regional Anesthesia* has won a lot of approval and recognition within the first month of publication in the German-speaking world. We thank Thieme Publisher's, notably Mrs A. C. Repnow and Mrs. A. Hollins, for their excellent cooperation and for making an English edition of this Atlas possible. We are proud to have acquired Dr. Dag Selander for revision of the translation. Dr. Selander is internationally renowned for his many publications in the field of regional anesthesia, including his article *Catheter technique in axillary plexus block* (Acta Anaesth Scand 1977;21:324-329). He was the first to describe continuous percutaneus axillary brachial plexus anesthesia. We are honored that Dr. Selander agreed, as a specialist in this field, to edit the translation and also supported us amicably with competent suggestions. We are grateful for this special support without which an English edition would have been impossible.

Panta rhei (Everything is in flux)
Heraklit (540-480 BC)

Oberammergau/Murnau

Gisela Meier and Johannes Buettner

Abbreviations

ASA	acetylsalicylic acid
b.w.	body weight
CAS	continuous anterior sciatic nerve block
CNB	central neuraxial block
CNS	central nervous system
COPD	chronic obstructive pulmonary disease
CRPS	complex regional pain syndrome
CT	computed tomography
ECG	electrocardiogram
G	Gauge
i.v.	intravenous
LA	local anesthetic
LOR	loss of resistance
PCA	patient-controlled analgesia
PNS	peripheral nerve stimulation
PTT	partial thromboplastin time
VIB	vertical infraclavicular block

Contents

Upper Limb

Lower Limb

General Considerations for Peripheral Nerve Blocks of the Limbs

Upper Limb

1   General Overview

1.1   Anatomy

The brachial plexus is formed by the anterior rami of the C5-C8 and T1 spinal nerves. The brachial plexus also contains contributions from C4 in over 60% of people, and from T2 in over 30% (Fig. 1.1). The roots of the spinal nerves exit from the spinal canal behind the vertebral artery and cross the transverse process of the corresponding vertebra. They then join to form three trunks and run together toward the first rib. The upper trunk arises from the union of the roots of C5/6, where the suprascapular nerve arises immediately as a lateral branch from the upper trunk. The middle trunk is formed by the root of C7, and the lower trunk by the roots of C8/T1. The trunks, which here lie on top of one another, pass between the scalenus anterior and scalenus medius muscles (the interscalene space). Just above the clavicle, the trunks each divide into an anterior and a posterior division. The three posterior divisions join to form the *posterior cord*, the anterior divisions of the upper and middle trunks form the *lateral cord*, and the *medial cord* is the continuation of the anterior division of the lower trunk. In the interscalene region, accordingly, we have the trunks initially, branching in the immediate supraclavicular and infraclavicular region, and then the cords. The cords lie very close together in the infraclavicular region. The *lateral cord* is the most superficial, the *posterior cord* is a little deeper and slightly lateral (!), and the *medial cord* lies deep. The cords lie craniolateral to the subclavian artery, which passes through the interscalene space

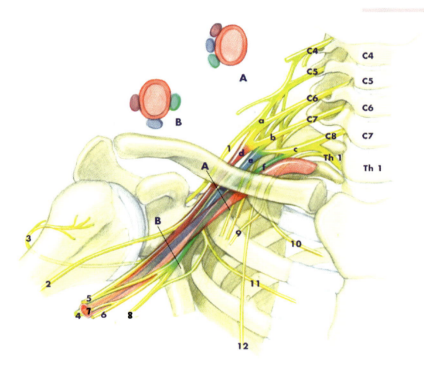

Fig. 1.**1**   Anatomy of the brachial plexus.

  a   Upper trunk (anterior rami of C5 and C6)
  b   Middle trunk (anterior ramus of C7)
  c   Lower trunk (anterior rami of C8 and T1)
  d   Lateral cord
  e   Posterior cord
  f   Medial cord
  1   Suprascapular nerve
  2   Musculocutaneous nerve
  3   Axillary nerve
  4   Radial nerve
  5   Median nerve
  6   Ulnar nerve
  7   Medial cutaneous nerve of forearm
  8   Medial cutaneous nerve of arm
  9   Intercostobrachial nerve I
  10 Intercostal nerve I
  11 Intercostal nerve II
  12 Long thoracic nerve

A and B: Sections in infraclavicular and axillary region (note position of cords)

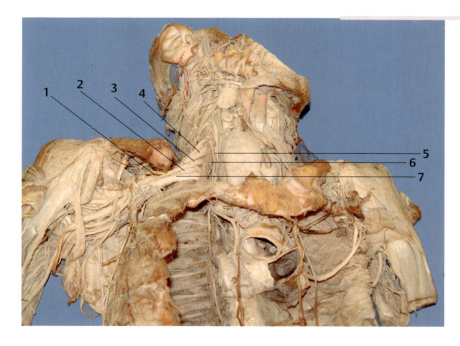

Fig. 1.**2**   Anatomy of the brachial plexus.

  1   Lateral cord
  2   Lower trunk
  3   Middle trunk
  4   Upper trunk
  5   Phrenic nerve
  6   Scalenus anterior
  7   Subclavian artery

together with the brachial plexus. The subclavian artery and brachial plexus pass into the axillary cavity inferior to the coracoid process (Figs. 1.**2**-1.**5**).

Overall, the cords rotate by about 90° around the axillary artery, with the medial cord passing under the artery and then combining with the lateral cord to form the *median nerve*. In the axilla the cords are actually located medially, laterally, and posteriorly in accordance with their names. The *ulnar nerve*, the medial cutaneous nerve of the arm and the medial nerve of the forearm,

and the medial root of the median nerve arise from the medial cord. After the *musculocutaneous nerve* has arisen from the lateral cord, this combines with parts of the medial cord to form the *median nerve* (Figs. 1.**6**-1.**8**). The posterior cord becomes the *radial nerve* after the origin of the axillary nerve (Figs. 1.**1** and 1.**5**). From its passage through the interscalene space as far as the axillary region, the entire brachial plexus is surrounded by a connective-tissue sheath (Fig. 1.**9**). Apart from the nerves, this also contains the blood vessels (axillary artery and vein). The subclavian

artery passes with the brachial plexus through the interscalene space, while the subclavian vein joins them medial to the anterior scalene muscle. There are connective-tissue septa inside this neurovascular sheath. However, in the majority of people, these do not appear to impede the steady spread of local anesthetic, so that a complete block of the brachial plexus is possible with a single injection, particularly in the supraclavicular, infraclavicular, and also axillary region.

Fig. 1.**3**   Anatomy of the brachial plexus.

1   Lateral cord
2   Lower trunk
3   Middle trunk
4   Upper trunk
5   Phrenic nerve
6   Scalenus anterior
7   Subclavian artery

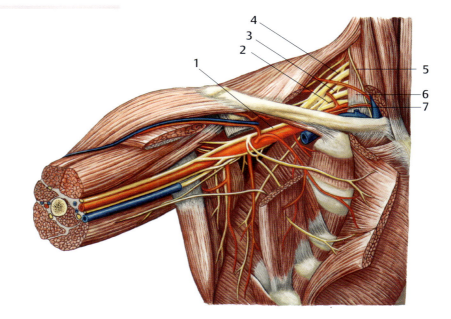

Fig. 1.**4**   Anatomy of the brachial plexus.

  1   Sternocleidomastoid
       (clavicular head divided)
  2   Scalenus anterior
  3   Scalenus medius
  4   Upper trunk
  5   Middle trunk
  6   Lower trunk
  7   Subclavian artery
  8   Posterior cord
  9   Medial cord
10   Lateral cord

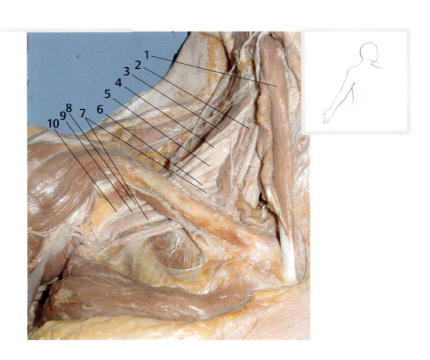

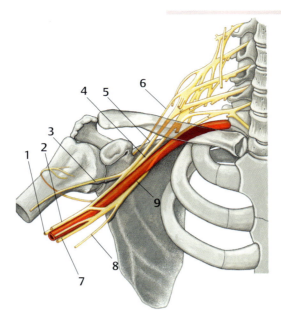

Fig. 1.**5**   Anatomy of the brachial plexus.

1   Radial nerve
2   Median nerve
3   Musculocutaneous nerve
4   Posterior cord
5   Lateral cord
6   Suprascapular nerve
7   Ulnar nerve
8   Medial cutaneous nerve of forearm
9   Medial cord

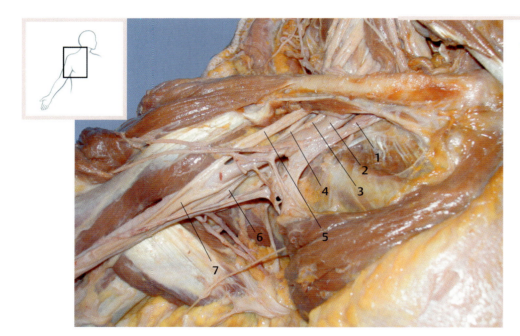

Fig. 1.**6**   Anatomy of the infraclavicular region.

1   Cephalic vein
2   Subclavian artery
3   Medial cord
4   Posterior cord
5   Lateral cord
6   Ulnar nerve
7   Median nerve

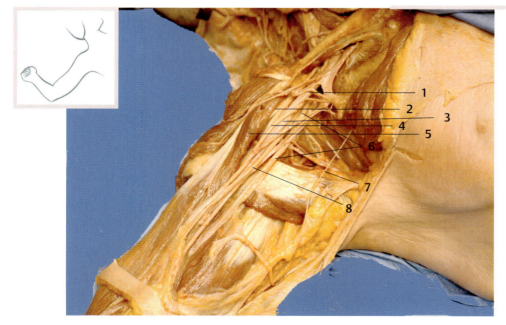

Fig. 1.**7**   Axillary plexus: anatomical overview.

1   Subclavian artery
2   Musculocutaneous nerve
3   Axillary artery
4   Median nerve with its two roots
5   Coracobrachialis
6   Ulnar nerve
7   Intercostobrachial nerve
8   Medial cutaneous nerve of forearm

Fig. 1.**8** Axillary plexus: anatomical overview.

1 Median nerve with its two roots
2 Musculocutaneous nerve
3 Lateral cord
4 Medial cutaneous nerve of forearm
5 Ulnar nerve
6 Medial cord contributing to the median nerve
7 Subclavian artery

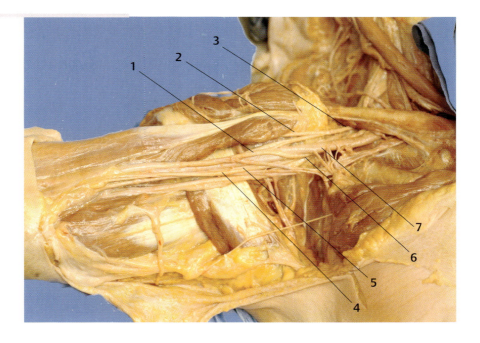

Fig. 1.**9** Neurovascular connective-tissue sheath of the brachial plexus.

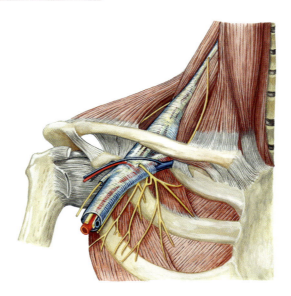

1.2 Important Topographical Anatomical Relations in the Region of the Brachial Plexus

The *phrenic nerve* runs on the belly of scalenus anterior (Figs. 1.**2**, 1.**3** and 1.**10**). If a response to stimulation of the phrenic nerve is triggered during interscalene block (contraction of the diaphragm), the position of the needle tip must be corrected laterally and posteriorly. Phrenic nerve paresis can be produced by the local anesthetic effect. *Recurrent nerve* block with hoarseness occurs occasionally (Fig. 1.**10**).

There are *cervical* and *thoracocervical sympathetic ganglia* in the immediate vicinity (Figs. 1.**10** and 1.**11**). Horner syndrome (miosis, ptosis, enophthalmos) can be produced by the local anesthetic effect. It is argued that bronchospasm can be triggered in asthmatic patients by the sympatholytic effect, but this is controversial. The *dome of the pleura* extends clearly above the first rib and is in the immediate vicinity of the structures described here (Fig. 1.**11**). The risk of

pneumothorax with the corresponding techniques in the supraclavicular and infraclavicular space must therefore be borne in mind. The *vertebral artery* lies anterior to the exit of the cervical spinal nerves through the intervertebral foramina (Fig. 1.**11**). If the needle is inserted in the wrong direction during interscalene block using the Winnie technique or in deep cervical plexus block, intravascular injection of the local anesthetic can occur. Only a few milliliters are suffi-

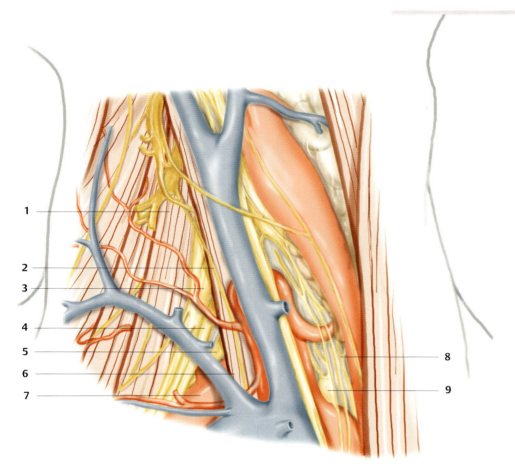

Fig. 1.**10**   Topographical anatomy of the brachial plexus.

1 Scalenus medius
2 Phrenic nerve
3 Upper trunk
4 Middle trunk
5 Lower trunk
6 Scalenus anterior
7 Subclavian artery
8 Recurrent laryngeal nerve
9 Stellate ganglion

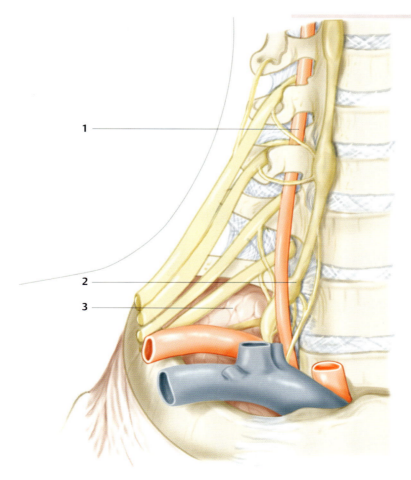

Fig. 1.**11**   Anatomy of the interscalene region.

1 Vertebral artery
2 Stellate ganglion
3 Dome of the pleura

cient to cause a seizure as the local anesthetic reaches the brain directly through the artery. The cervical *epidural and subarachnoid space can be punctured accidentally through the intervertebral foramina.* Cervical epidural or high spinal anesthesia can occur. Cervical spinal cord injuries with tetraplegia have also been described after interscalene plexus block, but only when this technique was used under general anesthesia.

1.3   Motor and Sensory Supply of the Upper Limb

Figure 1.**12** shows the different areas of sensory innervation of the skin.
The *motor responses* (Fig. 1.**13**) of the individual nerves are as follows:

- *Suprascapular nerve:* abduction and external rotation of the shoulder (supraspinatus and infraspinatus muscles).

- *Musculocutaneous nerve:* elbow flexion (biceps muscle).
- *Median nerve:* palmar flexion at the wrist, pronation of the forearm, flexion of the middle phalanges of the fingers, flexion of the distal phalanges of D II and D III, flexion of the thumb.

- *Ulnar nerve:* ulnar flexion of the wrist, flexion of the proximal phalanges of D III–V, adduction of the thumb.
- *Radial nerve:* extension of the elbow (triceps muscle), extension (and radial abduction) of the wrist, supination of the forearm and hand, extension of the fingers.

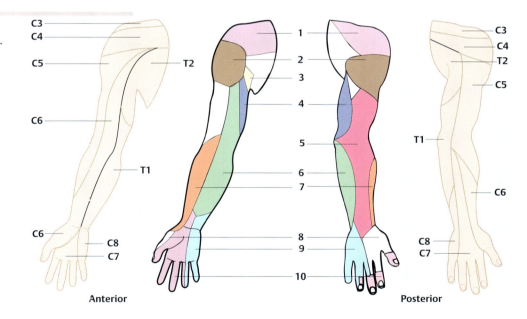

Fig. 1.12   Sensory supply of the upper limb.

1   Supraclavicular nerve
2   Axillary nerve (lateral cutaneous nerve of the arm)
3   Intercostobrachial nerve
4   Medial cutaneous nerve of arm
5   Dorsal cutaneous nerve of forearm (radial nerve)
6   Medial cutaneous nerve of forearm
7   Lateral cutaneous nerve of forearm (musculocutaneous nerve)
8   Radial nerve
9   Ulnar nerve
10   Median nerve

Anterior

Posterior

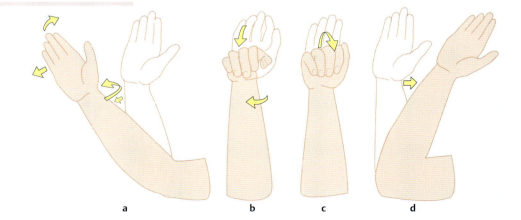

Fig. 1.13   Motor stimulus response of the individual nerves of the upper limb.

a   Radial nerve
b   Median nerve
c   Ulnar nerve
d   Musculocutaneous nerve

2   Interscalene Techniques of Brachial Plexus Block

2.1   Anatomy

The brachial plexus is formed by the anterior rami of spinal nerves C5-C8 and T1 and it sometimes receives contributions from C4 and T2. The roots of the spinal nerves exit from the spinal canal behind the vertebral artery and cross the transverse process of the corresponding vertebra. They then com-

bine to form three trunks and run together toward the first rib (Fig. 2.**1**). The *upper trunk* is formed by the junction of the roots of C5/6 and the *suprascapular nerve* arises immediately as a lateral branch from the upper trunk. The *middle trunk* is formed by the root of C7 and the *lower trunk* by the

roots of C8/T1. The trunks, which here lie on top of one another, cross the interscalene space between the scalenus anterior and scalenus medius muscles. Just above the clavicle, the trunks each divide into an anterior and a posterior division (Fig. 2.**2**). The three posterior divisions unite to form the

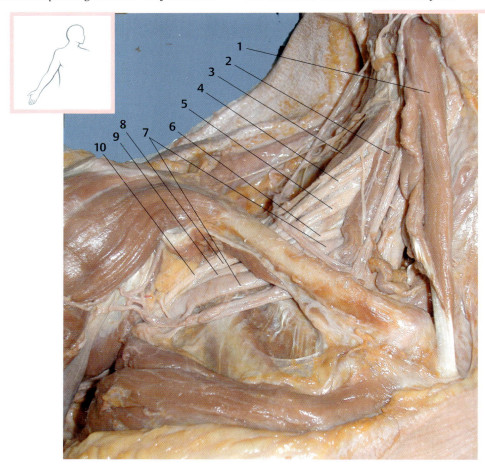

Fig. 2.**1**   Anatomy of the brachial plexus.

   1   Sternocleidomastoid
      (clavicular head divided)
   2   Scalenus anterior
   3   Scalenus medius
   4   Upper trunk
   5   Middle trunk
   6   Lower trunk
   7   Subclavian artery
   8   Posterior cord
   9   Medial cord
 10   Lateral cord

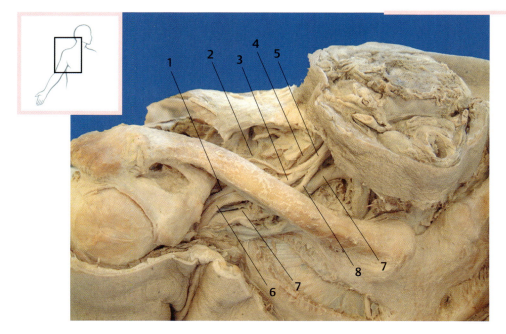

Fig. 2.**2**   Anatomy of the brachial plexus.

   1   Posterior cord
   2   Suprascapular nerve
   3   Upper trunk, posterior division
   4   Scalenus medius
   5   Upper trunk
   6   Lateral cord
   7   Subclavian artery
   8   Upper trunk, anterior division

Fig. 2.**3**   Anatomy of the brachial plexus (neurovascular sheath).

1   Sternocleidomastoid
2   Scalenus medius
3   Scalenus anterior with phrenic nerve
4   Neurovascular sheath (brachial plexus)

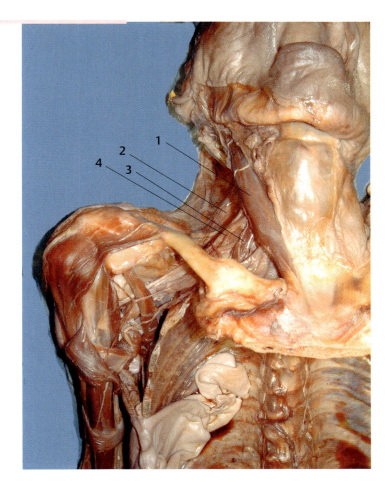

Fig. 2.**4**   Anatomy of the brachial plexus (neurovascular sheath).

1   Sternocleidomastoid
2   Scalenus medius
3   Scalenus anterior with phrenic nerve
4   Neurovascular sheath (brachial plexus)

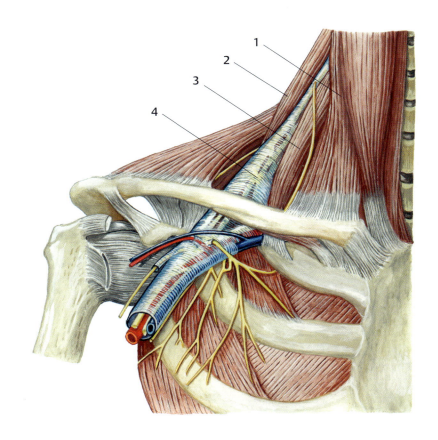

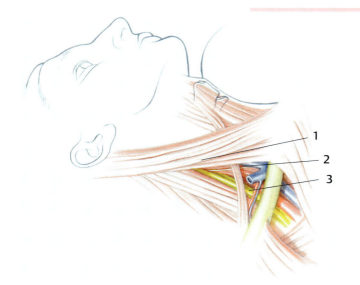

Fig. 2.**5**   Anatomy for orientation in inter-scalene plexus anesthesia.

1   Sternocleidomastoid
2   Scalenus anterior
    (with phrenic nerve)
3   Interscalene groove (with upper trunk
    and middle trunk)

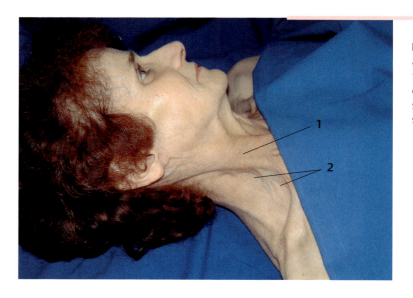

Fig. 2. **6**   Orientation in interscalene plexus anesthesia: Lifting the head, which is turned to the opposite side, makes the sternoclei-domastoid muscle stand out clearly, and in slim patients the scalene groove can be shown on deep inspiration.

1   Sternocleidomastoid
2   Interscalene groove

posterior cord, the anterior divisions of the upper trunk and middle trunk form the *lateral cord*, and the *medial cord* is the continuation of the anterior division of the lower trunk. In the interscalene region, accordingly, we have the trunks initially, dividing in the immediate supraclavicular and infraclavicular region, and then the *cords*.The lower trunk lies deepest and can be reached by an interscalene block only with difficulty (Fig. 2.**1**). At the caudal end of the interscalene space just above the clavicle, the subclavian artery emerges with the brachial plexus through the interscalene space, while the subclavian vein joins them

only after they emerge. Distally, the inter-scalene space is crossed by the omohyoid muscle, which can usually be palpated. The *phrenic nerve* (C3-C5) runs on the ventral surface of the anterior scalene muscle. The *cervical and thoracocervical sympathetic ganglia and the recurrent nerve* are in the immediate vicinity. The *vertebral artery* lies anterior to the exit of the cervical spinal nerves through the intervertebral foramina. The *cervical epidural and subarachnoid* space can be punctured accidentally through the intervertebral foramina. Cervical epidural or high spinal anesthesia can occur (Fig. 2.**8**).

From its entrance through the interscalene space as far as the axillary region, the entire brachial plexus is surrounded by a connective-tissue sheath (Figs. 2.**3**, 2.**4**). Connective-tissue septa may exist within this neurovascular sheath . However, in the majority of people, these do not appear to impede an even spread of local anesthetic.
The posterior border of the sternocleidomastoid muscle is used for orientation. It becomes prominent when the head is elevated ("sniffing position," Figs. 2.**5**, 2.**6**). In very thin patients, the interscalene groove can be palpated easily and it sometimes even becomes visible on deep inspiration.

2.2   General Overview

Interscalene block was first described in 1970 by Winnie. The puncture site is at the level of the cricoid cartilage in the interscalene groove. The needle direction is perpendicular

to the skin (medial, caudal, and dorsal) (Fig. 2.**7**). With this needle direction, the brachial plexus is no deeper than 2.5 cm. If the recommended needle direction is not strictly

observed, serious complications can occur (Fig. 2.**8**):

Fig. 2.**7**   Interscalene block, Winnie technique.

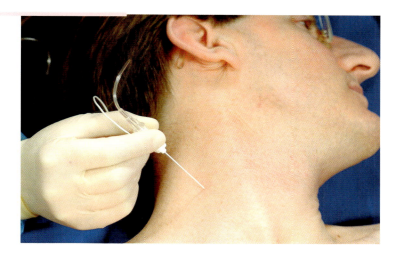

Fig. 2.**8**   Interscalene block: Winnie technique. Note: (1) Passing the needle vertical to the brachial plexus makes it difficult to advance an indwelling catheter. (2) Puncture of the vertebral artery is possible. (3) Puncture of the epidural or spinal space is possible.

1   Direction of the needle (Winnie technique)
2   Accidental puncture of the vertebral artery
3   Accidental subarachnoid (spinal) puncture
4   Vertebral artery
5   Stellate ganglion
6   Dome of the pleura

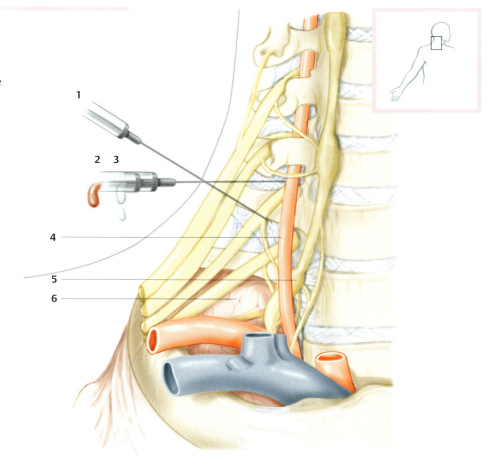

Fig. 2.**9**   Interscalene block, Meier technique.

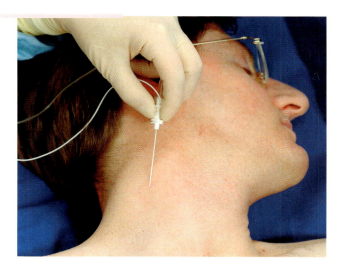

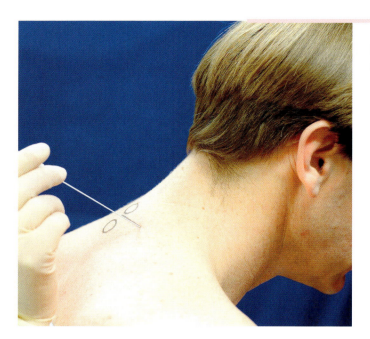

Fig. 2.**10** Interscalene block, Pippa technique.

- Puncture of the vertebral artery; injection of a few milliliters of the local anesthetic can cause a seizure.
- Puncture of the cervical epidural or subarachnoid space can result in cervical epidural or spinal anesthesia (Cook 1991).
- Incomplete permanent tetraplegia has been described after interscalene block due to injury of the cervical spine (Benumof 2000). In all cases the technique was performed under general anesthesia.

- A slightly caudal needle direction must be followed at all costs. A horizontal or even cranial direction of the needle enables the puncture needle to enter the intervertebral foramen.
- Because of the immediate vicinity of the pleural dome, pneumothorax has been described.

As the needle reaches the brachial plexus vertically, advancing an indwelling catheter for a continuous block is difficult or impossible.

The variant of the interscalene technique described by Meier et al. (1997, 2001) is considerably safer because the needle is inserted in the lateral direction (Fig. 2.**9**) and it also provides the possibility of inserting an indwelling catheter for continuous block. Besides the anterior approach to the interscalene brachial plexus, a posterior approach was described right at the start of the 20th century. This technique was taken up again by Pippa et al. (1990) (Fig. 2.**10**). This technique too can be employed as a continuous method.

2.3   Meier Technique

Position: The patient's head is turned to the opposite side and the needle direction corresponds to the course of the interscalene groove (lateral, caudal, dorsal). The target is the distal end of the interscalene groove lateral to the subclavian artery (Figs. 2.**11**, 2.**12**). (Note: an oxygen mask prevents the sterile drape from lying on the patient's mouth and nose!)
Note the phrenic nerve, which runs on the scalenus anterior muscle medial to the brachial plexus (Fig. 2.**13**). If this is stimulated (response: hiccup) the needle must be corrected in the lateral and dorsal direction. The suprascapular nerve is variable and can leave the upper trunk very far proximally (Fig. 2.**13**). If there is a motor response (abduction and external rotation in the shoulder region), the needle must be corrected in the medial and anterior direction.

The patient lies supine with the head turned slightly to the opposite side. The posterior border of the sternocleidomastoid muscle serves for orientation. This becomes prominent when the patient elevates the head slightly. The scalenus anterior muscle can be palpated behind the sternocleidomastoid and the fingers slide laterally over the scalenus anterior muscle into the interscalene groove, which is formed by the scalenus anterior and medius muscles.
The interscalene groove can usually be palpated easily, it runs posterolaterally from the sternocleidomastoid muscle in a slightly lateral direction. The subclavian artery is palpable directly above the clavicle and marks the distal medial end of the interscalene groove. The artery can also be imaged using a Doppler probe. The interscalene groove feels like the gap between

two fingers lying lightly next to one another. On deep inspiration, it sometimes becomes more visible. Distally, the interscalene groove is crossed by the omohyoid muscle, which is usually easy to palpate (Fig. 2.**17**). If the interscalene groove cannot be palpated, a horizontal line 3 cm long can be drawn at the level of the anular cartilage (level of C6) from the middle of the sternocleidomastoid muscle laterally (Fig. 2.**14**). The end of this line marks the interscalene groove (Meier et al. 2001).
The intersection of a horizontal line about 2 cm above the anular cartilage marks the puncture site, and this is therefore further cranial than the classical puncture site with the Winnie technique. The interscalene groove is palpated: the upper finger of the palpating hand slides cranially in the interscalene groove until this disappears under

Fig. 2.**11** Position, site of injection, and direction of needle in interscalene plexus anesthesia according to Meier.

1 Sternocleidomastoid
2 External jugular vein
3 Interscalene groove
4 Subclavian artery (medial boundary of the interscalene groove)

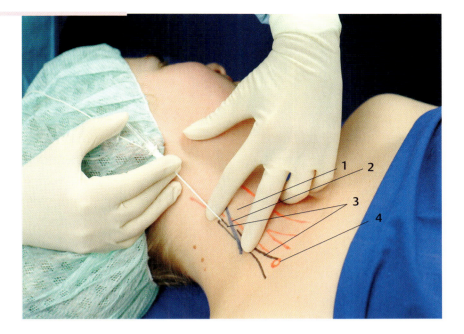

Fig. 2.**12** Position, site of injection, and direction of needle in interscalene plexus block according to Meier (traction on the upper arm facilitates anatomical orientation).

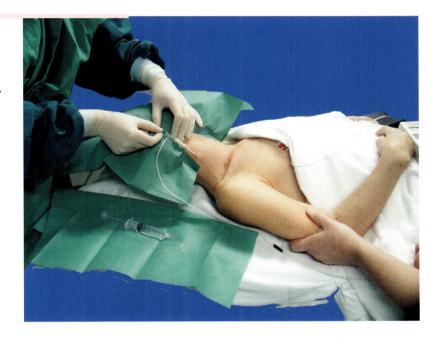

Fig. 2.**13** Anatomy of the interscalene region as seen by the person performing the block.

1 Sternocleidomastoid
2 Scalenus anterior (phrenic nerve marked)
3 Brachial plexus, upper trunk
4 Brachial plexus, middle trunk
5 Scalenus medius
6 Suprascapular nerve (marked)
7 Injection point for vertical infraclavicular plexus anesthesia
8 Omohyoid (reflected)

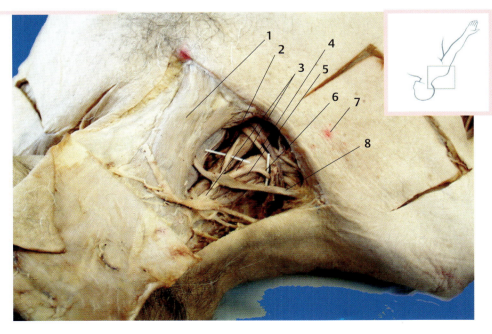

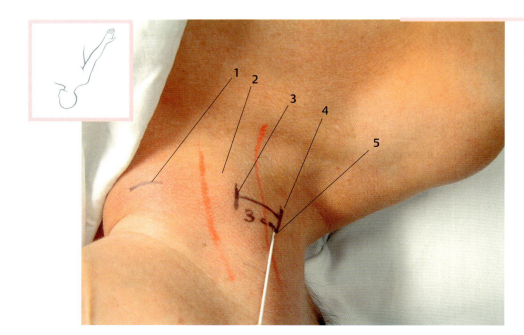

Fig. 2.**14** Interscalene plexus anesthesia (Meier technique): aids to orientation.

1 Cricoid cartilage
2 Sternocleidomastoid
3 Middle of the sternocleidomastoid belly
4 Line following the interscalene groove
5 Site of insertion

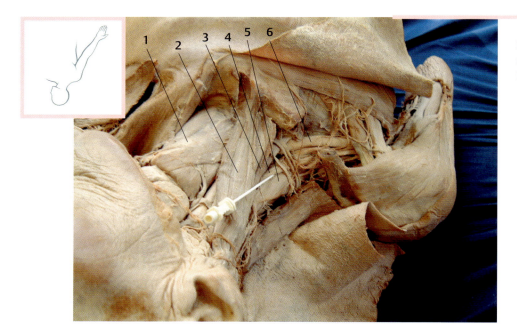

Fig. 2.**15** Interscalene plexus anesthesia (Meier technique): anatomy (clavicle partially removed).

1 Cricoid cartilage
2 Sternocleidomastoid
3 Scalenus anterior
4 Brachial plexus
5 Scalenus medius
6 Subclavian artery

the sternocleidomastoid. The posterior border of the sternocleidomastoid is pushed slightly cranially, while the lower finger lies further distally in the interscalene groove. The puncture site is as far cranial as possible, usually directly beneath the cranially palpating finger. The puncture is performed in the direction of the interscalene groove (Fig. 2.**18**). Depending on the angle of puncture (ca. 30 to the skin) the brachial plexus is reached after about 2.5 cm to a maximum of 5 cm. A clear click is often felt on penetration of the prevertebral fascia (Fig. 2.**22**). The use of a nerve stimulator is mandatory while performing this technique.

The motor response usually arises through stimulation of the upper trunk (deltoid or biceps muscle). This response is adequate and should be striven for (Silverstein et al. 2000; Urmey 2000).
If there is a motor response of the phrenic nerve (twitching of the diaphragm, "hiccup") the needle is too far medially and forward, and it must be corrected laterally and backward.
If there is a motor response of the suprascapular nerve (supraspinatus and infraspinatus: external rotation and abduction of the shoulder), the needle is at the outer border of the brachial plexus and correction in the

medial and anterior direction may be necessary. A motor response in the hand region should not be striven for.
This technique can be performed as a "single-shot" or as a continuous technique (Fig. 2.**23**).
Material
• Single-shot: insulated needle, 22gauge (G), 5-6 cm.
• Continuous technique: 19.5G, 5-6 cm needle with "pencil-point" tip and lateral opening.

Fig. 2.**16** Needle insertion for interscalene plexus anesthesia (Meier technique) before injection of the LA (see also Figs. 2.**21** and 2.**24**).

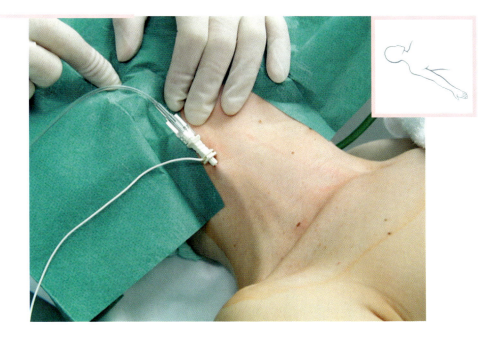

Fig. 2.**17** Interscalene plexus anesthesia (Meier technique): anatomy (lateral view), needle position, advancing an indwelling catheter.

1 Sternocleidomastoid
2 Scalenus anterior
3 Phrenic nerve
4 Brachial plexus with indwelling catheter
5 Scalenus medius
6 Omohyoid

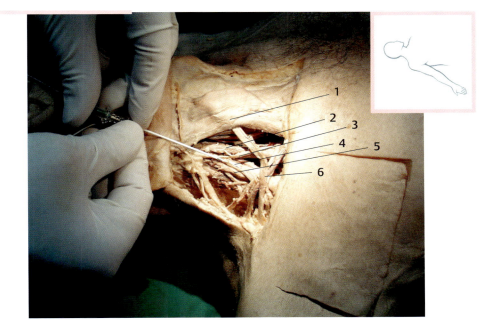

Practical Notes
- The technique should always be performed with a nerve stimulator.
- The motor response usually occurs due to stimulation of the upper trunk (deltoid or biceps). This response is sufficient and should be striven for (Silverstein et al. 2000, Urmey 2000).
- If there is a motor response of the phrenic nerve (twitching of the diaphragm, "hiccup"), the needle is too far medially and forward and must be corrected laterally and backward.
- If there is a motor response of the supras-capular nerve (supraspinatus and

infraspinatus: external rotation and abduction in the shoulder), the needle is at the outer border of the brachial plexus and correction medially and forward may be necessary.
- A motor response in the region of the hand does not have to be striven for.
- If performed correctly, a pneumothorax is ruled out.

With the continuous technique, use a pencil-point needle with lateral opening. The opening should point in the anterolateral direction after successful stimulation and injection of some of the local anesthetic, so that

the catheter can be advanced readily (Fig. 2.**23**). This usually slides along the upper trunk. The catheter tip should be advanced no more than 3-4 cm over the needle tip. The skin level of the catheter is usually 7-8 cm. The frequency of dislocation is extremely low.
Orientation aid for finding the interscalene groove (Figs. 2.**14**, 2.**15**): At the level of the cricoid, a 3 cm long horizontal line is drawn laterally from the middle of the belly of the sternocleidomastoid; the end of the line marks the interscalene groove, and the puncture site is ca. 2 cm further cranially at the intersection of the interscalene groove

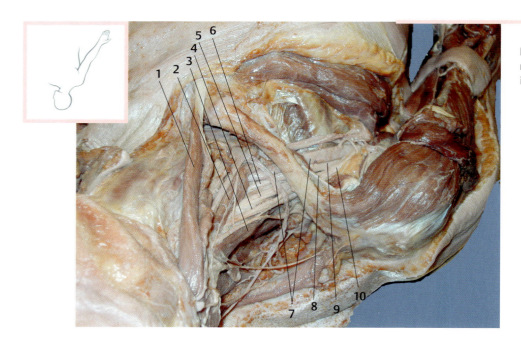

Fig. 2.**18** Anatomy of the interscalene region as seen by person performing the interscalene block.

1 Sternocleidomastoid (clavicular head divided)
2 Scalenus anterior
3 Scalenus medius
4 Upper trunk
5 Middle trunk
6 Lower trunk
7 Subclavian artery
8 Posterior cord
9 Medial cord
10 Lateral cord

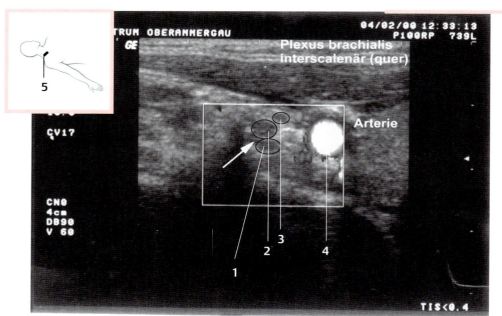

Fig. 2.**19** Ultrasonographic imaging of the interscalene region on right side of neck (cross section).

1 Lower trunk
2 Middle trunk
3 Upper trunk
4 Carotid artery
5 Position of transducer

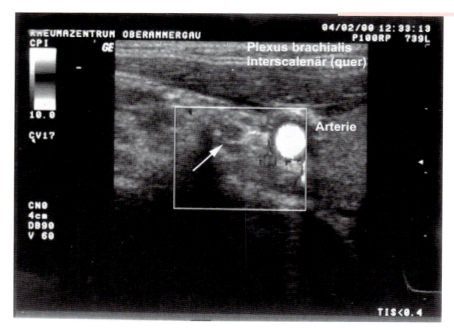

Fig. 2.**20** Ultrasonographic imaging of the interscalene region on the right side of the neck (same as Fig. 2.**19** but without marking of the trunks.)

Fig. 2.21 Interscalene plexus anesthesia (Meier technique). External view after injection of the LA (note the triangular swelling of the cervical fascia).

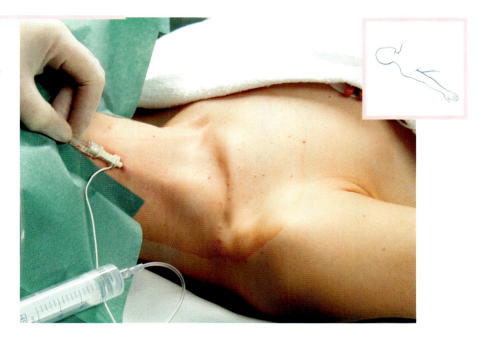

Fig. 2.22 Interscalene region (cervical fascia partially removed).

1 Cervical fascia
2 Brachial plexus (cervical fascia partially removed)
3 Omohyoid

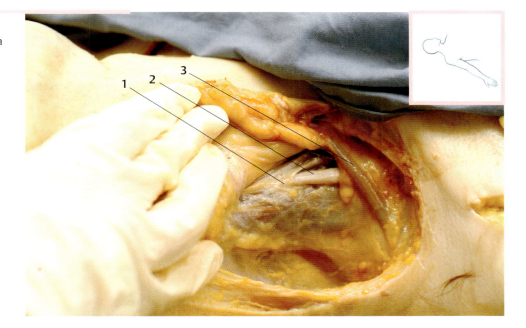

Fig. 2.23 Interscalene region with preserved plexus sheath (needle direction and course of catheter according to Meier interscalene technique).

1 Scalenus anterior
2 Brachial plexus with indwelling catheter in the course of the brachial plexus
3 Scalenus medius

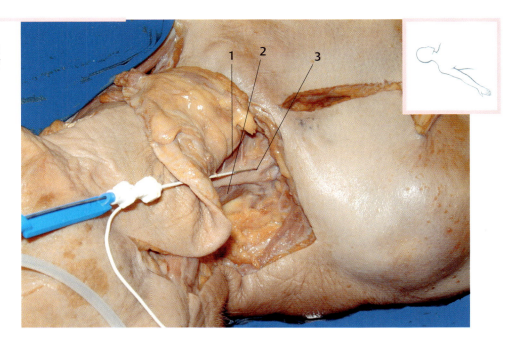

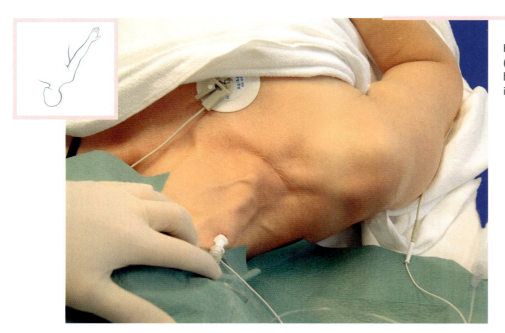

Fig. 2.**24**   Interscalene plexus anesthesia (Meier technique). External anatomy as seen by the person performing the block (after injection of the LA).

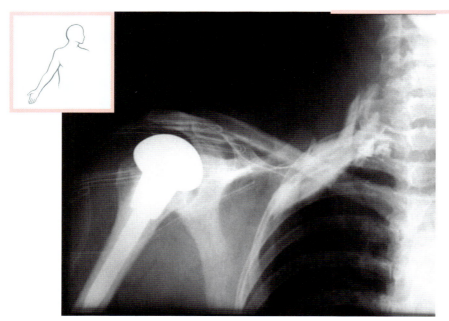

Fig. 2.**25**   Contrast imaging of the correctly spread LA in interscalene plexus anesthesia.

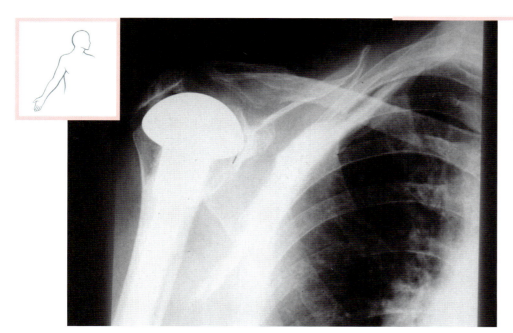

Fig. 2.**26**   Contrast imaging of the spread of LA when the interscalene plexus catheter is advanced too far: spread into the infraclavicular/axillary region with corresponding effects (complete anesthesia in the region of the arm and hand and inadequate anesthesia in the shoulder region).

with the posterior border of the sternoclei-domastoid.

The needle is advanced under stimulation until a response is obtained in the region of the upper trunk. An adequate response is contraction of the biceps and/or deltoid. A response should normally occur at 0.3-0.5 mA with a pulse width of 0.1 ms. Depending on the angle of the puncture and the patient's constitution, the plexus is reached after 2.5-5 cm (Figs. 2.**16**, 2.**17**). The nerve structures can be shown using ultrasound control (Figs. 2.**19**, 2.**20**). With adequate experience of this technique, ultrasound can be very helpful when the anatomical relations are difficult.

When the needle is in the correct position, a volume of 30-40 ml is injected. In slim patients a triangular distension of the cervical fascia becomes visible in the region of the interscalene groove (Figs. 2.**21**, 2.**24**).

Local Anesthetics

Initially: 30-40 ml of 1% mepivacaine or 1% lidocaine (10 mg/ml).

Alternatively: 30-40 ml of 0.75% (7.5 mg/ml) ropivacaine or 0.5% (5 mg/ml) of bupivacaine.

Continuous: 0.2-0.375% (2-3.75 mg/ml)of ropivacaine or 0.25% (2.5 mg/ml)of bupivacaine 6-8 ml/h.

With a suitable needle, a catheter can be introduced without difficulty. The catheter is

advanced in the line of the plexus. During the puncture, the person injecting is located at the patient's head end.

If the catheter is advanced too far, the local anesthetic spreads in the infraclavicular region (Fig. 2.**26**). This results in complete anesthesia in the region of the arm and hand, while the shoulder region may be insufficiently anesthetized. The catheter should then be withdrawn (Fig. 2.**25**). Depending on the depth of penetration of the puncture needle, the catheter is then advanced ca. 3-4 cm beyond the tip of the needle (6-8 cm skin level).

2.4   Dorsal Technique (Pippa Technique)

(Pippa et al. 1990)

Posterior approach (Figs. 2.**27**-2.**29**): The patient is in sitting position or lying on his or her side. The head should be in the axis of the body and the cervical spine should be flexed forward as far as possible (Fig. 2.**30**). The landmark is the spinous process of C7 (vertebra prominens), which is usually easily palpable. With maximum head flexion, the spinous process of C6 can also be palpated above the spinous process of C7. A horizontal line is drawn from midway between the two spinous processes (C6/C7) 3 cm laterally to

the side to be blocked. This is the puncture site.

The puncture is performed with a 10 cm needle strictly in the sagittal plane perpendicular to the skin (Fig. 2.**31**), aiming roughly at the level of the cricoid cartilage. Deviation in the medial direction must be avoided. After 4-7 cm the transverse process of C7 is encountered. After slight correction, the needle is advanced a further 1-2 cm in the cranial direction until the brachial plexus is reached.

Material: 22G, 10-12 cm long insulated needle; catheter technique is possible (19.5G insulated needle).

Practical notes: The technique must always be performed with the nerve stimulator. Major complications such as puncture of larger vessels (vertebral artery, carotid artery), puncture close to the spinal cord, or pneumothorax cannot safely be ruled out.

Fig. 2.**27**   Neck region at level of CVII, cadaver in prone position, cranial view.

  1 Scalenus anterior
  2 Scalenus medius
  3 Brachial plexus
  4 Vertebral artery
  5 Spinal cord
  6 Body of CVII vertebra
  7 Sternocleidomastoid
  8 Internal jugular vein
  9 Common carotid artery

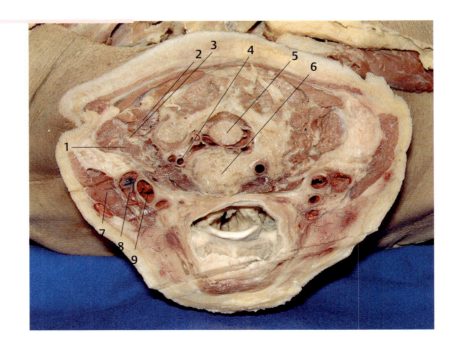

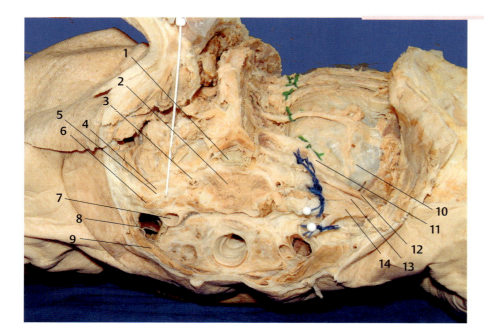

Fig. 2.**28**   Dorsal introduction of needle for brachial plexus block, Pippa technique.

1   Spinal cord
2   Body of CVII vertebra
3   Vertebral artery
4   Scalenus medius
5   Brachial plexus
6   Scalenus anterior
7   Common carotid artery
8   Internal jugular vein
9   Sternocleidomastoid
10 Dome of the pleura
11 Subclavian artery
12 Lower trunk
13 Middle trunk
14 Upper trunk

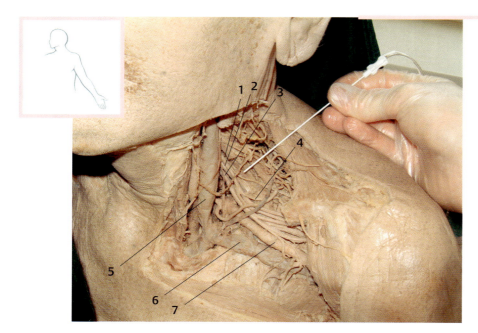

Fig. 2.**29**   Direction of needle in Pippa technique, inserted 3 cm lateral to midline between the spinous processes of CVI/VII.

1   Upper trunk
2   Middle trunk
3   Lower trunk
4   Suprascapular nerve
5   Internal jugular vein
6   Subclavian vein
7   Subclavian artery

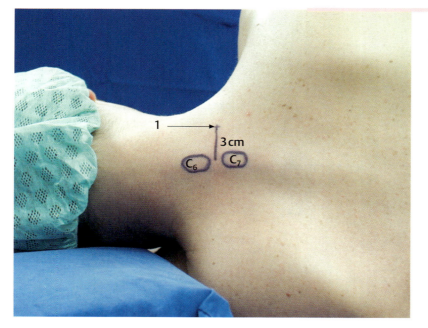

Fig. 2.**30**   Interscalene plexus block, Pippa method: posterior needle insertion in lateral position, anatomical landmarks.

1   Site of puncture
C6 Spinous process of CVI
C7 Spinous process of CVII

Fig. 2.**31**   Approach according to Pippa (in lateral position): direction of needle insertion.

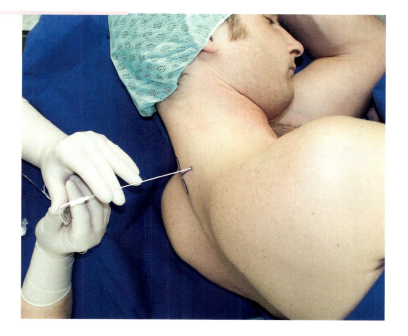

2.5   Sensory and Motor Effects of the Interscalene Block

In the normal case, there is sensory loss of segments C5-C7 (upper and middle trunk), while segments C8 and T1 are usually spared. A sensation of numbness in the thumb and the index and middle fingers is typical, while the ring and little fingers are often spared or are anesthetized after a delay (Fig. 2.**32**). If the incision in shoulder operations is in the anterior axillary line, the supraclavicular nerves (cervical plexus) may also have to be blocked by subcutaneous infiltration below the clavicle if the operation is to be performed under regional anesthesia alone (Fig. 2.**33**). Segments T2 and T3 are not included by interscalene block. There is motor block of the axillary nerve (C5/6) and musculocutaneous nerve (C5/6), and often also a partial block of the radial nerve and median nerve (C6/7).

Evidence that the block is adequate for operation is provided by the "deltoid sign" (abduction of the arm [axillary nerve] is no longer possible) (Wiener and Speer 1994) and the "money sign" (Brown 1996), when the thumb and middle finger can no longer be rubbed together.

Fig. 2.**32**   Sensory effects of complete interscalene plexus anesthesia.

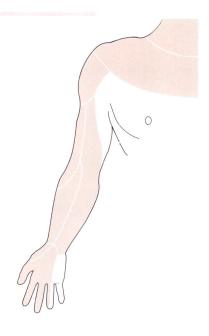

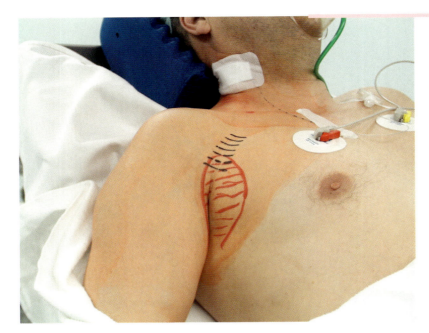

Fig. 2.**33**   Problem regions in open shoulder surgery under interscalene plexus anesthesia. *Black:* innervation area of the supraclavicular nerves (cervical plexus). *Red:* innervation area of T2.

2.6   Indications and Contraindications for the Interscalene Block

Indications
- Anesthesia and analgesia for arthroscopic and open procedures on the shoulder and proximal upper arm region
- Reduction of shoulder dislocation
- Physiotherapy treatment in the shoulder region postoperatively or in frozen shoulder

- Therapy of pain syndromes (CRPS, sympathetic block)

Contraindications
Besides the general contraindications to peripheral nerve blocks, the following special contraindications must be noted in the case of interscalene block:

- Contralateral phrenic nerve paresis
- Contralateral recurrent nerve paresis (Kempen et al. 2000)
- COPD/bronchial asthma (relative contraindication)

2.7   Supraclavicular Nerve Block (Cervical Plexus)

In open shoulder surgery, certain regions are not anesthetized even with well-positioned interscalene plexus block. These regions are innervated by the T2 segment or by the supraclavicular nerves, which derive from the cervical plexus. While an additional regional block (paravertebral T2) is difficult to carry out in the former, the supraclavicular nerves can be anesthetized easily using subcutaneous infiltration below the clavicle (Figs. 2.**34**-2.**37**).

Fig. 2.**34**   Cervical plexus with supraclavicular nerves.

1   Supraclavicular nerves from the cervical plexus

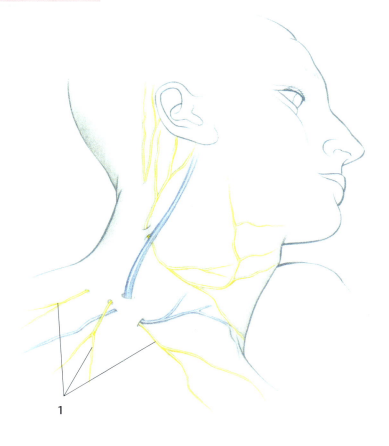

Fig. 2.**35**   Cervical plexus with supraclavicular nerves.

1   Supraclavicular nerves from the cervical plexus

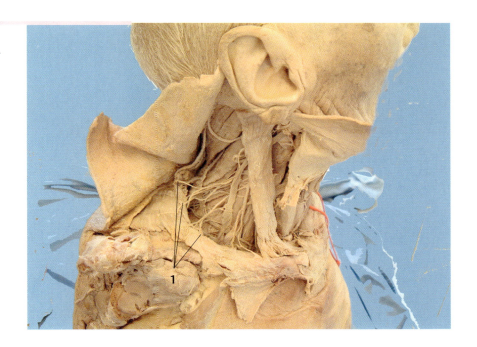

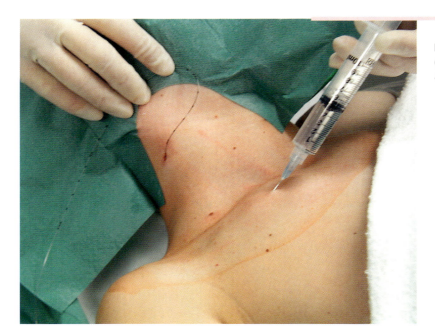

Fig. 2.**36** Block of the supraclavicular nerves (cervical plexus) by subcutaneous infiltration along the clavicle.

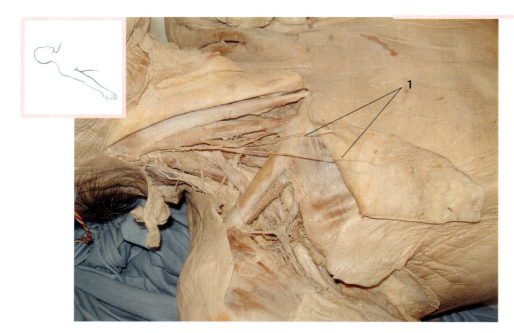

Fig. 2.**37** Cervical plexus. Note: the supraclavicular nerves extend to the infraclavicular region.

1   Supraclavicular nerves from the cervical plexus

2.8   Complications, Side Effects, Method-Specific Problems

Correct performance of the Meier technique eliminates the possibility of complications such as intravascular injection (vertebral artery), high spinal or epidural anesthesia, cervical spine injury, or pneumothorax.

Side effects intrinsic to the method

- *Horner syndrome:* miosis, ptosis, enophthalmos (Fig. 2.**38**). The reported incidence varies between 12.5% and 75%.
- *Hearing loss:* a reversible impairment of hearing can occur, also caused by sympathetic block (Rosenberg et al. 1995).
- *Bronchospasm:* the upper thoracic sympathetic ganglia supply the smooth muscle

of the bronchi. Bronchospasm produced by sympathetic block in the course of an interscalene block has been described (Lim 1979; Thiagarajah et al. 1984) but appears to be an extremely rare event so that the risk and benefit should be weighed carefully.

- *Recurrent nerve paresis:* in 6-8% of cases ipsilateral recurrent nerve paresis has to be expected (hoarseness). Simultaneously existing contralateral recurrent nerve paresis can cause an acute respiratory distress syndrome, which necessitates immediate intubation (Kempen et al. 2000).

- *Phrenic nerve paresis* (Fig. 2.**39**): phrenic nerve paresis in association with interscalene plexus block is described in up to 100% of cases (Urmey et al. 1991). In the case of interscalene block performed according to the Meier technique (Meier et al. 1997, 2001) clinical signs of phrenic nerve paresis occurred in only 7% and clinically relevant respiratory insufficiency was not observed.
- *Bezold-Jarisch reflex:* a fall in blood pressure associated with bradycardia was observed in about 10% of the patients after they were placed in the "beach chair position" (Fig. 2.**40**). The event occurred

Fig. 2.**38** Side effects of interscalene plexus anesthesia: Horner syndrome on patient's right (miosis, ptosis, enophthalmos).

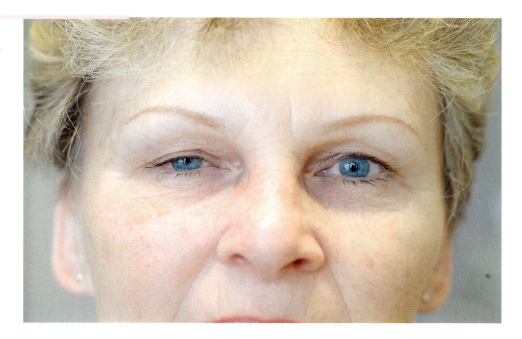

Fig. 2.**39** Side effects of interscalene plexus anesthesia: Phrenic paresis on patient's right with elevated diaphragm.

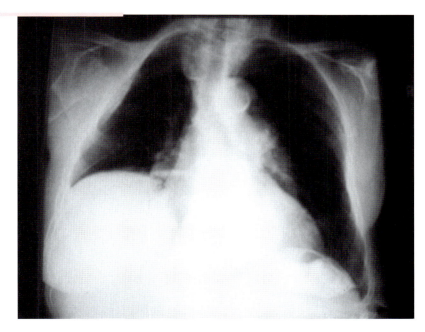

Fig. 2.**40** "Beach chair position" in shoulder surgery.

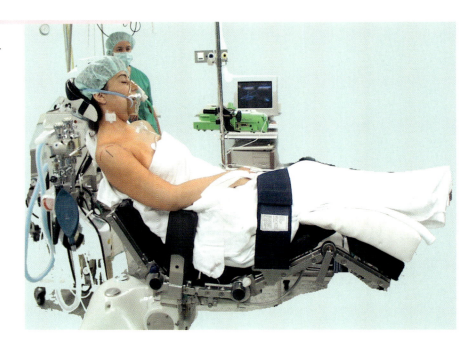

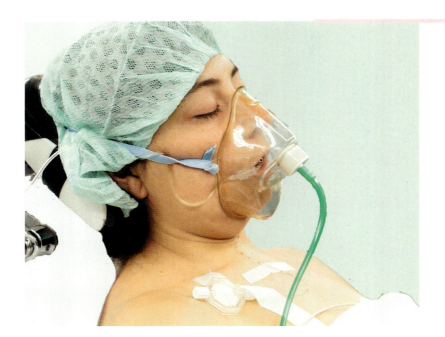

Fig. 2.**41**   Oxygen mask, capnometry to monitor ventilation safely.

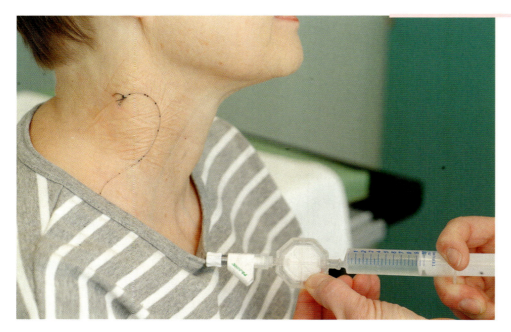

Fig. 2.**42**   Transparent film dressing to monitor injection site. Note the correct catheter tip position at 8 cm from skin level.

on average about 60 minutes after setting up the block (D'Alessio et al. 1995; Ligouri et al. 1998; Roch and Sharrock 1991). Cardiocirculatory arrest requiring resuscitation can occur. Treatment consists of administration of an adrenergic stimulating drug (e.g., ephedrine), and possibly lowering the patient's head and volume administration. Prophylactic administra-

tion of metoprolol is recommended (D'Alessio et al. 1995; Ligouri et al. 1998). This phenomenon was not described and was not observed during continuous administration of local anesthetic for postoperative pain therapy. In this connection, the necessity of continuous monitoring of the patients during an operative procedure should be stressed;

capnometric monitoring of spontaneous respiration has proved useful for monitoring a trend. The patient should always be given O_2 through a mask (Fig. 2.**41**). A transparent dressing allows the injection site to be inspected daily without changing the dressing. Note the 8 cm distance from the tip of the catheter to skin level (Fig. 2.**42**)!

References

Benumof JL. Permanent loss of cervical spinal cord function associated with interscalene block performed under general anesthesia. Anesthesiology. 2000;93:1541-4.

Brown A. Early sign of successful bupivacaine interscalene block: "The money sign." Reg Anesth. 1996;21:166-7.

Cook LB. Unsuspected extradural catheterization in an interscalene block. Br J Anaesth. 1991;67:473-5.

D'Alessio JG, Weller RS, Rosenblum M. Activation of the Bezold-Jarisch reflex in the sitting position for shoulder arthroscopy using interscalene block. Anesth Analg. 1995;80:1158-62.

Kempen PM, O'Donnell J, Lawler R. Acute respiratory insufficiency during interscalene plexus block. Anesth Analg. 2000; 90:1415-6.

Ligouri GA, Kahn RL, Gordon J. The use of metoprolol and glycopyrrolate to prevent hypotension/bradycardic events during shoulder arthroscopy in the sitting position under interscalene block. Anesth Analg. 1998;87:1320-5.

Lim EK. Interscalene brachial plexus block in asthmatic patients. Anesthesia. 1979;34:370.

Meier G, Bauereis C, Heinrich C. Der interscalenäre Plexuskatheter zur Anästhesie und postoperativen Schmerztherapie. Anaesthesist. 1997;46:715-9.

Meier G, Bauereis C, Maurer H. Interscalenäre Plexusblockade. Anaesthesist. 2001;50:333-41.

Pippa P, Cominelli E, Marinelle C. Brachial plexus block using the posterior approach. Eur J Anaesth. 1990;7:411-20.

Roch J, Sharrock NE. Hypotension during shoulder arthroscopy in the sitting position under interscalene block. Reg Anesth. 1991;1S(Suppl):64

Rosenberg PH, Lamberg TS, Tarkkila P. Auditory disturbance associated with interscalene brachial plexus block. Br J Anaesth. 1995;74:89-91.

Silverstein WB, Saiyed MU, Brown AR. Interscalene block with a nerve stimulator: A deltoid motor response is a satisfactory endpoint for successful block. Reg Anesth. 2000;25:356-9.

Thiagarajah S, Lear E, Azar I. Bronchospasm following interscalene brachial plexus block. Anesthesiology. 1984;61:759-61.

Urmey WF. Interscalene block: The truth about twitches. Reg Anesth. 2000;25:340-2.

Urmey WF, Talts KH, Sharrock NE. One hundred percent incidence of hemidiaphragmatic paresis associated with interscalene brachial plexus anesthesia as diagnosed by ultrasonography. Anesth Analg. 1991;72:498-503.

Wiener D, Speer K. The deltoid sign. Anesth Analg. 1994;79:192.

Winnie AP. The interscalene brachial plexus block. Anesth Analg. 1970;49:455-66.

3   Infraclavicular Techniques of Brachial Plexus Block

3.1   Anatomical Basis

Just above the clavicle, each of the trunks divides into an anterior and a posterior division. The three posterior divisions combine to form the *posterior cord*, the anterior divisions of the upper and middle trunks form the *lateral cord*, and the *medial cord* is the continuation of the anterior division of the lower trunk (Fig. 3.**1**, 3.**2**). The cords are located very close to one another in the

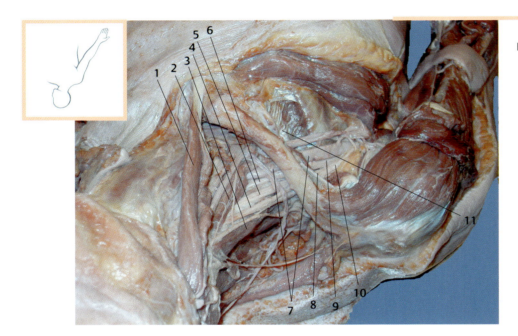

Fig. 3.**1**   Anatomy of the brachial plexus.

   1 Sternocleidomastoid
      (clavicular part divided)
   2 Scalenus anterior
   3 Scalenus medius
   4 Upper trunk
   5 Middle trunk
   6 Lower trunk
   7 Subclavian artery
   8 Posterior cord
   9 Medial cord
  10 Lateral cord
  11 Intercostal space

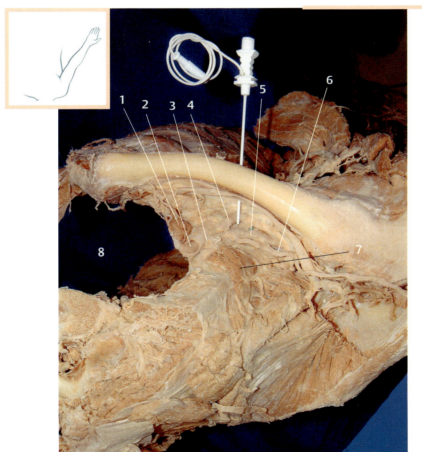

Fig. 3.**2**   Anatomy of the infraclavicular region, seen from cranial aspect.

   1 Scalenus anterior
   2 Subclavian artery
   3 Medial cord
   4 Lateral cord
   5 Posterior cord
   6 Suprascapular nerve
   7 Scalenus medius
   8 Pleural cavity

infraclavicular region. The *lateral cord* lies most superficially, the *posterior cord* is found a little deeper and slightly lateral(!), and the *medial cord* lies deep (Figs. 3.**3**, 3.**4**). The

cords lie cranial and lateral to the subclavian artery, which passes through the interscalene space together with the brachial plexus. The subclavian artery and brachial

plexus pass into the axilla caudal to the coracoid process.
Note the rotation of the cords through 90° around the subclavian artery from the infra-

Fig. 3.**3**   Brachial plexus, infraclavicular region.

1   Subclavian vein
2   Subclavian artery
3   Pectoral nerves
4   Brachial plexus
5   Cephalic vein

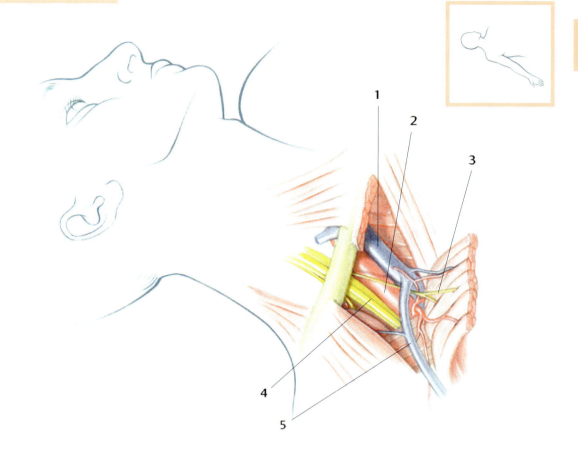

Fig. 3.**4**   Brachial plexus, infraclavicular region.

1   Subclavian artery
2   Lateral cord
3   Posterior cord
4   Medial cord
5   Pectoral nerves
6   Cephalic vein

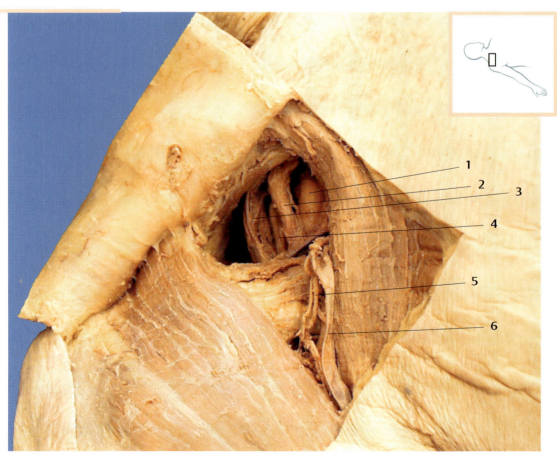

clavicular region to the axillary region. While the posterior cord is furthest laterally (but deeper) compared to the lateral cord in the infraclavicular region, in the axillary region the names of the cords correspond to their actual positions relative to one another. The medial cord passes under the artery and then unites with the lateral cord to form the median nerve (Figs. 3.5-3.8).

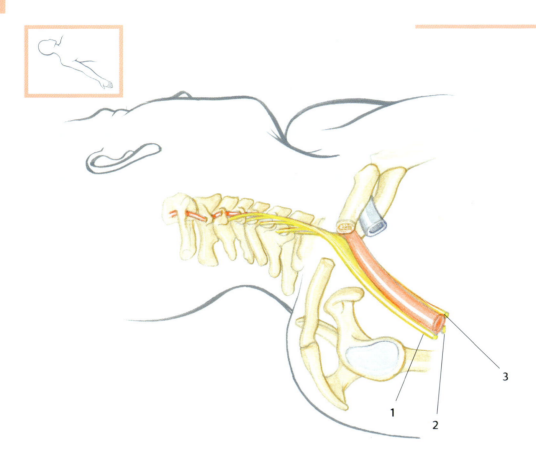

Fig. 3.**5**   Brachial plexus in relation to the subclavian (axillary) artery. Note that the cords rotate 90° around the subclavian artery from the infraclavicular region to the axillary region.
While the posterior cord is furthest laterally (but deeper) compared to the lateral cord in the infraclavicular region, in the axillary region the names of the cords correspond to their actual positions relative to one another.

  1 Lateral cord
  2 Posterior cord
  3 Medial cord

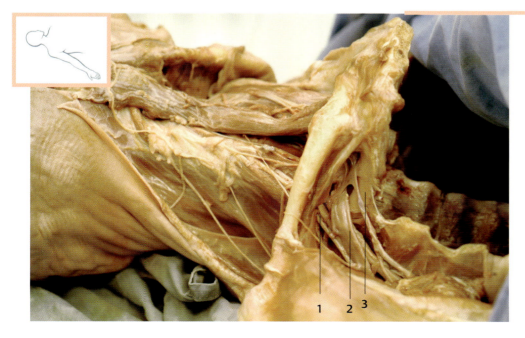

Fig. 3.**6**   Anatomy of the brachial plexus.

  1 Brachial plexus
  2 Subclavian artery
  3 First rib

Fig. 3.**7** Anatomy of the brachial plexus.

1 Radial nerve
2 Median nerve
3 Musculocutaneous nerve
4 Posterior cord
5 Lateral cord
6 Suprascapular nerve
7 Ulnar nerve
8 Medial cutaneous nerve of the forearm
9 Medial cord

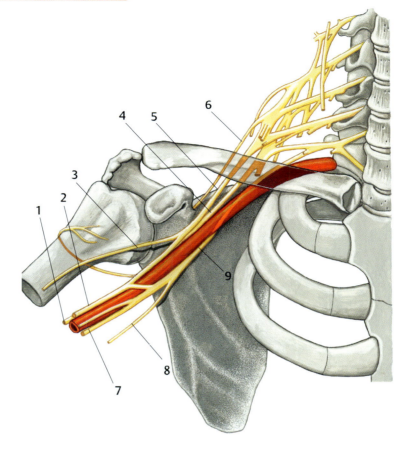

Fig. 3.**8** Anatomy of the infraclavicular region.

1 Cephalic vein
2 Subclavian artery
3 Medial cord
4 Posterior cord
5 Lateral cord
6 Ulnar nerve
7 Median nerve with its two roots

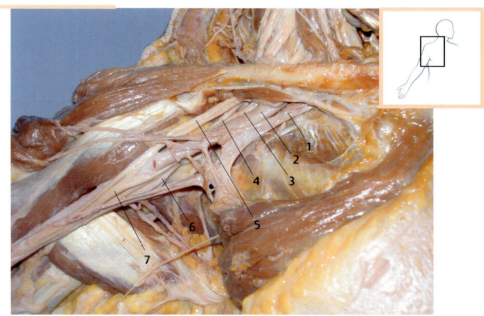

3.2   Vertical Infraclavicular Block (VIB) according to Kilka, Geiger, and Mehrkens

(Kilka et al. 1995)

In contrast to the other infraclavicular techniques, this technique has clear landmarks. These landmarks are the anterior end of the acromion and the middle of the jugular notch. The midpoint of the line connecting these two points marks the injection site, which here lies just below the clavicle (Fig. 3.**9**, 3.**10**).

The patient lies supine; special positioning of the arm is not necessary. If possible, the patient's hand should lie comfortably on his or her abdomen (Fig. 3.**11**).

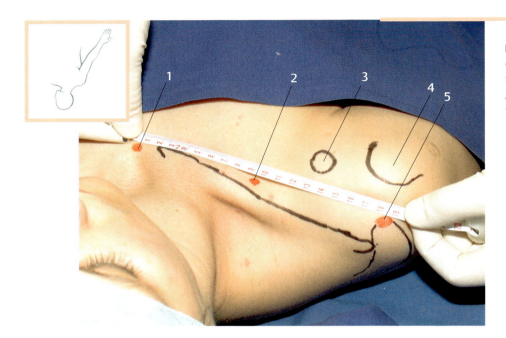

Fig. 3.**9** Orientation points for vertical infraclavicular plexus anesthesia. (The puncture site is half way between the middle of the jugular notch and the anterior part of the acromion.)

1   Middle of the jugular notch
2   Puncture site
3   Coracoid process
4   Head of humerus
5   Anterior part of the acromion

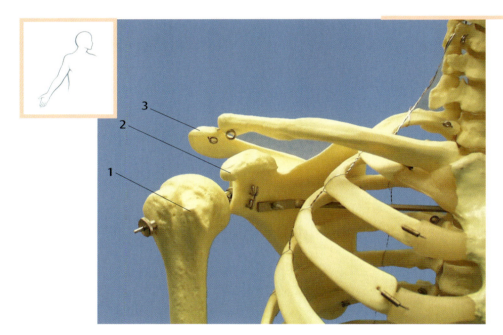

Fig. 3.**10**   Overview of the bony structures for performing vertical infraclavicular plexus anesthesia.

1   Head of humerus
2   Coracoid process
3   Anterior part of the acromion

The puncture is performed just below the clavicle strictly vertical (perpendicular) to the surface the patient is lying on (Figs. 3.**12**-3.**14**). After penetrating the often very tough clavipectoral fascia, there is a stimulus response after 2.5-4 cm. Peripheral muscle contractions in the fingers are striven for as a response indicating success (posterior cord/radial nerve, lateral cord/median nerve, medial cord/ulnar nerve). Stimulation of the lateral cord only, which leads to contraction of the biceps muscle and/or pronator teres, may result in an incomplete block. In order to obtain a successful response, the needle in this case must be withdrawn to a subcutaneous position, and after moving the skin

slightly more lateral (0.5-1.0 cm) it should be advanced again vertically to the underlying surface. The desired response is about 0.5 cm deeper and is then usually in the region of the posterior cord, which here lies laterally(!) and deeper than the lateral cord.
Puncture needle: 4-6 cm long insulated needle; a catheter technique is possible. The puncture is performed just below the clavicle strictly vertical (perpendicular) to the surface the patient is lying on.
Practical Notes:
● Because of the potential danger of a pneumothorax, a medial needle direction, a puncture site too far medially, and excessively deep puncture should be

avoided at all costs (Figs. 3.**15**, 3.**16**). The depth of puncture must never be more than 6 cm even in large patients. In asthenic patients where the distance between the acromion and the jugular notch is short (<20 cm) the risk of a pneumothorax is increased, as the plexus is sometimes located at a depth of only < 3 cm (Neuburger et al. 2001) (Fig. 3.**17**). Even when all the rules are followed, a pneumothorax cannot absolutely be avoided (Neuburger et al. 2000).
● When the distance from the acromion to the jugular notch is < 20 cm it is advisable to move the puncture site further laterally by 0.3 mm for each centimeter by which

Fig. 3.**11**   VIB puncture site: vertical to surface on the horizontal supine patient.

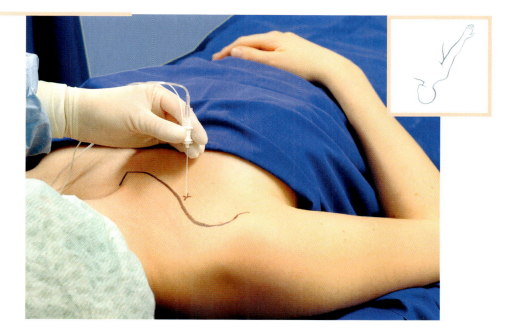

Fig. 3.**12**   Anatomy of the brachial plexus,
VIB puncture site.

  1   Lower trunk
  2   Middle trunk
  3   Upper trunk, site of division into
        anterior and posterior divisions
  4   Suprascapular nerve
  5   Anterior division of the upper trunk,
        joins with the anterior division of
        the middle trunk to form the lateral
        cord (9)
  6   Posterior division of the upper
        trunk, joins with posterior divisions
        of the middle and inferior trunks to
        form the posterior cord (8)
  7   Subclavian artery
  8   Posterior cord
  9   Lateral cord
 10   Intercostal space

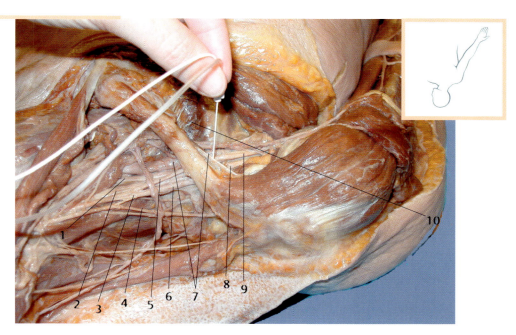

Fig. 3.**13**   VIB puncture site, vertical to surface on the horizontal supine patient. Note
the relation to the supraclavicular region.

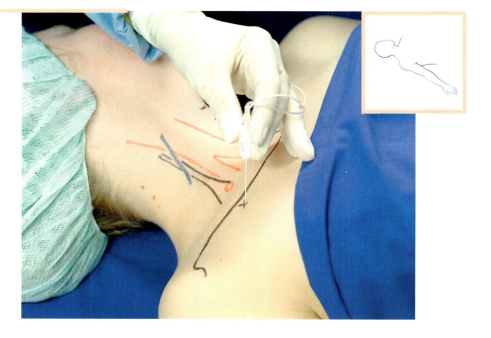

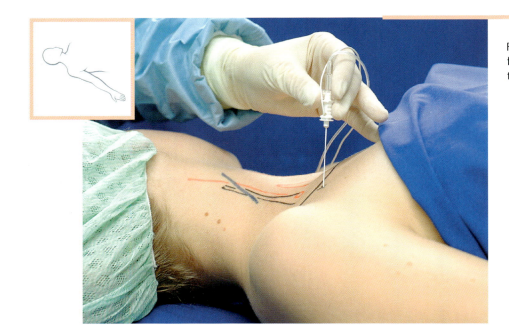

Fig. 3.**14**   VIB puncture site, vertical to surface on the horizontal supine patient. Note the relation to the supraclavicular region.

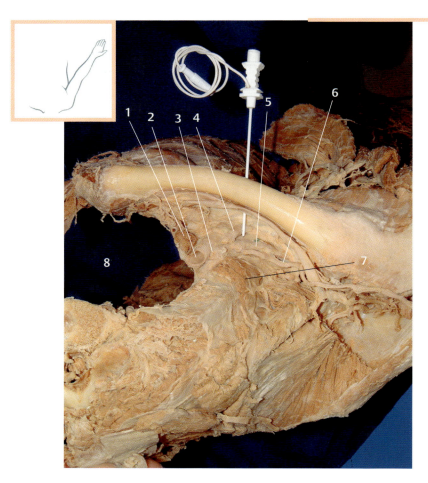

Fig. 3.**15**   Anatomy of the infraclavicular region, view from above.

1   Scalenus anterior
2   Subclavian artery
3   Medial cord
4   Lateral cord
5   Posterior cord
6   Suprascapular nerve
7   Scalenus medius
8   Pleural cavity

the distance falls below 20 cm (e.g., jugular-acromion distance 17 cm; puncture site not 8.5 cm but 7.6 cm from the anterior end of the acromion or 9.4 cm from the middle of the jugular notch on the J-A line) (Neuburger et al. 2003) (Fig. 3.**18**).

• The injection point is largely identical with the medial boundary of the "infraclavicular fossa" (clavipectoral trigone or Mohrenheim's fossa). The plexus emerges under the clavicle exactly at the lateral margin of the superficial part of pectoralis major. The so-called "finger point" acts as an additional orientation and thus provides certainty that the correct injection site has been defined. The anesthetist's index finger (right index finger when the right limb is to be blocked, left index finger when the left limb is to be blocked) is placed in the gap between the deltoid and pectoralis major muscles and pressed laterally on the coracoid process. The tip of this finger encounters the clavicle and its ulnar border marks the medial margin of the infraclavicular fossa and thus the puncture site (Neuburger et al. 2003) (Fig. 3.**19**).

Fig. 3.**16** With a jugular notch–acromion distance of ca. 20 cm or more, the needle direction has to be changed considerably in the medial direction to cause a pleural injury when vertical infraclavicular plexus anesthesia is performed. The "shortest route" to the pleura is 6.3 cm here.

1 Puncture site, indicated by radiodense nitrocapsule
2 Clavicle
3 Brachial plexus
4 Lung
5 Vessels

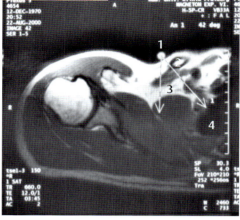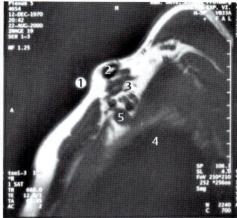

MRI: transverse plane   MRI: sagittal plane

Fig. 3.**17** In asthenic, slim patients with a jugular notch–acromion distance of 18–20 cm or less, there is a risk of injuring the lung even if the basic rules are followed. In the case illustrated, the pleura could be hit after only 4.2 cm. The first rib would protect the pleura in this case. The brachial plexus is reached after only 1.7 cm!

1 Puncture site, indicated by radiodense nitrocapsule
2 Clavicle
3 Brachial plexus
4 Lung
5 Vessels
6 First rib

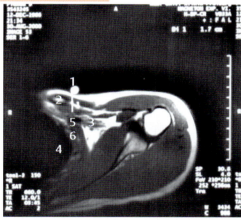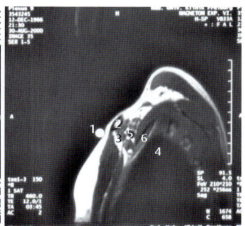

MRI: transverse plane   MRI: sagittal plane

Fig. 3.**18** Determining the puncture site for vertical infraclavicular plexus anesthesia: With a jugular notch (J)–acromion (A) distance of d ≥ 20 cm, the puncture site is at the halfway point (d/2). According to Neuburger and Kaiser, with an J–A distance < 20 cm, the puncture site is moved 0.3 cm laterally for each centimeter by which the J–A distance is less than 20 cm (see example).

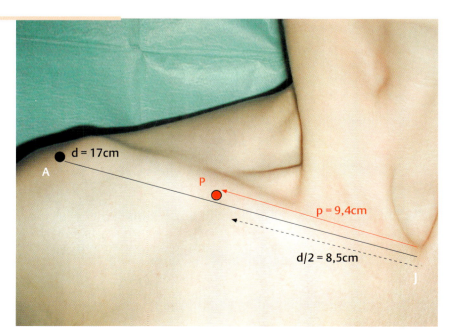

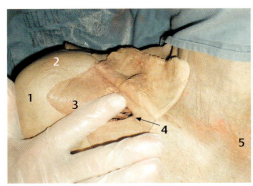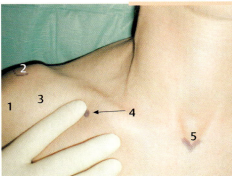

Fig. 3.**19**   The so-called "finger point" is helpful in finding the puncture site for vertical infraclavicular plexus anesthesia. To do this, the index finger of the person administering the plexus anesthesia (right index finger with plexus anesthesia on the right) is placed in the patient's infraclavicular fossa. The puncture site determined this way is usually on the ulnar side of this finger. If there are greater deviations, the measurement must be repeated.

1   Head of humerus
2   Acromion
3   Coracoid process
4   Brachial plexus (puncture site)
5   Jugular notch

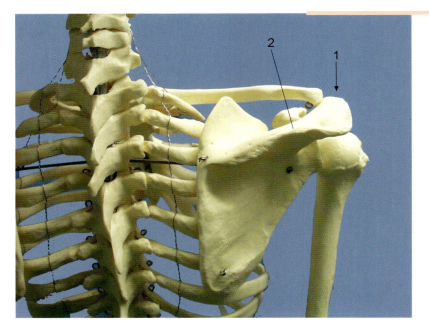

Fig. 3.**20**   Scapula, orientation to the anterior part of the acromion over the spine of the scapula.

1   Anterior part of the acromion
2   Spine of the scapula

Identification of the anterior end of the acromion often causes difficulty. It is advisable to look for the lateral margin of the spine of the scapula from behind (Fig. 3.**20**). This is where the lateral boundary of the acromion commences, and it passes forward at a right angle to the spine of the scapula. If one feels forward along the lateral boundary, one comes automatically to the anterior end of the acromion (Fig. 3.**21**). If the acromion is now followed over the "vertex" (= anterior end), the acromioclavicular joint is reached, which is medial and slightly dorsal to the anterior end. On no account should the anterior end be confused with the head of the humerus or coracoid process. The humerus moves under the palpating finger during rotation of the arm and so can be well demarcated from the acromion (Fig. 3.**21**).

Contrary to expectations, a catheter can often be introduced here although the opening of the needle is relatively vertical to the brachial plexus (Figs. 3.**22**, 3.**23**).
Use of a needle with a "pencil-point" tip and lateral opening would be desirable, but the needle has proved to be "too blunt" for this technique as considerable pressure is required to penetrate the clavipectoral fascia, which does not allow controlled advance. The loss of resistance when the clavipectoral fascia is penetrated does not indicate that the needle is in the correct position, so that this technique is not a "loss-of-resistance" method. A nerve stimulator is essential for performing this technique.
Vascular puncture occurs relatively frequently (10-30%) (Kilka et al. 1995; Neuburger et al. 1998). Usually it is not the

subclavian artery that is punctured but the cephalic vein, which crosses the puncture site in this region (Figs. 3.**24**, 3.**25**). Vascular puncture indicates that the puncture site is too medial.
If there is a response in the pectoralis muscle, the puncture site is likewise too far medial (the pectoral nerves run medial to the cords) (Fig. 3.**25**), and local contractions of the infraclavicular muscles should not be interpreted as a correct stimulus response.
Local anesthetics (LA), dosages: Initially, 30-50 ml of a short/medium-acting (e.g., mepivacaine 1% [10 mg/ml]) or long-acting (e.g., ropivacaine 0.5-0.75% [5-7.5 mg/ml]) LA; continuous block 5-10 ml/h of ropivacaine 0.2-0.375% (2-3.75 mg/ml). Complete block of all nerves supplying the arm is usually achieved with this volume (Fig. 3.**26**).

Fig. 3.**21** Overview of the bony structures for performing vertical infraclavicular plexus anesthesia.

1   Head of humerus
2   Coracoid process
3   Anterior part of the acromion

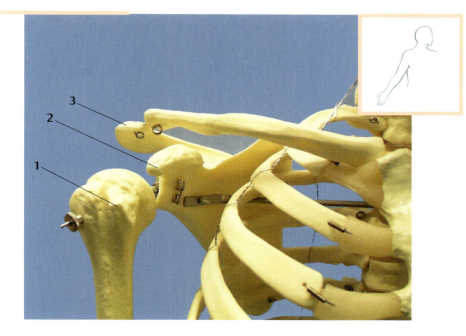

Fig. 3.**22** Insertion of an indwelling catheter in vertical infraclavicular plexus block.

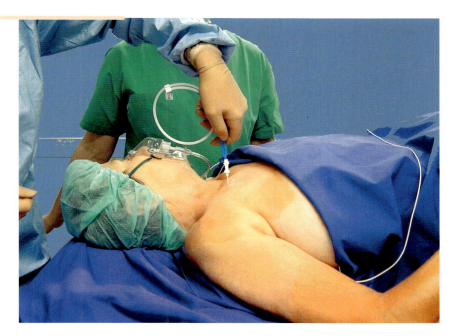

Fig. 3.**23** Infraclavicular plexus catheter in situ.

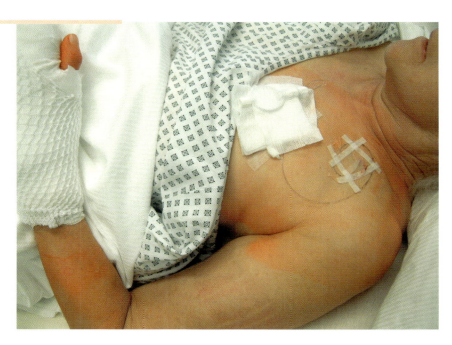

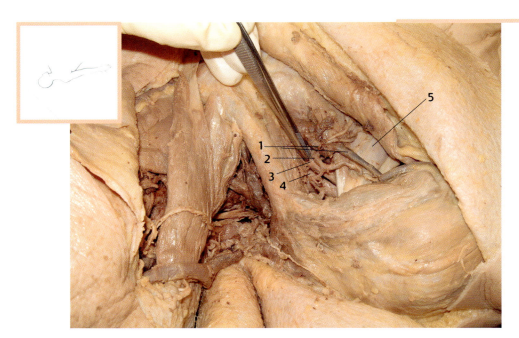

Fig. 3.**24** Anatomy of the brachial plexus (infraclavicular region), relation to neighboring vessels.

1 Cephalic vein
2 Thoracoacromial artery
3 Lateral cord
4 Posterior cord
5 Pectoralis minor

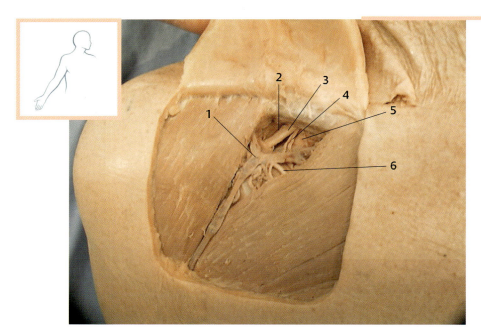

Fig. 3.**25** Brachial plexus, infraclavicular region.

1 Cephalic vein
2 Posterior cord
3 Lateral cord
4 Pectoral nerves
5 Subclavian artery
6 Thoracoacromial artery

In two studies (Kilka et al. 1995; Neuburger et al. 1998) the success rate for operative anesthesia is reported as 88% and 94%, respectively; 9% and 5.2%, respectively, were successfully supplemented and 3% and 0%, respectively, were classified as complete failures. In the two studies cited, no pneumothorax was described, although there are case reports of such a complication. A pneumothorax risk of 0.2-0.7% can be assumed (Neuburger et al. 2000).

Comparison of the vertical infraclavicular technique with the axillary technique: The range of indications for the two approaches to the brachial plexus is largely identical. With complex injuries of the arm, abduction can be very painful. If there has been previous surgery (breast surgery with axillary lymph node clearance) (Fig. 3.**27**) or frozen shoulder (Fig. 3.**28**) axillary blockade is not feasible. In this case, techniques close to the clavicle, which can be performed without

abduction of the arm, are of benefit (vertical infraclavicular plexus anesthesia). The vertical infraclavicular technique is characterized by a faster onset of effect and a greater success rate, particularly compared to the perivascular axillary technique (Neuburger et al. 1998).

Fig. 3.**26**   Spread of contrast in the infraclavicular region with vertical infraclavicular
plexus block technique.

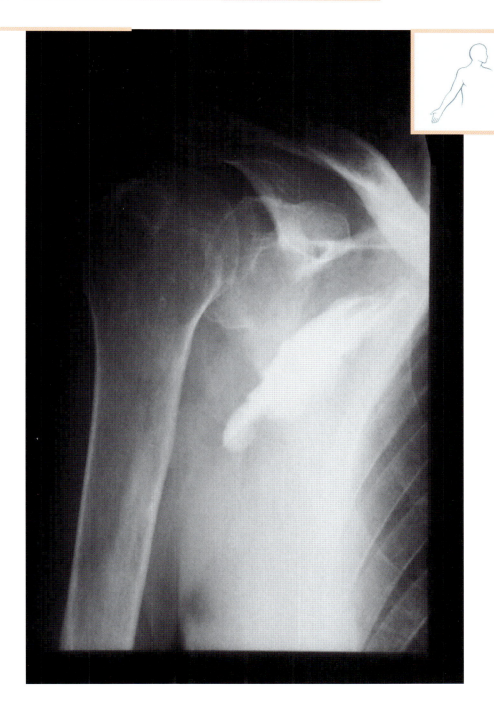

Fig. 3.**27**   Differential indication for infraclavicular plexus block vs. axillary plexus
block: previous mastectomy with axillary
lymph node clearance.

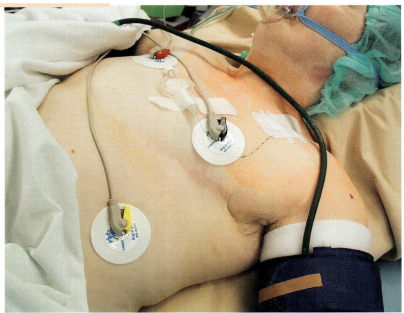

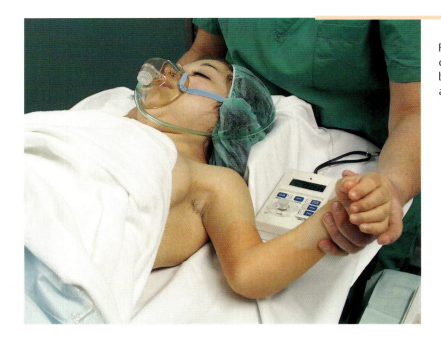

Fig. 3.**28**   Differential indication for infra-clavicular plexus block vs. axillary plexus block: frozen shoulder with inability to abduct the arm.

3.3   Raj Technique, Modified by Borgeat

(Raj et al. 1973; Borgeat et al. 2001)
The patient lies supine with the head turned to the opposite side. The puncture site is identical with the puncture site for vertical infraclavicular plexus anesthesia. The injection point is half way between the anterior part of the acromion and the middle of the jugular notch about 1 cm below the clavicle (Figs. 3.**29**, 3.**30**). The injection point is determined with the arm adducted. For puncture, the arm is abducted 90° and elevated about 30°. The needle is directed later-ally to the most proximal point at which the axillary artery can still just be palpated in the axilla (Figs. 3.**31**-3.**34**). The angle to the skin is ca. 45-60°. After ca. 3-8 cm a response is obtained in the arm, wrist, or hand. In order to obtain a satisfactory

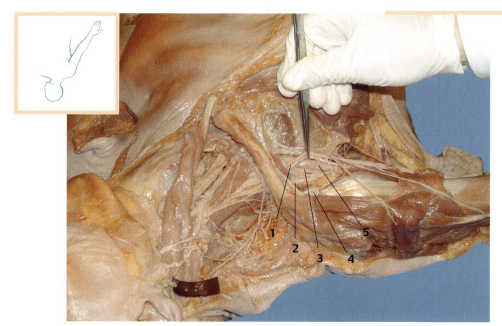

Fig. 3.**29**   Anatomy of the infraclavicular region: Raj technique (view from above).

1   Lateral cord
2   Posterior cord
3   Medial cord
4   Coracoid process
5   Subclavian artery

Fig. 3.**30** Orientation points for infraclavicular plexus anesthesia with Raj technique. (The puncture site is half way between the jugular notch [1] and the anterior part of the acromion, about 1 cm below the clavicle, with the needle pointing toward the most proximal point at which the axillary artery can be palpated in the axilla.)

1 Middle of the suprasternal notch
2 Puncture site
3 Anterior part of acromion
4 Axillary artery

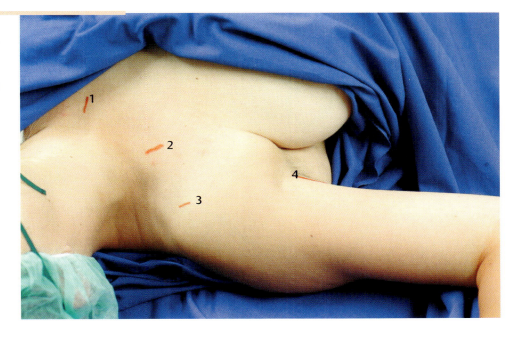

Fig. 3.**31** Raj technique, needle direction.

1 Subclavian artery
2 Medial cord
3 Lateral cord
4 Coracoid process
5 Musculocutaneous nerve

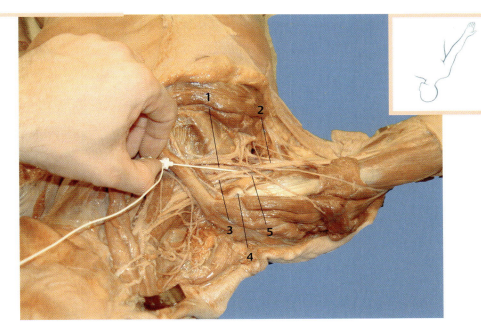

Fig. 3.**32** Raj technique, needle direction.

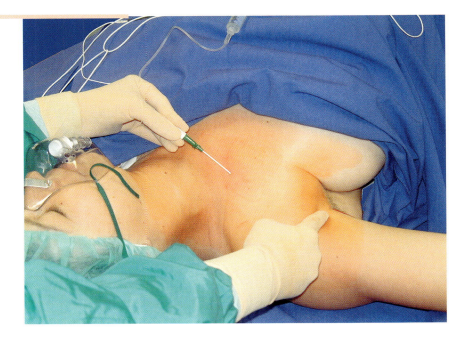

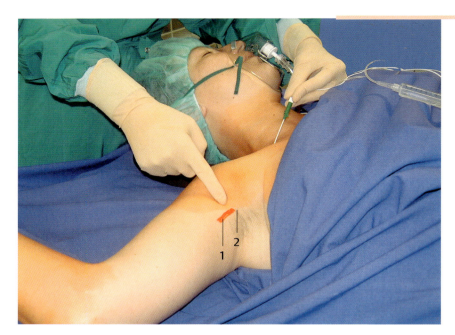

Fig. 3.**33**   Raj technique, needle direction.

    1   Axillary artery
    2   Needle target

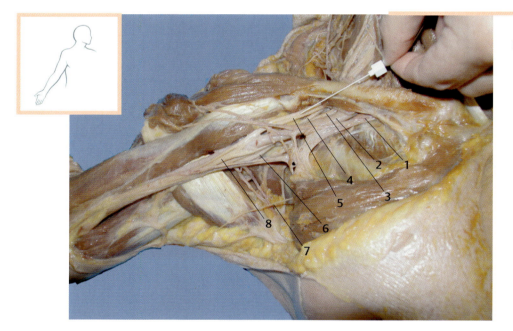

Fig. 3.**34**   Raj technique, needle direction.

    1   Cephalic vein
    2   Subclavian artery
    3   Medial cord
    4   Posterior cord
    5   Lateral cord
    6   Ulnar nerve
    7   Intercostobrachial nerve
    8   Median nerve

success rate, a distal response in the hand or fingers should be striven for.

Material: 22G, 8-10 cm long insulated needle; a continuous technique is possible (e.g., 19.5G × 10 cm Plexolong with catheter [Pajunk]).

Practical notes: Because of the lateral direction of the needle, the danger of pneumothorax is lower.

Vascular puncture (usually venous, cephalic vein) is observed.

Because of the tangential approach to the plexus, a catheter can be advanced readily (Figs. 3.**35**, 3.**36**).

Local anesthetics, dosages: Initially 30-50 ml of a short/medium-acting (e.g., mepivacaine 1 %, lidocaine 1 % [10 mg/ml]) or long-acting (e.g., ropivacaine 0.5-0.75 % [5-7.5 mg/ml])

LA. This volume usually results in adequate block of all nerves supplying the arm (Figs. 3.**37**, 3.**38**).

Continuous block: e.g., ropivacaine 0.2-0.375 % (2-3.75 mg/ml), 5-10 ml/h.

Fig. 3.**35**   Raj technique, insertion of a catheter.

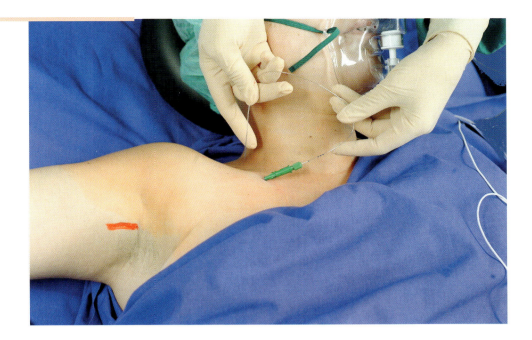

Fig. 3.**36**   Raj technique, needle direction.

1   Subclavian artery
2   Brachial plexus
3   Axillary artery

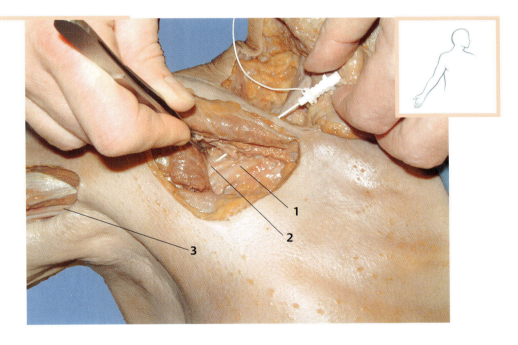

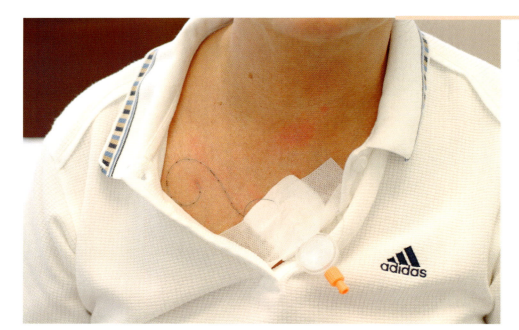

Fig. 3.**37** Infraclavicular plexus catheter, Raj technique.

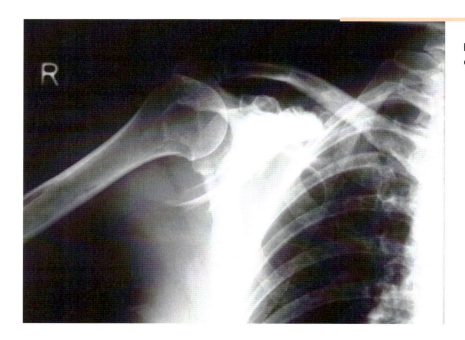

Fig. 3.**38** Spread of contrast with infra-clavicular plexus block using Raj technique.

The following applies generally for all infraclavicular blocks:

3.4   Sensory and Motor Effects

In the region of the clavicle, the divisions and cords of the brachial plexus lie very close together so that profound sensory and motor block of all the nerves supplying the arm can be expected here. The nerves that leave the plexus further cranially (e.g., suprascapular nerve) are not included. An interscalene block should be performed for anesthesia and analgesia in the region of the shoulder and proximal upper arm. Because of the similar indications for axillary and infraclavicular brachial plexus block, the risks and benefits of these techniques must be weighed up against one another.

3.5   Indications and Contraindications

Indications
Anesthesia or analgesia and sympathetic block in the distal upper arm, elbow, fore-arm, and hand.

Contraindications
Contralateral phrenic nerve paresis: while a varying incidence of phrenic nerve paresis is reported with supraclavicular blocks (Neal et al. 1998), this complication is less likely with infraclavicular block (Rodriguez et al. 1998) but can occur (Stadlmeyer et al. 2000). For this reason, contralateral phrenic nerve pare-

sis should be regarded as a contraindication to infraclavicular plexus anesthesia also, particularly in the case of the vertical technique. *Contralateral recurrent nerve paresis*: similarly to phrenic nerve paresis, recurrent nerve paresis can be expected potentially because of the anatomical vicinity in both supraclavicular and infraclavicular block, although

there have been no reports of this in association with the infraclavicular technique. Marked *respiratory insufficiency* is regarded as a relative contraindication.
Chest deformities and clavicular fractures that have healed with dislocation make anatomical orientation difficult, so the risk of a pneumothorax is increased.

A bilateral block is also regarded as contraindicated due to the risk of pneumothorax, as it is in the case of an existing contralateral pneumothorax, or status after contralateral pneumonectomy.

3.6   Complications, Side Effects, Method-Specific Problems

Horner syndrome: An incidence between 1% and 6.9% is reported with the infraclavicular vertical technique (Kilka et al. 1995; Neuburger et al. 1998).
Hoarseness and a foreign body sensation in the throat are presumably caused by block of the recurrent laryngeal nerve.
Horner syndrome and hoarseness are side effects rather than complications. These phenomena are usually of shorter duration than the actual block effect and are rarely observed to be lasting with a continuous block.
Phrenic nerve paresis: there have been reports of acute respiratory insufficiency in association with vertical infraclavicular block, due to unilateral *phrenic nerve paresis* (Stadlmeyer et al. 2000). For this reason, marked *respiratory insufficiency* is regarded as a relative contraindication.
Pneumothorax is a feared complication of all blocks performed close to the clavicle. The reported incidence varies between 0.2% and 6% (Jankovic et al. 2000; Neuburger et al. 1998), depending on the block technique. This complication must always be antici-

pated and the patient must be informed accordingly. Particularly in conjunction with general anesthesia with positive-pressure ventilation (e.g., incomplete block for operation with subsequent intubation), the development of a life-threatening tension pneumothorax must be considered. A unilateral decrease in breath sounds after the block is given must be distinguished in the differential diagnosis from ipsilateral phrenic nerve paresis. Particularly because of the danger of pneumothorax, ambulant regional anesthesia in this region is regarded as a relative contraindication and requires special informed consent.

References

Borgeat A, Ekatodramis G, Dumont C. An evaluation of the infraclavicular block via a modified approach of the Raj technique. Anesth Analg. 2001;93:436-41.

Jankovic D. Regionalblockaden in Klinik und Praxis. 2 nd ed. Berlin: Blackwell; 2000:58-86.

Kilka HG, Geiger P, Mehrkens HH. Die vertikale infraklavikuläre Blockade des Plexus brachialis. Anaesthesist. 1995;44:339-44.

Neal JM, Moore JM, Kopacz DJ. Quantitative analysis of respiratory, motor, and sensory function after supraclavicular block. Anesth Analg. 1998;86:1239-44.

Neuburger M, Kaiser H, Rembold-Schuster I. Vertikale infraklavikuläre Plexus-brachialis-Blockade. Anaesthesist. 1998;47:595-9.

Neuburger M, Landes H, Kaiser H. Kasuistik: Pneumothorax bei der vertikalen infraklavikulären Blockade des Plexus brachialis. Fallbericht einer seltenen Komplikation. Anaesthesist. 2000:49:901-4.

Neuburger M, Kaiser H, Uhl M.Biometrische Daten zum Pneumothoraxrisiko bei der vertikalen infraklavikulären Plexus-brachialis-Blockade (VIP). Anaesthesist. 2001;50:511-6.

Neuburger M, Kaiser H, Äss B. Vertikal-Infraklavikuläre Plexus-brachialis-Blockade (VIP) - Eine modifizierte Methode der Punktionsortbestimmung unter Berücksichtigung des Pneumothoraxrisikos. Anaesthesist. 2003;52:619-24.

Raj PR, Montgomery SJ, Nettles D. Infraclavicular brachial plexus block—A new approach. Anesth Analg. 1973;52:897-903.

Rodríguez J, Bárcena M, Rodríguez V. Infraclavicular brachial plexus block effects on respiratory function and extent of the block. Reg Anesth Pain Med. 1998;23:564-8.

Stadlmeyer W, Neubauer J, Finkl RO. Unilaterale Phrenikusparese bei vertikaler infraklavikulärer Plexusblockade (VIP). Anaesthesist. 2000;49:1030-3.

4 Suprascapular Nerve Block

4.1 Anatomical Basis

The upper trunk is formed by the roots of C5/C6. The suprascapular nerve branches from the brachial plexus in the region of the upper trunk (Figs. 4.1, 4.2). It continues along the lateral border of the brachial plexus in the supraclavicular fossa as far as the scapular notch. After passing through the notch, it reaches the supraspinous fossa (Fig. 4.3). The supraspinous fossa is shaped like a tub. On the floor of this fossa, the nerve runs laterally and then passes through the neck of the scapula to reach the infraspinous fossa and shoulder. It divides into a motor branch to the supraspinatus and infraspinatus muscles and gives a sensory branch to the shoulder (Figs. 4.4-4.6).

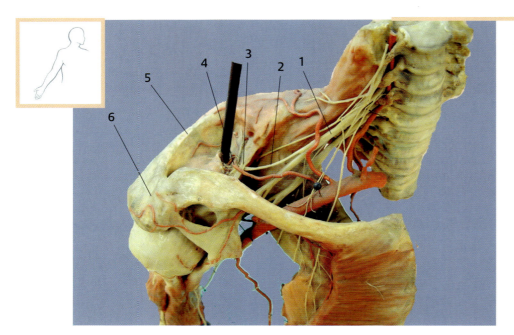

Fig. 4.**1**   Course of the suprascapular nerve.

1 Upper trunk
2 Suprascapular nerve
3 Transverse ligament
4 Suprascapular artery
5 Spine of scapula
6 Acromion

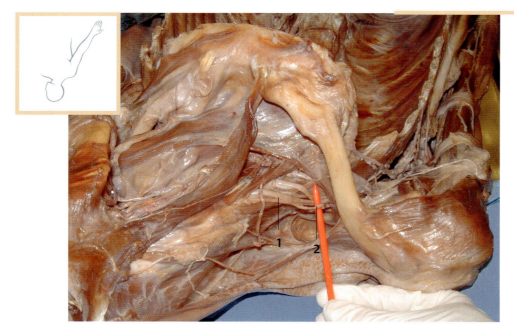

Fig. 4.**2**   Course of the suprascapular nerve, origin from upper trunk.

1 Upper trunk
2 Suprascapular nerve

Fig. 4.**3**   Scapula, seen from behind.

1   Suprascapular artery and vein
2   Suprascapular nerve
3   Acromion
4   Infraspinatus
5   Spine of the scapula
6   Transverse ligament

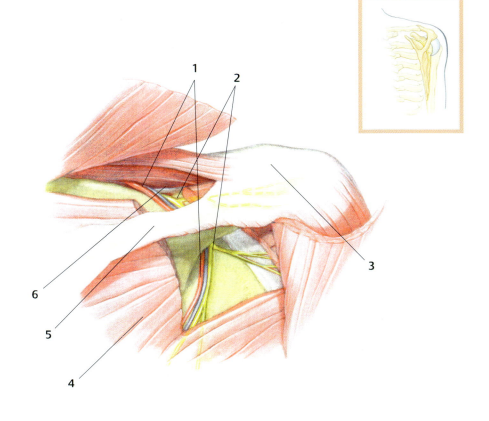

Fig. 4.**4**   Suprascapular nerve block, Meier technique (seen from behind).

1   Spine of the scapula
2   Acromion
3   Branch of the suprascapular nerve innervating the infraspinatus muscle.
4   Infraspinatus (partially divided from bone)

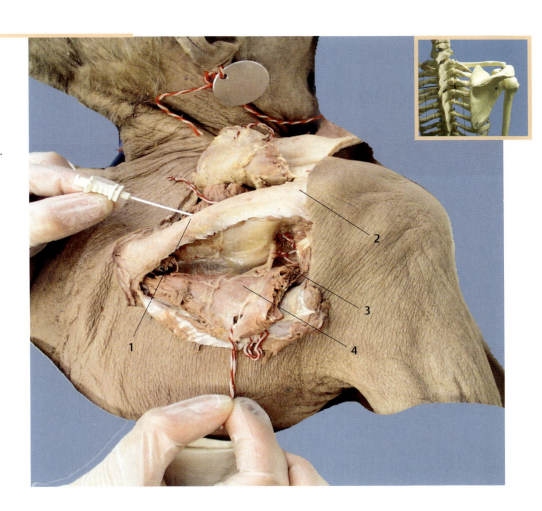

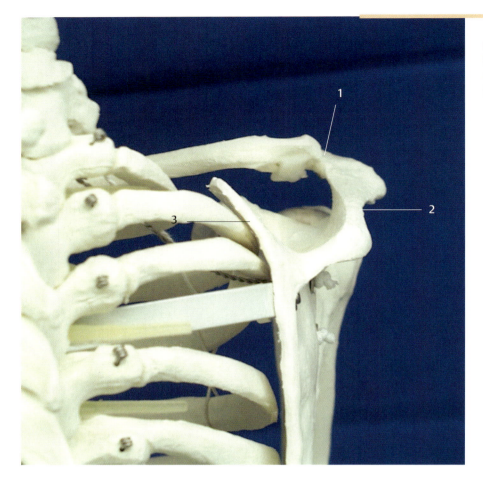

Fig. 4.**5**   Scapula, seen obliquely from behind. Note "tub" shape between the scapula and the spine of the scapula (supraspinous fossa).

1   Acromion
2   Spine of the scapula
3   Scapula

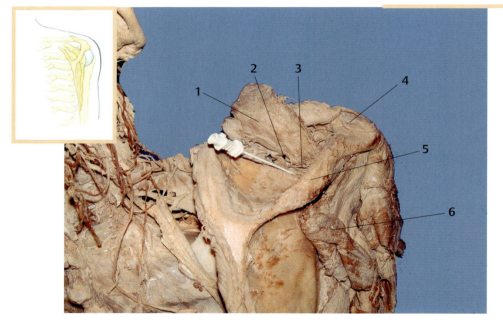

Fig. 4.**6**   Suprascapular nerve block, Meier technique (view from behind).

1   Supraspinatus
2   Scapular notch with transverse ligament
3   Suprascapular nerve
4   Acromion
5   Spine of the scapula
6   Infraspinatus

4.2   Meier Technique

Meier and Bauereis (2002) were able to show from anatomical studies that dye, when injected on the floor of the fossa, drains out through the notch and thus definitely reaches the suprascapular nerve (Fig. 4.**7**). Dangoisse et al. (1994) also arrived at similar results.

The patient is in sitting position with the head bent slightly forward. A line is drawn from the medial end of the spine of the scapula to the lateral posterior border of the acromion. After halving this line, the injection site is established 2 cm medial and 2 cm cranial from this point (Figs. 4.**8**, 4.**9**).

Fig. 4.**7** Right shoulder region, seen from above after injection of dye into the supraspinous fossa. Note the passage of the dye through the scapular notch with staining of the suprascapular nerve. Dissection in prone position.

1   Dye in the supraspinous fossa
2   Transverse ligament with scapular notch
3   Suprascapular nerve before its passage through the scapular notch, bathed in dye

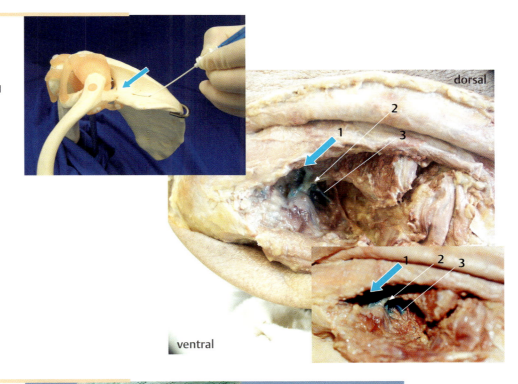

Fig. 4.**8** Site of injection and needle direction for suprascapular block using Meier method.

1   Middle of spine of the scapula
2   Injection site (2 cm cranial and 2 cm medial to the middle of the spine of the scapula)

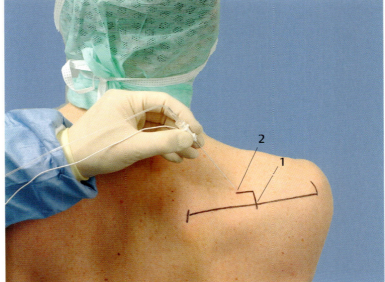

Fig. 4.**9** Scapula, seen from behind. Note "tub" shape of fossa supraspinata.

1   Acromion
2   Scapular notch

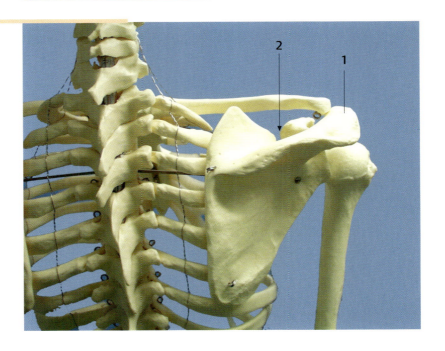

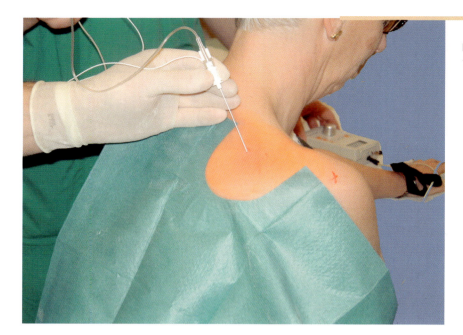

Fig. 4.**10**   Suprascapular nerve block, Meier technique: direction of injection needle.

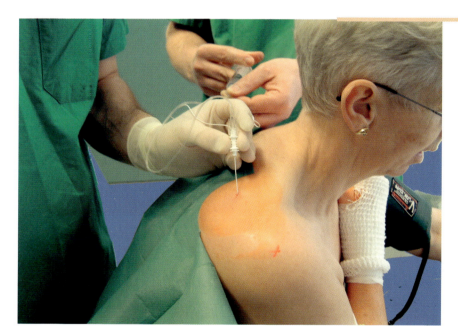

Fig. 4.**11**   Suprascapular nerve block, Meier technique: direction of injection needle.

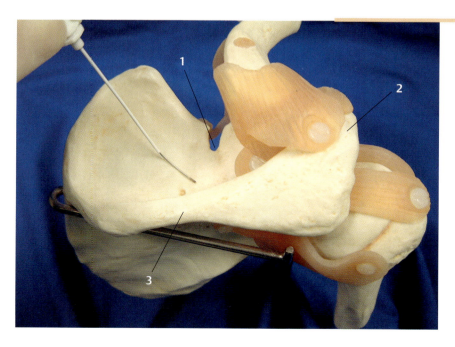

Fig. 4.**12**   Supraspinous fossa, seen from above: position of indwelling catheter.

1   Scapular notch
2   Acromion
3   Spine of the scapula

With the aid of a 22G, 6 cm long insulated needle and using the nerve stimulator, the needle is advanced in a lateral direction on the floor of the fossa at an angle of 75° to the skin surface. The needle should be directed roughly toward the head of the humerus (Figs. 4.**10**, 4.**11**). The presence of a motor response at 0.3-0.5 mA and 0.1 ms shows that the needle is in the correct position. A continuous technique is possible without problems (Fig. 4.**12**).

Material
22G, 6 cm insulated needle.
Continuous technique: Pencil-point needle (catheter-through-needle technique). (E.g., 19.5G, 6 cm (Plexolong Pajunk or Contiplex B. Braun.)

Practical Notes
If no response is obtained on bone contact, the needle is withdrawn and corrected slightly laterally (lower angle to the skin). A catheter can be advanced beyond the tip of the needle (3-5 cm) without difficulty using a pencil-point needle with lateral opening, which should be facing laterally.

Local Anesthetics [LA]
Initially: 10-15 ml of a long-acting LA (e.g., ropivacaine 0.5-0.75 % [5-7.5 mg/ml] or bupivacaine 0.5 % [5 mg/ml]) is administered in the adult. An adequate block can be achieved with this volume (Fig. 4.**13**).
Continuous: 0.2-0.375 % (2 -3.75 mg/ml) ropivacaine or 0.25 % (2.5 mg/ml) bupivacaine, 6-8 ml/h.

Fig. 4.**13**   Suprascapular nerve block, Meier method: spread of contrast in the supraspinous fossa.

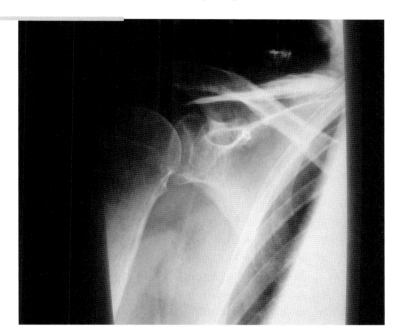

4.3   Sensory and Motor Effects

The suprascapular nerve is responsible for ca. 70 % of the sensory innervation of the shoulder (Ritchie et al. 1997). As it does not innervate any area of skin, this block on its own is inadequate for operative purposes. In pain therapy it is an alternative to the interscalene technique. The motor effect is impairment in the shoulder region (abduction, external rotation).

4.4   Indications and Contraindications

Indications
Pain therapy in shoulder pain of any cause (Fig. 4.**14**).

Contraindications
No special contraindications.

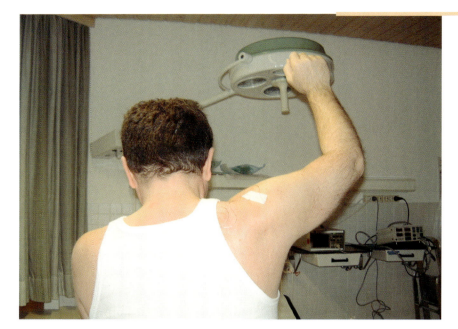

Fig. 4.**14**   Successful suprascapular nerve block for pain therapy in "frozen shoulder" syndrome.

4.5   Complications, Side Effects, Method-Specific Problems

The risk profile of the technique described is much better than that of the classical technique of suprascapular nerve block. In particular, there is a much lower risk of pneumothorax. The problem of difficulty in inserting an indwelling catheter with the risk of a bottleneck syndrome in the region of the scapular notch does not exist with this technique.

Compared to interscalene block there is no motor impairment in the arm and hand with the exception of the muscles innervated by the suprascapular nerve. The suprascapular block has proved very effective for perioperative pain therapy in conjunction with general anesthesia (Ritchie et al. 1997). Numerous articles confirm its effectiveness in pain syndromes due to trauma (Breen and Haigh 1990), in shoulder pain and restriction of movement of rheumatic origin (Brown et al. 1988; Emery et al. 1989; Gado and Emery 1993; Vecchio et al. 1993), and in shoulder pain associated with hemiplegia (Hecht

1992; Lee and Khunadorn 1986). In direct contrast, however, interscalene block for immediate postoperative pain therapy after shoulder operations is markedly superior to suprascapular block (Lhotel et al. 2001). Both blocks were significantly more effective than intra-articular injection of local anesthetics or systemic intravenous pain therapy (Lee and Khunadorn 1986).

References

Breen TW, Haigh JD. Continuous suprascapular nerve block for analgesia of scapular fracture. Can J Anaesth. 1990;37:786-8.

Brown DE, James DC, Roy S. Pain relief by suprascapular nerve block in gleno-humeral arthritis. Scand J Rheumatol. 1988;17:411-5.

Dangoisse MJ, Wilson DJ, Glynn CJ. MRI and clinical study of an easy and safe technique of suprascapular nerve blockade. Acta Anaesth Belg. 1994;45:49-54.

Emery P, Bowman S, Wedderburn L. Suprascapular nerve block for chronic shoulder pain in rheumatoid arthritis. BMJ. 1989;299:1079-80.

Gado K, Emery P. Modified suprascapular nerve block with bupivacaine alone effectively controls chronic shoulder pain in patients with rheumatoid arthritis. Ann Rheum Dis. 1993;52:215-8.

Hecht JS. Suprascapular nerve block in the painful hemiplegic shoulder. Arch Phys Med Rehabil. 1992;73:1036-9.

Lee KH, Khunadorn F. Painful shoulder in hemiplegic patients: A study of the suprascapular nerve. Arch Phys Med Rehabil. 1986;67:818-20.

Lhotel L, Fabre B, Okais I. Postoperative analgesia after arthroscopic shoulder surgery: suprascapular nerve block, intraarticular analgesia or interscalene brachial plexus block. Reg Anesth Pain Med. 2001;26(2, Suppl):34.

Meier G, Bauereis C. Die kontinuierliche N.-suprascapularis-Blockade zur Schmerztherapie der Schulter. Anaesthesist. 2002;51:747-53.

Ritchie ED, Tong D, Chung F. Suprascapular nerve block for postoperative pain relief in arthroscopic shoulder surgery: a new modality? Anesth Analg. 1997;84:1306-12.

Vecchio PC, Adebajo AO, Hazleman BL. Suprascapular nerve block for persistent rotator cuff lesions. J Rheumatol. 1993;20:453-5.

5   Axillary Block

5.1   Anatomical Basis

In the axilla the cords are medial, lateral, and posterior, corresponding to their names (Fig. 5.**1**).

The *ulnar nerve*, the cutaneous nerve of the arm and the medial nerve of the forearm, and also part of the median nerve arise from the medial cord. After the *musculocutaneous nerve* has arisen from the lateral cord, this combines with parts of the medial cord to form the *median nerve*. The posterior cord forms the radial nerve after the axillary nerve has arisen (Figs. 5.**2**, 5.**3**).

From where it passes through the interscalene space as far as the axillary region, the entire brachial plexus is surrounded by a connective-tissue sheath. Besides the nerves, this also contains the blood vessels (axillary artery and vein) (Figs. 5.**4**, 5.**5**). There are connective-tissue septa within this neurovascular sheath (Fig. 5.**6**). However, in the majority of people, these do not appear to hinder the uniform spread of local anesthetic so that block of the entire brachial plexus is possible with a single injection in the axillary region.

The musculocutaneous nerve and the axillary nerve leave the neurovascular sheath very far proximally (Figs. 5.**7**, 5.**8**). The axillary nerve is included in the axillary block only in a few cases and the *musculocutaneous* nerve only if the technique extends very far proximally and an appropriate volume of local anesthetic is used. The radial nerve lies in the axillary region behind the axillary artery and thus, depending on the technique employed, represents the second "problem nerve" in axillary block in addition to the musculocutaneous nerve.

Fig. 5.**1**   Brachial plexus in relation to the subclavian (axillary) artery. Note that the cords rotate through 90° around the subclavian artery from the infraclavicular region to the axillary region. While the posterior cord is furthest laterally (but deeper) compared to the lateral cord in the infraclavicular region, in the axillary region the names of the cords correspond to their actual positions relative to one another.

   1   Lateral cord
   2   Posterior cord
   3   Medial cord

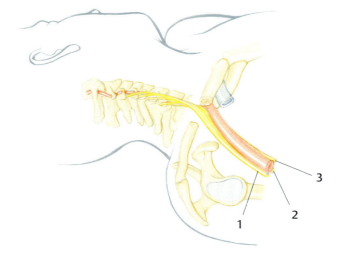

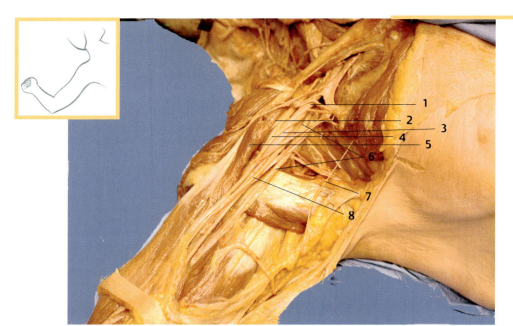

Fig. 5.**2**   Axillary plexus: anatomical overview.

1   Subclavian artery
2   Musculocutaneous nerve
3   Axillary artery
4   Median nerve with its two roots
5   Coracobrachialis
6   Ulnar nerve
7   Intercostobrachial nerve
8   Medial cutaneous nerve of the forearm

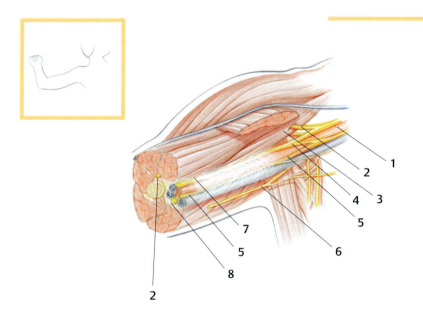

Fig. 5.**3**   Axillary plexus: anatomical overview. (Note the neurovascular connective-tissue sheath.)

1   Subclavian artery
2   Musculocutaneous nerve
3   Coracobrachialis
4   Median nerve with its two roots
5   Ulnar nerve
6   Intercostobrachial nerve
7   Median nerve
8   Radial nerve

Fig. 5.**4**   Connective-tissue sheaths in the axillary neurovascular region.

1   Coracobrachialis
2   Axillary artery
3   Median nerve
4   Ulnar nerve

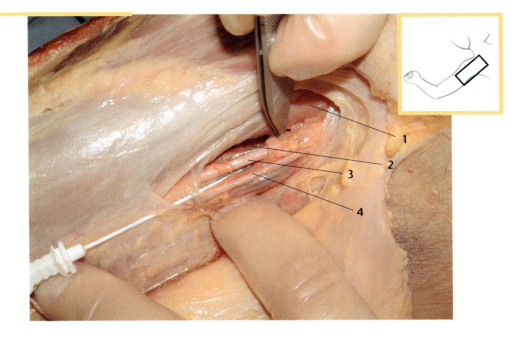

Fig. 5.**5**   Axillary plexus: anatomical over-view.

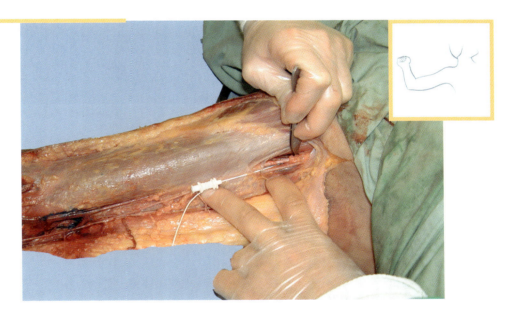

Fig. 5.**6**   Axillary plexus with connective-tissue septation.

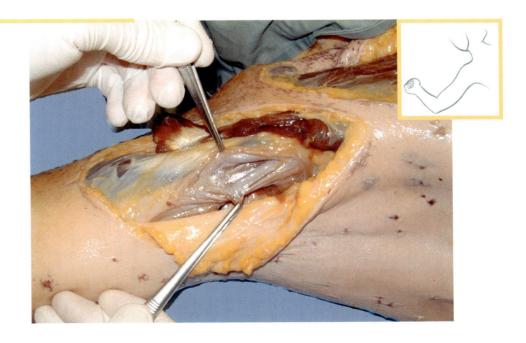

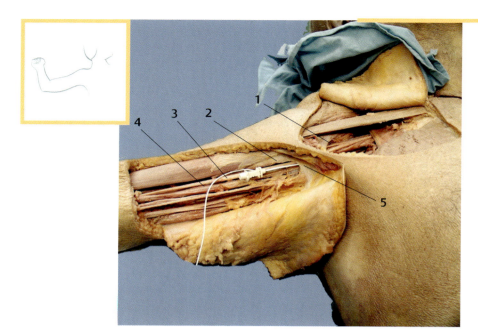

Fig. 5.**7**   Axillary plexus anesthesia, anatomical relations.

1 Musculocutaneous nerve
2 Coracobrachialis
3 Median nerve
4 Axillary artery
5 Neurovascular connective-tissue sheath

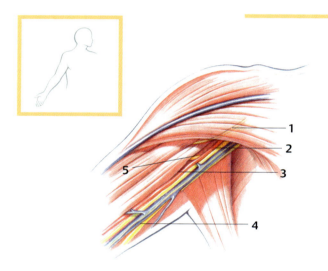

Fig. 5.**8**   Anatomy of the axillary region.

1 Musculocutaneous nerve
2 Median nerve
3 Axillary artery
4 Ulnar nerve
5 Axillary nerve (situated deeply)

5.2   Perivascular "Single-Injection" Technique

The patient lies supine, the arm is abducted about 90° and the elbow is flexed about 90° and externally rotated. The axillary artery, which is usually palpated readily, acts as a landmark. The coracobrachialis muscle runs cranial to the axillary artery. The palpating fingers find the gap between the axillary artery and coracobrachialis somewhat distal to the axillary crease. The injection site is located where the lateral edge of pectoralis major crosses the axillary artery (Fig. 5.**9**). Following intracutaneous local anesthetic

(LA) infiltration, a prepuncture is made through the skin. The needle used for the block should have a short bevel (Fig. 5.**10**) for optimal identification of the neurovascular sheath. The needle is inserted at an angle of ca. 30-45° parallel to the artery in the palpated gap (Fig. 5.**9**); after a few millimeters, noticeable resistance is felt, which can be overcome with controlled pressure. Immediately after overcoming this resistance, the needle is lowered and advanced proximally as far as it will go in the neurovascular

sheath. A nerve stimulator can now be used to check that the needle is in the correct position. Using small "wobbling movements" different nerves can often be stimulated (median nerve, ulnar nerve, radial nerve) (Figs. 5.**11**, 5.**12**). The tip of the needle is occasionally behind the median nerve, so it can be helpful to back the needle tip toward the skin (anteriorly) to obtain a response. In contrast to all other blocks, there is no correlation here between the amplitude of the stimulus and the success rate.

Fig. 5.**9** Technique of "perivascular" axillary
plexus anesthesia.

1 Coracobrachialis
2 Axillary artery
3 Site of injection

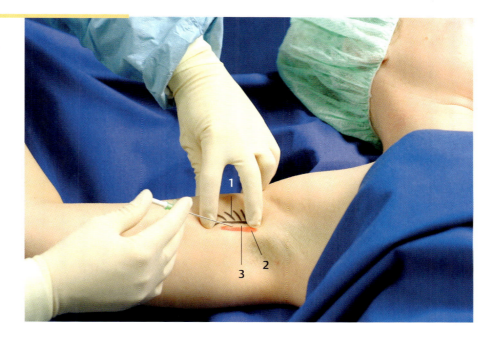

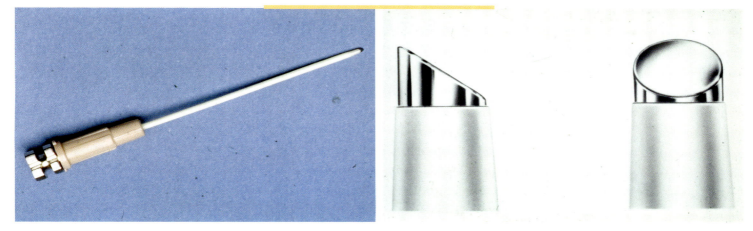

Fig. 5.**10** Atraumatic cannula for technique of perivascular axillary block.

Fig. 5.**11** Axillary plexus anesthesia. (Note:
the tip of the needle extends almost to the
musculocutaneous nerve.)

1 Lateral cord
2 Subclavian artery (axillary)
3 Musculocutaneous nerve

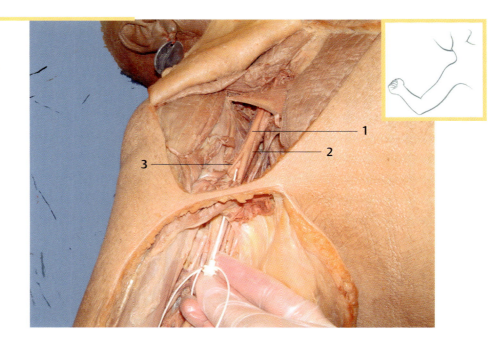

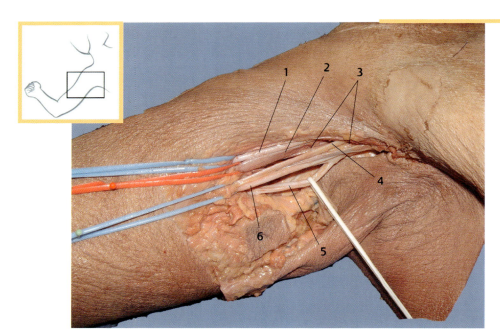

Fig. 5.**12**   Axillary plexus.

1   Musculocutaneous nerve
2   Axillary vein
3   Axillary artery
4   Median nerve
5   Radial nerve (pulled forward)
6   Ulnar nerve

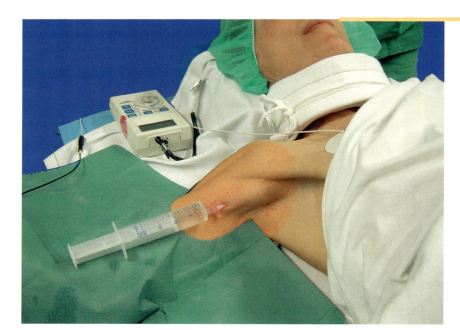

Fig. 5.**13**   Axillary plexus anesthesia, perivascular technique. Note the tubelike distension due to the injected local anesthetic.

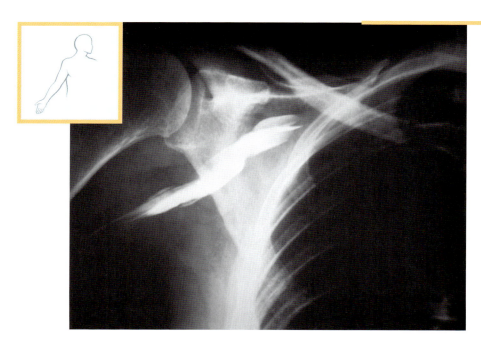

Fig. 5.**14**   Spread of contrast with perivascular axillary plexus anesthesia technique. (Note tubelike spread of local anesthetic.)

Fig. 5.**15** Inserting an axillary plexus ind-welling catheter.

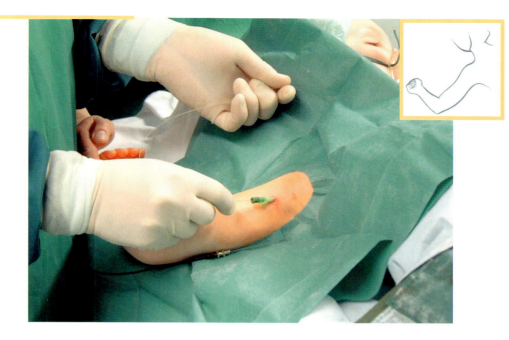

Fig. 5.**16** Axillary plexus indwelling catheter.

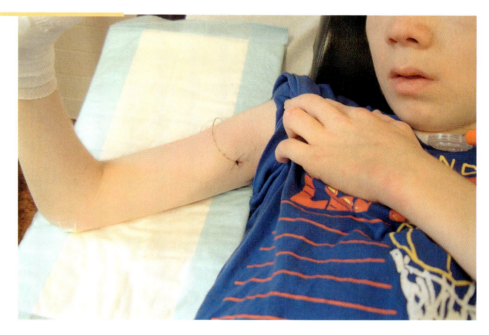

Material

"Single-shot" technique: 22G, 5-6 cm long insulated needle with blunt bevel; pencil-point tip is also possible.

Continuous technique: 18G indwelling needle with blunt stylet (e.g., 45° bevel) (Fig. 5.**10**). After successful placement, remove the sty-let, advance a flexible catheter through the introducing cannula (Fig. 5.**15**), and remove the needle.

For children: 20G needle with solid steel sty-let.

Practical Notes

A response from the musculocutaneous nerve indicates that the needle is in the wrong position (runs in the coracobrachialis muscle after leaving the brachial plexus) (Fig. 5.**3**). As an alternative to the use of a nerve stimulator, the correct needle position can also be verified by the production of paresthesia using refrigerator-chilled isotonic saline. In terms of effectiveness, this method is similar to the use of a nerve stimulator (Aul 2000; Rodriguez et al. 1996), but for patients it is associated with unpleasant paresthesia. Paresthesia should not be pro-duced deliberately with the needle because of the increased risk of nerve injury. Axillary plexus anesthesia performed by this method is one of the few techniques that can also be performed without the use of a nerve stimu-lator. For this, an 18G needle with a solid steel stylet, 45° bevel, and rounded edges is helpful as the loss of resistance can be felt clearly.

Apart from cold paresthesia and/or a response through the nerve stimulator, the following criteria are regarded as evidence that the needle is in the correct position:
- Clear loss of resistance
- Smooth advancement of the needle

If the needle is in the correct position, there will be a tubelike distension of the neu-rovascular sheath due to the injected local anesthetic (Figs. 5.**13**, 5.**14**).

The commonest mistakes in puncture are incorrect orientation (artery not located cor-rectly) and too-deep puncture. The needle must not be advanced beyond the point of loss of resistance. (Lower the needle and advance it tangentially according to the pro-cedure in peripheral venipuncture.)

This technique is excellently suited to a continuous catheter technique (Figs. 5.**15**, 5.**16**).

5.3   Sensory and Motor Effects

When this technique is performed correctly, there is reliable sensory and motor block of the median, ulnar, and *musculocutaneous* nerve (Fig. 5.**17**) (Aul 2000; Büttner and Klose 1991; Büttner et al. 1987). The radial nerve occasionally demonstrates incomplete block.

The incidence of complete block with this technique is 70-75% (Büttner et al. 1988; Neuburger et al. 1998); ca. 20-25% can be supplemented (see below) and ca. 5% can be classified as complete failures. Using a volume of 50 ml of, for example, mepivacaine 1%, the incidence of complete block will be 80-85% (Büttner et al. 1987; Büttner and Klose 1991; Vester-Andersen 1989): The success rate depends among other things on the volume of LA (Vester-Andersen 1984). While the musculocutaneous nerve does not usually pose a problem when an indwelling needle and an adequate volume of LA are used (Fig. 5.**11**) (Aul 2000; Büttner and Klose 1991; Büttner et al. 1987), the *commonest failures* can be attributed to incomplete block of the radial nerve. The assumption that placing the arm close to the body while the LA is being given increases the likelihood of a successful block of the radial nerve (a requirement for this is insertion of an indwelling cannula or catheter), (Vester-Andersen et al. 1986), was not confirmed in a clinical study (Koscielniak-Nielsen et al. 1995b).

Local Anesthetic, Dosages
Initially: In adults, 40-50 ml of a medium-acting (e.g., mepivacaine or lidocaine 1% (10 mg/ml) or a long-acting (ropivacaine 0.5-0.75% [5-7.5 mg/ml]) LA is given. An adequate volume is required to sufficiently load the entire neurovascular sheath with the single-shot technique (Fig. 5.**18**). If the LA is given through an indwelling catheter, spread as far as the supraclavicular region can be achieved (Figs. 5.**19**, 5.**20**). If the catheter is in the wrong position, the LA is distributed diffusely in the tissue without effect (Fig. 5.**21**). Advancing the catheter too far (> 4-5 cm beyond the tip of the needle) or advancing it against resistance should be avoided.
Continuous: 0.2-0.375% (2-3.75 mg/ml) ropivacaine, 6-8 ml/h.

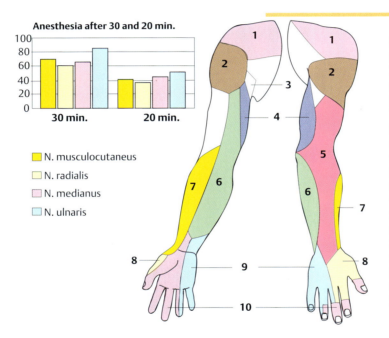

Fig. 5.**17**   Percentages of patients who have reached the stage of anesthesia after 30 and 20 minutes, respectively, after axillary plexus anesthesia with 400 mg mepivacaine 1% (10 mg/ml) (Aul 2000; Büttner and Klose 1991; Büttner et al. 1987). Note that the musculocutaneous nerve, which is often described as a problem nerve, is anesthetized with the same frequency as the median nerve, and the radial nerve is not significantly worse. The ulnar nerve together with the medial cutaneous nerve of the forearm tends to be anesthetized best. 1 and 2 are usually not included in the axillary block, and 3 and 4 can be anesthetized by subcutaneous infiltration on the inside of the upper arm as they are purely cutaneous nerves.
Sensory innervation of the upper limb:

1   Supraclavicular nerve
2   Axillary nerve (lateral cutaneous of arm)
3   Intercostobrachial nerve
4   Medial cutaneous nerve of the arm

5   Posterior cutaneous nerve of the forearm (radial nerve)
6   Medial cutaneous nerve of the forearm
7   Lateral cutaneous nerve of the forearm (musculocutaneous nerve)

8   Radial nerve
9   Ulnar nerve
10   Median nerve

Fig. 5.**18**   Axillary plexus block, perivascular technique. Note the tubelike distension due to the injected local anesthetic.

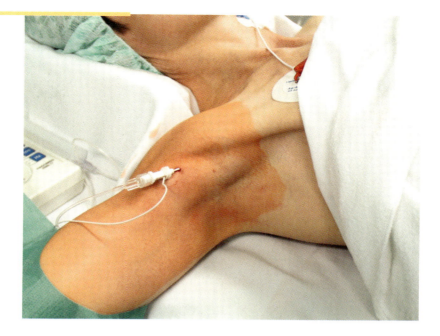

Fig. 5.**19**   Spread of contrast through the axillary plexus indwelling catheter.

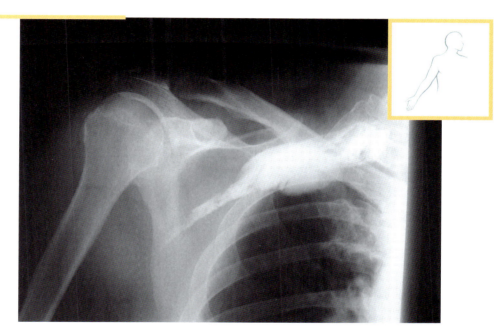

Fig. 5.**20**   Axillary plexus: anatomical overview.

  1 Subclavian artery
  2 Musculocutaneous nerve
  3 Axillary artery
  4 Coracobrachialis
  5 Median nerve with its two roots
  6 Ulnar nerve
  7 Axillary artery
  8 Median nerve

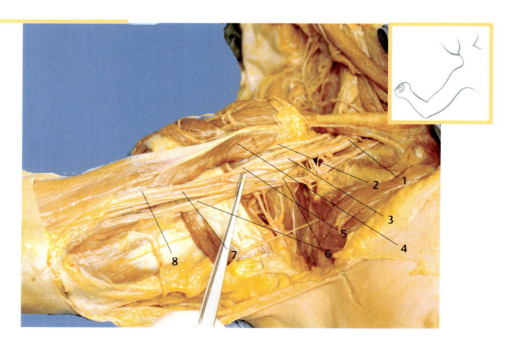

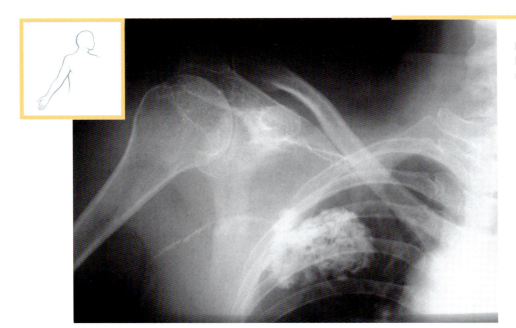

Fig. 5.**21**   Spread of contrast when an axillary plexus indwelling catheter is in an incorrect position.

5.4   Indications and Contraindications

Indications

All operative procedures on the elbow, forearm, and hand. In the distal upper arm and elbow region, too, excellent analgesia and anesthesia can be obtained with the axillary block (Schroeder et al. 1996). Continuous axillary block is suitable for postoperative pain therapy, physiotherapeutic treatment (e.g., mobilization of stiff joints), prophylaxis and treatment of chronic pain states (CRPS, postamputation pain), sympathetic block (e.g., after replantation of amputated limbs), frostbite, and vasospasm after accidental intra-arterial injection (e.g., of thiopentone).

Contraindications

- General contraindications to peripheral blocks
- No special contraindications

5.5   Complications, Side Effects, Method-Specific Problems

- The brachial plexus lies directly subcutaneously, and puncture is often performed too deep in the tissue.
- If there are difficulties in identifying the axillary artery, a Doppler probe can be used for assistance.
- An indwelling cannula (18G) with a solid stylet has proved to be useful even when a "single-shot" block is performed. If a continuous block is not required, the cannula can at least be left in place until the end of the operation in order to supplement or prolong the block by further injection of local anesthetic (Selander 1977).

- The indwelling needle shifts the injection point for the LA proximally so that the likelihood of successfully blocking the musculocutaneous nerve is high (Figs. 5.**11**, 5.**20**).
- An adequate volume (40-50 ml in adults) of an adequately concentrated LA should be used in order to obtain a successful block (Vester-Andersen 1984).
- When an indwelling needle and an adequate volume are used, there are very few problems with the tourniquet (6.1 %) (Büttner et al. 1988).
- Vascular puncture with this technique is very rare (1.1 %) (Büttner et al. 1988).

- Nerve injuries are extremely rare with this technique (Büttner et al. 1988; Krebs and Hempel 1984).
- An additional block of the superficial cutaneous nerves supplying the inside of the upper arm, particularly the intercostobrachial nerve, in the form of subcutaneous infiltration is recommended.
- A tourniquet or compression distal to the injection site does not appear to confer any additional advantage (Koscielniak-Nielsen et al. 1995a).

5.6 Multistimulation Technique, "Mid-Humeral Approach" According to Dupré

(Dupré 1994)

Dupré described the "bloc du plexus brachial au canal huméral" in 1994, which is translated incorrectly in the Anglo-American literature as "mid-humeral approach." In fact, this is technique is performed at the junction of the proximal and middle thirds of the upper arm (Fig. 5.**22**).

Positioning, Landmarks

The patient lies supine, the arm is abducted 80° and extended on an arm table. The brachial artery is found at the junction of the proximal and middle thirds of the upper arm. The principle is to find and separately block the four main nerves innervating the arm from one injection site by withdrawing the needle under the skin and advancing it in different directions (Fig. 5.**22**).

Method

The *median nerve* is found first. While palpating the brachial artery, the needle is advanced tangentially to the skin proximally and cranially and parallel to the artery under the brachialis fascia; after a typical median nerve motor response is produced, 8-10 ml of the local anesthetic is injected (Figs. 5.**23**-5.**25**).

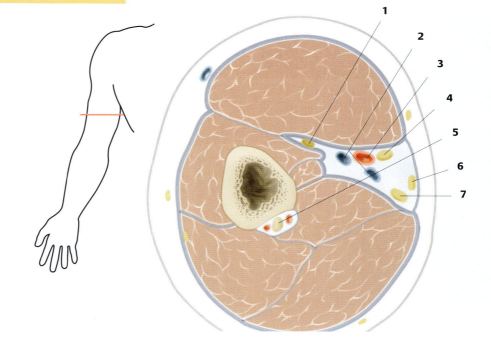

Fig. 5.**22**   Anatomy of axillary block using Dupré method (mid-humeral approach).

1   Musculocutaneous nerve
2   Axillary veins
3   Axillary artery
4   Median nerve
5   Radial nerve
6   Medial cutaneous nerve of the forearm
7   Ulnar nerve

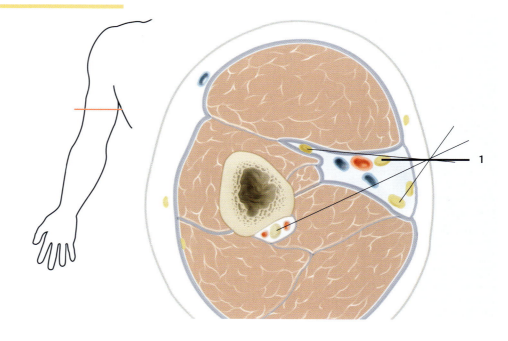

Fig. 5.**23**   Direction of needle for median nerve block (mid-humeral approach).

1   Median nerve block (direction of needle)

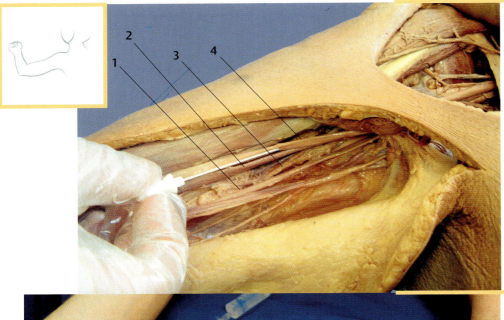

Fig. 5.**24**   Direction of needle for median nerve block (mid-humeral approach).

1   Ulnar nerve
2   Axillary artery
3   Radial nerve
4   Median nerve

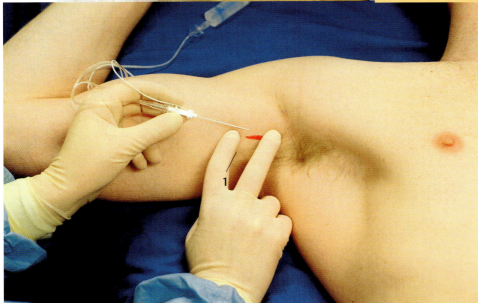

Fig. 5.**25**   Direction of needle for median nerve block (mid-humeral approach).

1   Course of the axillary artery

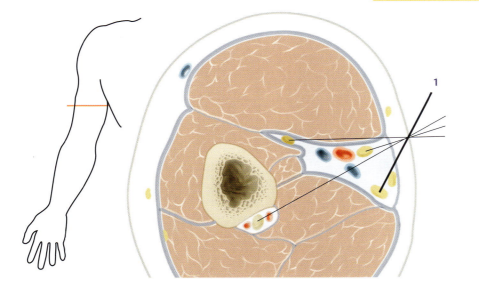

Fig. 5.**26**   Direction of needle for ulnar nerve block (mid-humeral approach).

1   Ulnar nerve block (direction of needle)

After blocking the median nerve, the needle is drawn back under the skin. By directing the needle anterior-posterior (toward the surface on which the patient is lying) the *ulnar nerve* is now found (Figs. 5.**26**-5.**28**).

After withdrawal of the needle it is advanced toward the lower edge of the humerus until a motor response is produced in the region of the *radial nerve* (extension of the hand/fingers). A muscle response in the triceps is regarded as unsatisfactory (Figs. 5.**29**-5.**32**).

Fig. 5.**27**   Direction of needle for ulnar nerve
block (mid-humeral approach).

1 Ulnar nerve
2 Axillary artery
3 Radial nerve
4 Median nerve

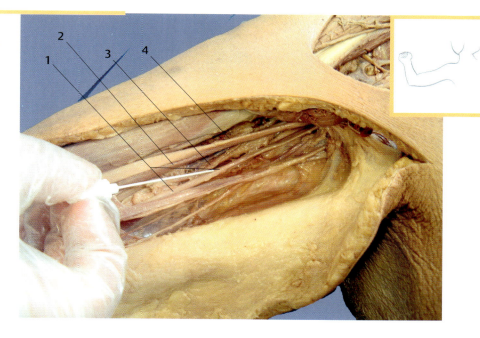

Fig. 5.**28**   Direction of needle for ulnar nerve
block (mid-humeral approach); the needle
passes between the skin and the axillary
artery in front of the axillary artery.

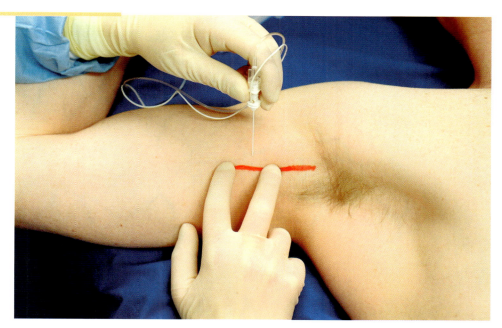

Fig. 5.**29**   Direction of needle for radial
nerve block (mid-humeral approach).

1 Radial nerve block (direction of
   needle)

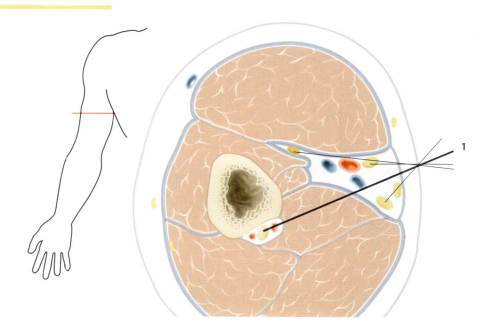

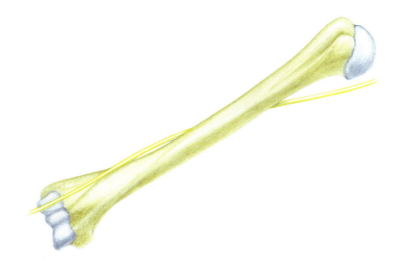

Fig. 5.**30** Course of the radial nerve around the humerus.

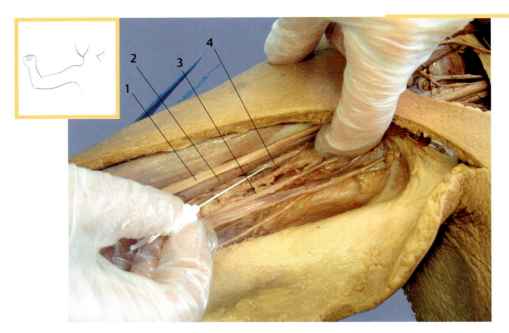

Fig. 5.**31** Direction of needle for radial nerve block (mid-humeral approach).

1 Median nerve
2 Axillary artery
3 Ulnar nerve
4 Radial nerve

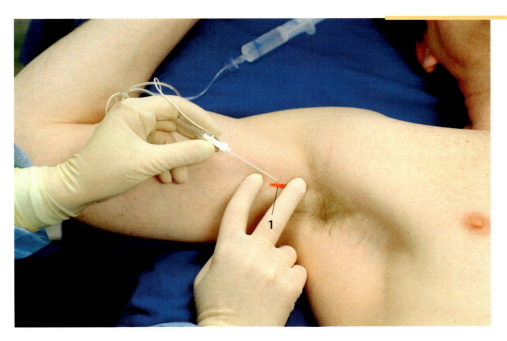

Fig. 5.**32** Direction of needle for radial nerve block (mid-humeral approach); the needle passes between the skin and the axillary artery, that is, below the axillary artery directed toward the humerus.

1 Course of the axillary artery

The *musculocutaneous nerve* is found by advancing the needle horizontally below the belly of the biceps. It is helpful here to elevate the muscle belly a little by pinching it (Figs. 5.**33**-5.**35**). 8-10 ml of local anesthetic per nerve is injected.

All nerves are found with the aid of the nerve stimulator according to the usual criteria. At the end, the medial cutaneous nerve of the arm is blocked by subcutaneous infiltration.

Puncture Needle

22G, 5-8 cm long insulated needle.

Practical Notes

- This method is not suitable as a continuous technique.
- The *success rate* is reported as 82.1% (Gaertner et al. 1999), 88% (Bouaziz et al. 1997), and 95% (Carles et al. 2001).
- Completion by selective blocks at the elbow is possible with the aid of the nerve stimulator.
- In addition to the "mid-humeral approach," a multistimulation technique in the axilla has been described (Koscielniak-Nielsen et al. 1997, 1999 a, 1999 b). Onset of effect (15 ± 7 minutes),

success rate (ca. 90%), and the time required to perform the block (5-10 minutes) are similar for the two techniques (Sia et al. 2002). An advantage of the distal "mid-humeral approach" compared to a "multistimulation technique" performed directly in the axilla is the fact that the nerves here lie widely separated from each other, so that a nerve injury due to injection into an already anesthetized nerve becomes more unlikely.

- The success rate in blocking the ulnar nerve is somewhat lower than for the other nerves with this technique (Bouaziz et al. 1997).

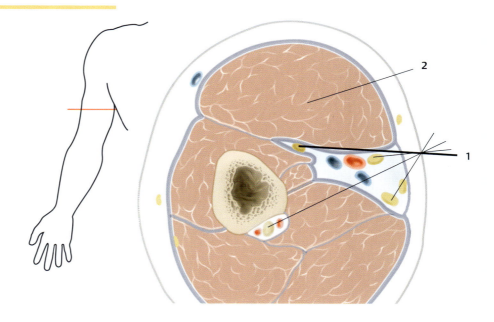

Fig. 5.**33**   Direction of needle for musculocutaneous nerve block (mid-humeral approach).

1   Musculocutaneous nerve block (direction of needle)
2   Biceps

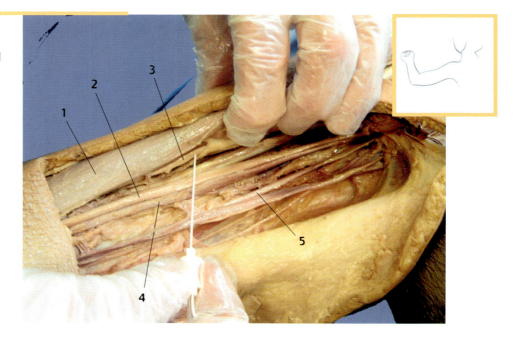

Fig. 5.**34**   Direction of needle for musculocutaneous nerve block (mid-humeral approach).

1   Biceps
2   Median nerve
3   Musculocutaneous nerve
4   Brachial artery
5   Ulnar nerve

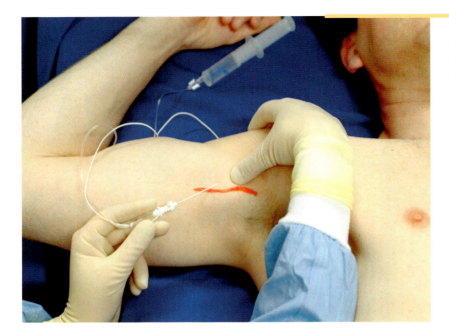

Fig. 5.**35**   Direction of needle for musculocutaneous nerve block (mid-humeral approach); the biceps muscle is grasped and elevated slightly.

- The technique allows a differentiated block of the individual nerves. Thus the nerve in whose innervation region the postoperative pain is to be expected can be anesthetized with a long-acting local anesthetic for postoperative pain therapy, while a shorter-acting local anesthetic enables early postoperative restoration of sensation and motor function.

References

Aul A. Untersuchungen zur Erfolgsrate der axillären Plexus-brachialis-Blockade [Dissertation]. Mannheim/Heidelberg; 2000.

Bouaziz H, Narchi P, Mercier FJ, et al. Comparison between conventional axillary block and a new approach at the midhumeral level. Anesth Analg. 1997;84:1058-62.

Büttner J, Klose R. Alkalinisierung von Mepivacain zur axillären Katheterplexusanästhesie. Reg Anaesth. 1991;14:17-24.

Büttner J, Klose R, Dreesen H. Vergleichende Untersuchung von Prilocain 1% und Mepivacain 1% zur axillären Plexusanästhesie. Reg Anaesth. 1987;10:70-5.

Büttner J, Kemmer A, Argo A. Axilläre Blockade des Plexus brachialis. Reg Anaesth. 1988;11:7-11.

Carles M, Pulcini A, Macchi P. An evaluation of the brachial plexus block at the humeral canal using a neurostimulator (1417 patients): The efficacy, safety, and predictive criteria of failure. Anesth Analg. 2001;92:194-8.

Dupré LJ. Bloc du plexus brachial au canal huméral. Cah Anesthesiol. 1994;42:767-9.

Gaertner E, Kern O, Mahoudeau G. Block of the brachial plexus branches by the humeral route. A prospective study in 503 ambulatory patients. Proposal of a nerve-blocking sequence. Acta Anaesthesiol Scand. 1999;43:609-13.

Koscielniak-Nielsen ZJ, Christensen LQ, Pedersen HL. Effect of digital pressure on the neurovascular sheath during perivascular axillary block. Br J Anaesth. 1995 a;75:702-6.

Koscielniak-Nielsen ZJ, Horn A, Nielsen PR. Effect of arm position on the effectiveness of perivascular axillary nerve block. Br J Anaesth. 1995 b;74:387-91.

Koscielniak-Nielsen ZJ, Stens-Pedersen HL, Lippert FK. Readiness for surgery after axillary block: Single or multiple injection techniques. Eur J Anaesthesiol. 1997;14:164-71.

Koscielniak-Nielsen ZJ, Nielsen PR, Nielsen SL. Comparison of transarterial and multiple nerve stimulation techniques for axillary block using a high dose of mepivacaine with adrenaline. Acta Anaesthesiol Scand. 1999 a;43:398-404.

Koscielniak-Nielsen ZJ, Nielsen PR, Sørensen T. Low dose axillary block by targeted injec-

tions of the terminal nerves. Can J Anaesth. 1999 b;46:658-64.

Krebs P, Hempel V. Eine neue Kombinationsnadel für die hohe axilläre Plexus-brachialis-Anästhesie. Anasth Intensivmed. 1984;25:219.

Neuburger M, Kaiser H, Rembold-Schuster I. Vertikale infraklavikuläre Plexus-brachialis-Blockade. Anaesthesist. 1998;47:595-9.

Rodríguez J, Bárcena M, Alvarez J. Axillary brachial plexus anesthesia: Electrical versus cold saline stimulation. Anesth Analg. 1996;83:752-4.

Schroeder LE, Horlocker TT, Schroeder DR. The efficacy of axillary block for surgical procedures about the elbow. Anesth Analg. 1996;83:747-51.

Selander D, Catheter technique in axillary plexus block. Acta Anaesthesiol. Scand. 1977;21:324-9.

Sia S, Lepri A, Campolo MC. Four-injection brachial plexus block using peripheral nerve stimulator: a comparison between axillary and humeral approaches. Anesth Analg. 2002;95:1075-9.

Vester-Andersen T, Husum B, Lindeburg T, Borrits L, Gothgen I: Perivascular Axillary Block IV: Blockade following 10, 50 or 60 ml of mepivacaine 1% with adrenaline. Acta Anaesthesiol. Scand. 1984;28:99-105.

Vester-Andersen T, Broby-Johansen U, Bro-Rasmussen F. Perivascular axillary block VI: the distribution of gelatine solutions injected into the axillary neurovascular sheath of cadavers. Acta Anaesthesiol Scand. 1986;30:18-22.

6   Selective Block of Individual Nerves in the Upper Arm, at the Elbow and Wrist

6.1   Radial Nerve Block (Middle of Upper Arm)

Anatomical Basis

The radial nerve passes under the middle of the humerus in the radial nerve sulcus to reach the outside of the upper arm and then enters the elbow on the radial side of the flexor aspect (Figs. 6.**1**-6.**3**).

Method

The arm is positioned as for perivascular axillary plexus anesthesia (Figs. 6.**4**, 6.**5**). In the middle of the upper arm, the furrow between the flexors and extensors is found. The posterior border of the humerus is pal-pated. Coming from below (below the brachial artery), the posterior border of the humerus is found with a 4-8 cm long insulated needle (Fig. 6.**2**). On bone contact, an attempt is made to advance the needle a little further under the humerus. The technique should generally be performed with

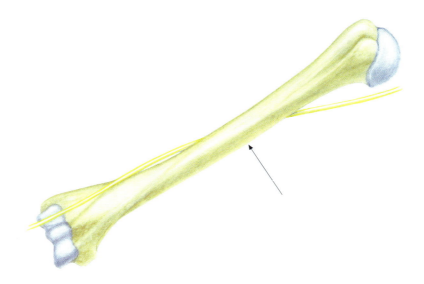

Fig. 6.**1**   Selective radial nerve block in the mid-upper arm. The posterior border of the humerus is sought.

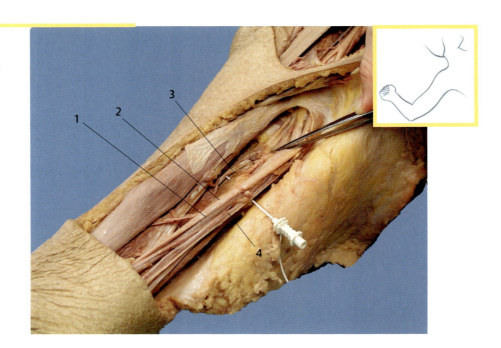

Fig. 6.**2**   Selective radial nerve block in the mid-upper arm. The posterior border of the humerus is found below the brachial artery and the other nerves supplying the arm.

1   Brachial artery
2   Median nerve
3   Radial nerve
4   Ulnar nerve

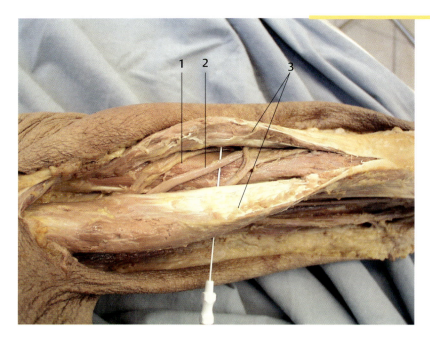

Fig. 6.**3** Selective radial nerve block in the right mid-upper arm, view from behind, dissection in prone position, triceps muscle split. The cannula has been advanced too far (for technical photographic reasons).

1 Humerus
2 Radial nerve
3 Triceps

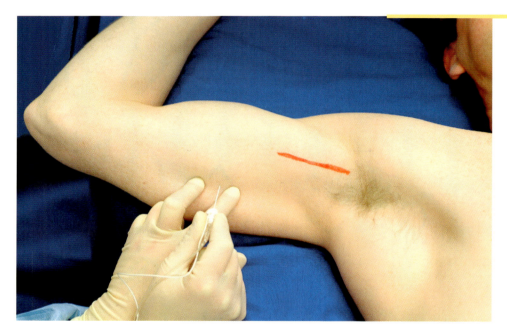

Fig. 6.**4** Selective radial nerve block in the mid-upper arm. The posterior border of the humerus is found below the brachial artery and the other nerves supplying the arm.

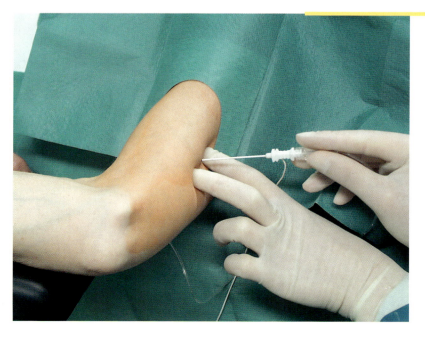

Fig. 6.**5** Selective radial nerve block in the mid-upper arm with peripheral nerve stimulation.

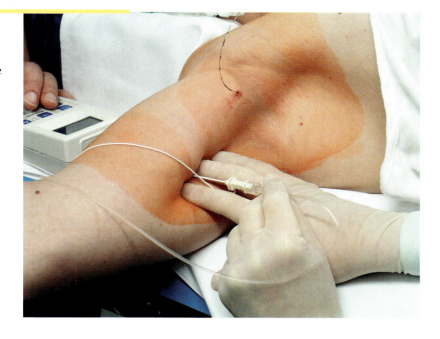

Fig. 6.**6**   Selective radial nerve block in the mid-upper arm. This block can be used to supplement a brachial plexus block. Note the in situ axillary plexus catheter.

the nerve stimulator and an insulated needle, particularly if an axillary block has already been performed. When there is a clear response to a corresponding stimulus and pulse duration (0.3-0.5 mA, 0.1 ms), 8-10 ml of the local anesthetic (LA) is injected with repeated aspiration.

Material
22G, 4-8 cm insulated needle.

Practical Notes
The response should be in the hand (extension of the wrist or fingers).

Sensory and Motor Effects
Sensory and motor loss in the region of the radial nerve distal to the injection site.

Indications
Supplement to brachial plexus anesthesia. It has proved useful to perform this block in

combination with a perivascular block (Fig. 6.**6**) if the radial nerve was not specially stimulated when the axillary block was performed. This is probably better from the aspects of the risk of nerve damage, the time required for its performance, and patient acceptance. (NB: The effectiveness of the multistimulation technique.)

6.2   Blocks at the Elbow

Anatomy

After passing under the humerus, the *radial nerve* appears at the elbow on the radial side between the brachioradialis and the brachialis muscles lateral to the biceps tendon (Fig. 6.**7**). Here it divides into a (sensory) superficial branch and a thicker (mainly motor) deep branch (Fig. 6.**8**).
The lateral cutaneous nerve of the forearm is the sensory terminal branch of the *musculocutaneous* nerve and provides the sensory innervation of the radial side of the forearm. It lies on the radial side; since it is already epifascial lateral to the biceps tendon it is very superficial(!) (Fig. 6.**8**).
The *median nerve* passes through the elbow medial to the brachial artery (on the ulnar side) (mnemonic: **m**edian nerve-**m**edial) (Figs. 6.**7**, 6.**8**).

The *ulnar nerve* passes through the ulnar sulcus (on the back of the medial epicondyle of the humerus) (Figs. 6.**9**, 6.**10**).

Radial Nerve Block (Elbow)

The extended arm is abducted and externally rotated and the forearm is supinated. The biceps tendon can be palpated easily. The puncture site is 1-2 cm lateral (radial) to the biceps tendon at the level of the intercondylar line (Figs. 6.**11**, 6.**12**). The insulated needle is advanced slightly proximally and laterally in the direction of the lateral epicondyle (Fig. 6.**13**). If the radial nerve responds to stimulation with a current less than 0.5 mA, 5-10 ml of LA is injected. If no response is produced, the needle is inserted until it makes contact with bone, and after

injection of 3-4 ml of LA this process is repeated in a fan pattern.
While withdrawing the needle, the lateral cutaneous nerve of the forearm (sensory terminal branch of the musculocutaneous nerve) can also be blocked with the same injection by subcutaneous injection in a fan pattern (Fig. 6.**11**; see Musculocutaneous Nerve Block).

Musculocutaneous Nerve Block (Elbow)

The lateral cutaneous nerve of the forearm, a sensory terminal branch of the musculocutaneous nerve, is already very superficial in the elbow region. It is blocked by subcutaneous infiltration lateral to the biceps tendon in the direction of the lateral epicondyle

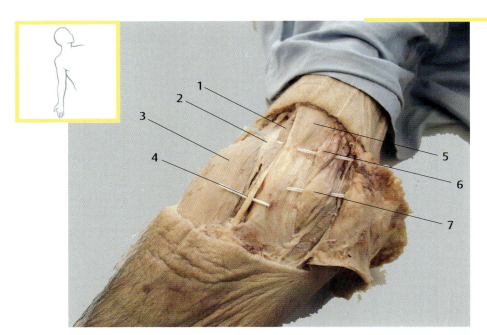

Fig. 6.**7**   Anatomy of the right elbow.

1   Brachialis
2   Radial nerve
3   Brachioradialis
4   Lateral cutaneous nerve of the fore-
    arm
5   Biceps
6   Brachial artery
7   Median nerve

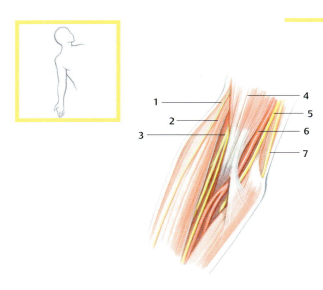

Fig. 6.**8**   Cubital fossa, right arm.

1   Posterior cutaneous nerve of the fore-
    arm
2   Brachioradialis
3   Radial nerve
4   Biceps
5   Median nerve
6   Brachial artery
7   Ulnar nerve

with a 24G or 25G needle about 5 cm in length (Figs. 6.**14**-6.**16**).
The technique can be readily combined with the technique of radial nerve block at the elbow.

Median Nerve Block (Elbow)

The extended arm is abducted and externally rotated and the forearm is supinated. The pulse of the brachial artery is palpated on the intercondylar line. Medial to the artery, a 24G needle is advanced parallel to the artery in a cranial direction at an angle of about 45° to the skin with stimulation (Figs. 6.**17**-6.**19**). When there is a corresponding response after 1-2 cm, ca. 5 ml of the LA is injected.

Fig. 6.**9**   Ulnar nerve in the ulnar sulcus,
right arm.

1   Medial epicondyle of the humerus
2   Ulnar nerve
3   Olecranon

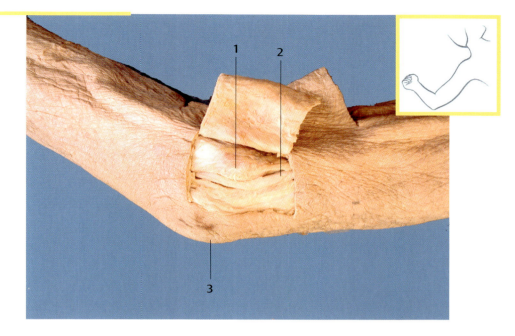

Fig. 6.**10**   Ulnar nerve in the ulnar sulcus.

1   Medial epicondyle of the humerus
2   Ulnar nerve
3   Olecranon

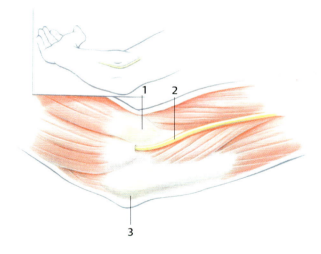

Ulnar Nerve Block (Elbow)

The extended arm is abducted and externally rotated and the elbow is flexed through 90°. The ulnar sulcus is located between the medial epicondyle and the olecranon. The ulnar nerve is often palpated easily here. The ulnar nerve is in the ulnar sulcus only when the elbow is flexed (Figs. 6.**20**-6.**22**). Because of the risk of pressure injury, the puncture should not be directly into the ulnar sulcus but about 1-2 cm cranial to it (Fig. 6.**23**). The needle should be introduced tangentially to the nerve. Using a 3.5-5 cm 24-25G insulated needle and a nerve stimulator, ca. 5 ml of the LA is injected when there is a corresponding motor response.

The ulnar nerve is very sensitive to irritation. Neuritis has been observed after puncture of the ulnar nerve.

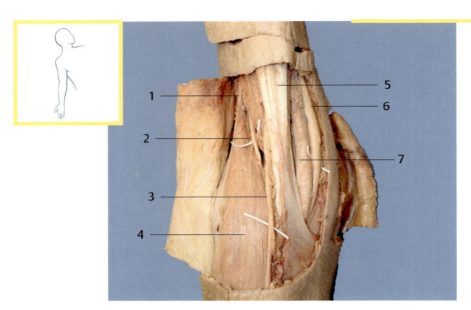

Fig. 6.**11** Cubital fossa, right arm.

1 Posterior cutaneous nerve of the forearm
2 Radial nerve
3 Lateral cutaneous nerve of the forearm (musculocutaneous nerve)
4 Brachioradialis
5 Biceps
6 Median nerve
7 Brachial artery

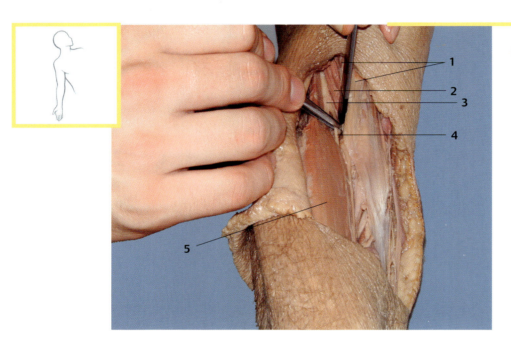

Fig. 6.**12** Radial nerve, right elbow.

1 Biceps
2 Brachialis
3 Radial nerve
4 Superficial branch of radial nerve
5 Brachioradialis

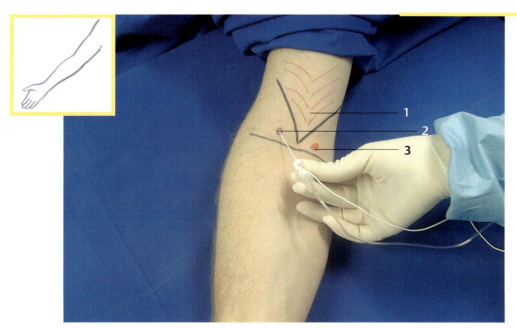

Fig. 6.**13** Block of the radial nerve, right elbow.

1 Biceps
2 Site of puncture, radial nerve block
3 Brachial artery

Fig. 6.**14**   Cubital fossa, right arm.

1   Posterior cutaneous nerve of the fore-
    arm
2   Radial nerve
3   Lateral cutaneous nerve of the fore-
    arm (musculocutaneous nerve)
4   Brachioradialis
5   Biceps
6   Median nerve
7   Brachial artery

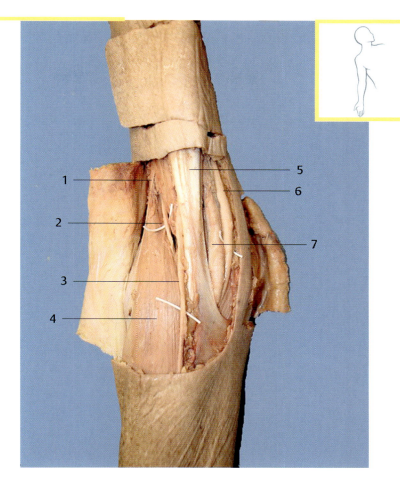

Fig. 6.**15**   Block of the right lateral
cutaneous nerve of the forearm (terminal
branch of the musculocutaneous nerve),
right arm, here subcutaneously located.

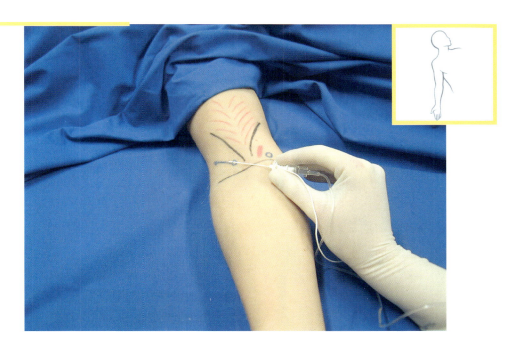

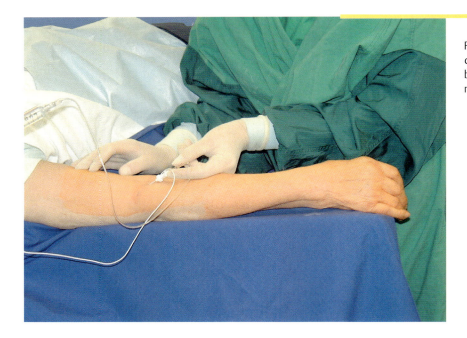

Fig. 6.**16** Block of the right lateral cutaneous nerve of the forearm (terminal branch of the musculocutaneous nerve), right arm, here subcutaneously located.

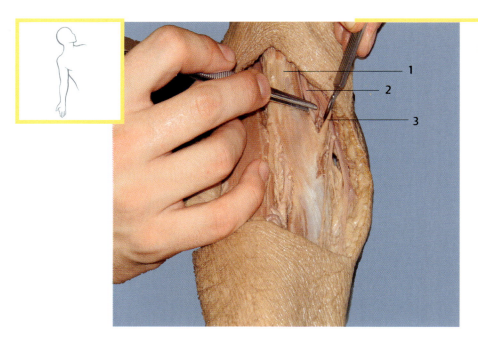

Fig. 6.**17** Median nerve, right elbow.

1 Biceps
2 Brachial artery
3 Median nerve

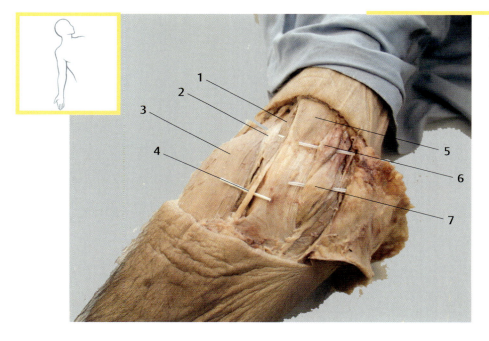

Fig. 6.**18** Anatomy of the right elbow.

1 Brachialis
2 Radial nerve
3 Brachioradialis
4 Lateral cutaneous nerve of the forearm (musculocutaneous nerve)
5 Biceps
6 Brachial artery
7 Median nerve

Fig. 6.**19**   Block of the median nerve in the
cubital fossa medial to the brachial artery.

1   Biceps
2   Brachial artery

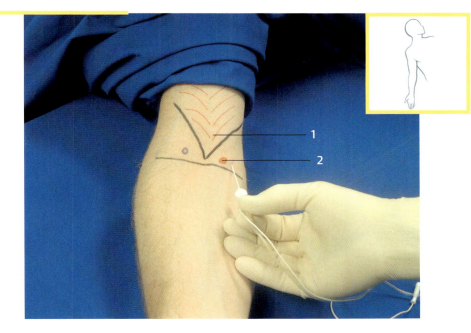

Fig. 6.**20**   Ulnar nerve, operative appearance
with ulnar sulcus syndrome of the right arm.

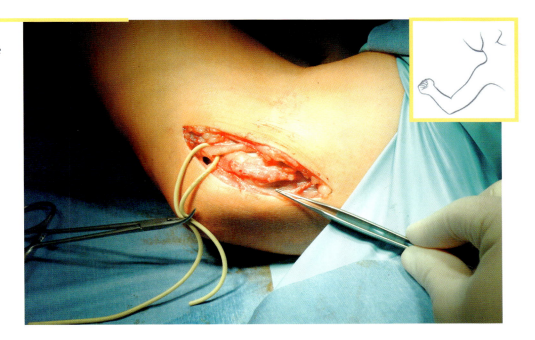

Fig. 6.**21**   Ulnar nerve in the ulnar sulcus.

1   Medial epicondyle of the right
    humerus
2   Ulnar nerve
3   Olecranon

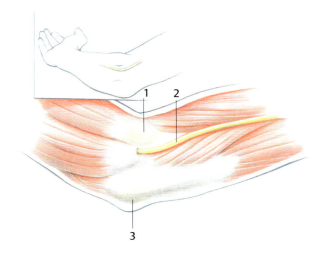

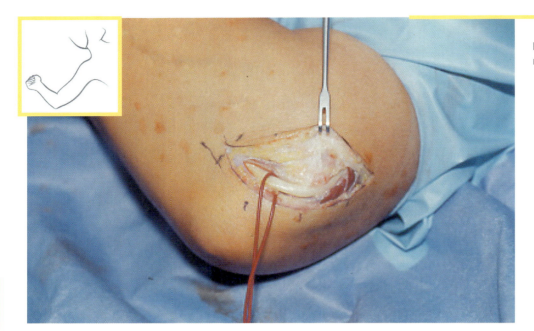

Fig. 6.**22**   Right ulnar nerve in the ulnar nerve sulcus.

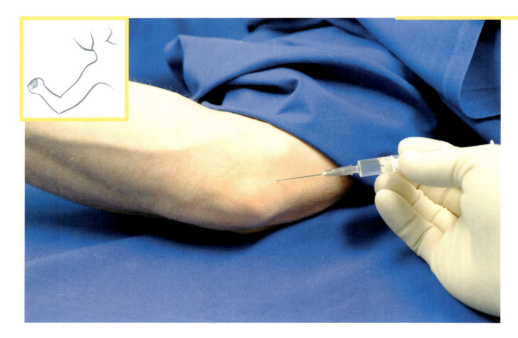

Fig. 6.**23**   Block of the right ulnar nerve proximal to the ulnar sulcus.

6.3   Blocks at the Wrist (Hand Block)

Anatomy

The *median nerve* at the wrist is on the palmar side between the tendon of flexor carpi radialis (radial side) and the palmaris longus tendon. It passes through the carpal tunnel into the palm of the hand (Figs. 6.**24**, 6.**25**). The *ulnar nerve* runs on the palmar side beside the tendon of flexor carpi ulnaris and passes here into the palm of the hand. In order from medial (ulnar) to lateral, the tendon of flexor carpi ulnaris, the ulnar nerve, and the ulnar artery lie immediately next to one another (Figs. 6.**24**, 6.**25**).

The *radial nerve* has only sensory fibers at the wrist. About 7-8 cm proximal to the wrist, the nerve that has been on the flexor surface until then passes under the brachioradialis tendon and now crosses the outer border of the wrist to reach the extensor side of the forearm (Fig. 6.**26**). In essence it is here epifascial and subcutaneous and can accordingly be blocked by subcutaneous infiltration.

Median Nerve Block (Wrist)

Abducted extended arm, forearm supinated. When the patient's fist is clenched tightly, the tendons of flexor carpi radialis and palmaris longus are readily shown. Directing the needle tangentially toward the nerve, a short 24G or 25G needle is introduced between the two tendons in the region of the wrist crease (Figs. 6.**27**, 6.**28**). When paresthesia is produced, the needle is withdrawn minimally and ca. 3 ml of the LA is injected. Occasionally the palmaris longus muscle has not developed. In these cases the

Fig. 6.**24**   Anatomy of the wrist region on the right, palmar aspect, focusing on the median and ulnar nerves.

1   Ulnar artery
2   Flexor carpi ulnaris
3   Ulnar nerve
4   Flexor carpi radialis (tendon)
5   Median nerve
6   Palmaris longus (tendon)

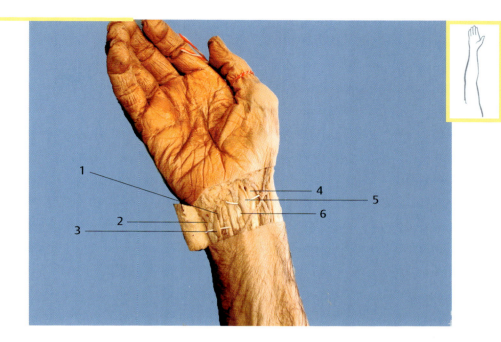

Fig. 6.**25**   Close-up of the anatomy of the wrist region on the right, palmar aspect, focusing on the median and ulnar nerves.

1   Palmaris longus (tendon)
2   Flexor carpi radialis (tendon)
3   Median nerve
4   Ulnar artery
5   Flexor carpi ulnaris
6   Ulnar nerve

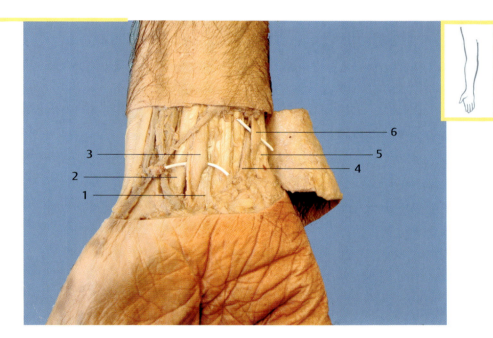

Fig. 6.**26**   Terminal branches of the superficial branch of the radial nerve, right wrist.

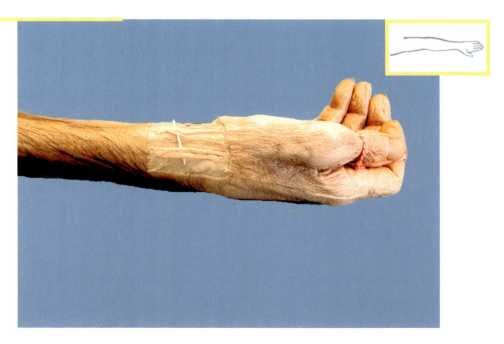

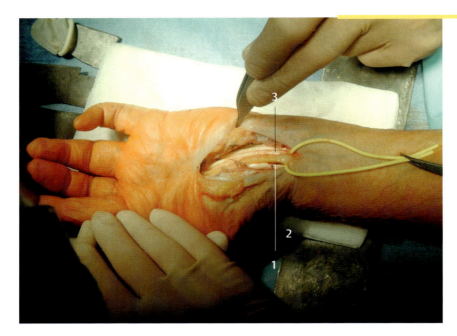

Fig. 6.**27** Median nerve, left wrist, exposed in situ.

1 Tendon of flexor carpi radialis
2 Median nerve
3 Tendon of palmaris longus

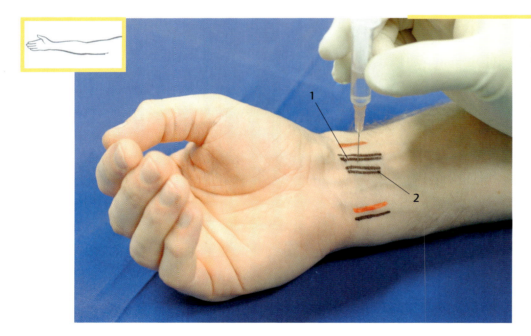

Fig. 6.**28** Block of the median nerve at the wrist.

1 Tendon of flexor carpi radialis
2 Tendon of palmaris longus

puncture must be made on the ulnar side of the flexor carpi radialis tendon. Subsequent subcutaneous infiltration in the radial and ulnar direction ensures a pain-free block of the ulnar and radial nerves.

Ulnar Nerve (Wrist)

The puncture is performed 3-4 fingers proximal to the wrist directly radial to the tendon of flexor carpi ulnaris; a 25G needle is advanced slowly tangentially toward the nerve (Figs. 6.**29**, 6.**30**); when paresthesia is produced, the needle is withdrawn mini-

mally and ca. 3 ml of the LA is injected. If no paresthesia is produced, a depot is injected under the tendon of flexor carpi ulnaris. In every case, the block should be supplemented with a subcutaneous injection medial to the tendon of flexor carpi ulnaris in the direction of the styloid process in order to block the dorsal branch as well.

Fig. 6.**29** Anatomy of the wrist region on the right, palmar aspect, for block of the median nerve and ulnar nerve.

1 Palmaris longus (tendon)
2 Flexor carpi radialis (tendon)
3 Median nerve
4 Ulnar artery
5 Flexor carpi ulnaris
6 Ulnar nerve

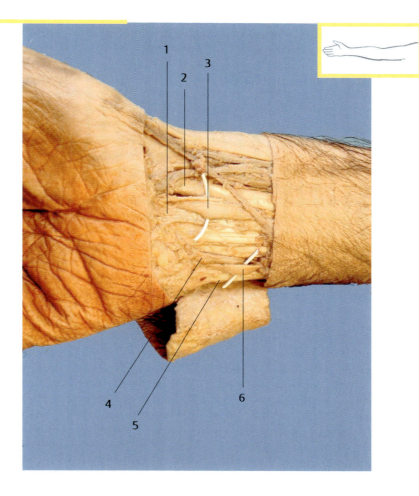

Fig. 6.**30** Block of the ulnar nerve at the wrist.

1 Ulnar artery
2 Flexor carpi ulnaris

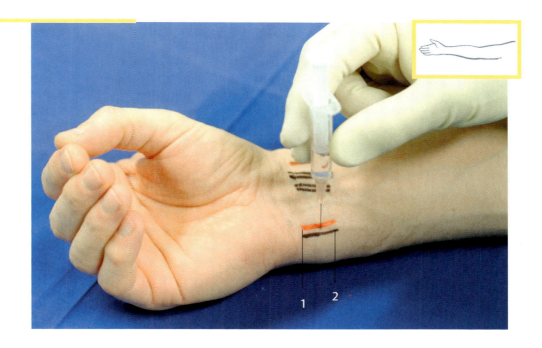

Radial Nerve (Wrist)

Starting from the "anatomical sniffbox," subcutaneous infiltration is performed with 5 ml of LA along the tendon of extensor pollicis longus in the direction of the dorsum of the wrist. After withdrawing the needle, further subcutaneous infiltration is performed at a right angle to the previous needle direction toward the palm. A further 5 ml of LA is given.

Alternatively, a subcutaneous ring infiltration can be injected with local anesthetic on the radial side (Figs. 6.**31**-6.**33**).

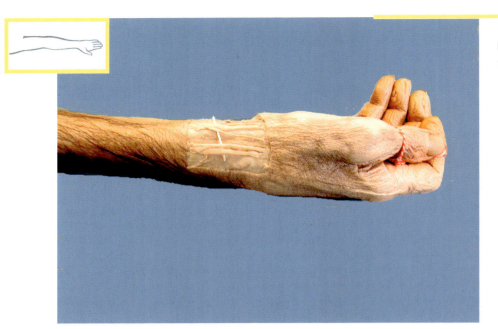

Fig. 6.**31** Terminal branches of the superficial branch of the radial nerve, right wrist.

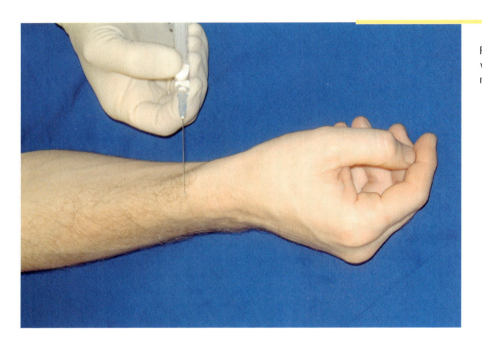

Fig. 6.**32** Block of the radial nerve in the wrist region: subcutaneous infiltration on the radial side.

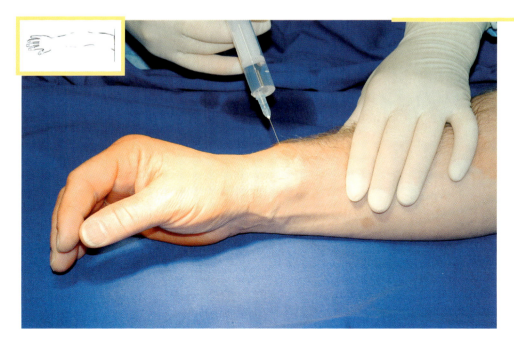

Fig. 6.**33** Block of the radial nerve in the wrist region: subcutaneous infiltration on the radial side.

Lower Limb

7   General Overview

7.1   Lumbosacral Plexus

The anterior rami of the lumbar, sacral, and coccygeal spinal nerves together form the lumbosacral plexus (Figs. 7.1, 7.2). The lumbar plexus and the sacral plexus are connected by the fourth lumbar nerve to the lumbosacral plexus. This nerve is bifurcated (nervus furcalis) and belongs to both the lumbar plexus and the sacral plexus (Fig. 7.3). In contrast to the upper limb, there is no technique that allows the entire lumbosacral plexus to be anesthetized with one injection, so that for complete "one-legged anesthesia" the lumbar plexus and the sacral plexus (or the parts of them relevant for the leg) must be anesthetized separately.

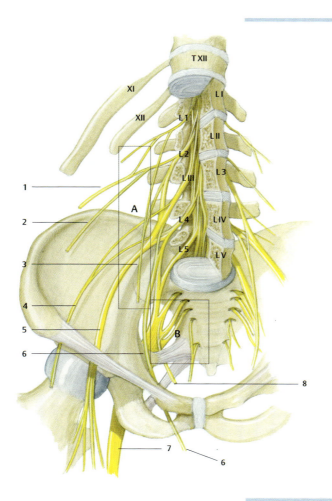

Fig. 7.**1**   Lumbosacral plexus, anterior view.

   A Lumbar plexus
   1 Iliohypogastric nerve
   2 Ilioinguinal nerve
   3 Genitofemoral nerve
   4 Lateral cutaneous nerve of the thigh
   5 Femoral nerve
   6 Obturator nerve
   B Sacral plexus
   7 Sciatic nerve
   8 Pudendal nerve

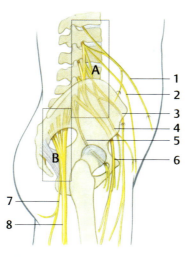

Fig. 7.**2**   Lumbosacral plexus, lateral view.

   A Lumbar plexus
   1 Iliohypogastric nerve
   2 Ilioinguinal nerve
   3 Lateral cutaneous nerve of the thigh
   4 Genitofemoral nerve
   5 Obturator nerve
   6 Femoral nerve
   B Sacral plexus
   7 Posterior cutaneous nerve of the thigh
   8 Sciatic nerve

Fig. 7.**3**   The nervus furcalis arises from the root of L4 and gives divisions to the lumbar plexus and the sacral plexus.

1   Lumbar plexus
2   Sacral plexus
3   Root from L4
4   Nervus furcalis (note division into a branch to the lumbar plexus and a branch to the sacral plexus)
5   Root of L5

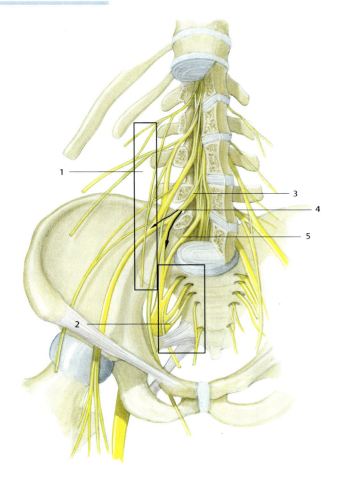

The parts of the *lumbar plexus* relevant for anesthesia of the leg are the femoral nerve, the lateral cutaneous nerve of the thigh, and the obturator nerve (Fig. 7.**4**). The sciatic nerve with its terminal branches and the posterior cutaneous nerve of the thigh are the parts of the sacral plexus that are important for the innervation of the leg (Fig. 7.**5**). This means that two injections have to be given, as complete anesthesia cannot be achieved reliably by one injection (Gligori-jevic 2000).

Lumbar Plexus

The lumbar plexus is formed by fibres from the 12th thoracic segment and the anterior rami of the 1st to 4th lumbar nerves. Segments L2-L4 are usually involved in the formation of the femoral nerve, the obturator nerve and the lateral cutaneous nerve of the thigh. The plexus passes peripherally after its exit from the intervertebral foramina, usually covered by the psoas muscle (Fig. 7.**4**). The genitofemoral nerve and the lateral cutaneous nerve of the thigh leave the plexus soon after the iliohypogastric and ilioinguinal nerves have split off.

The individual nerves of the lumbar plexus relevant for anesthesia are as follows:
- The *lateral cutaneous nerve of the thigh (L2/3)* passes over the iliacus muscle medial to the anterior superior iliac spine under the inguinal ligament and is a purely sensory nerve innervating the skin on the lateral side of the thigh.
- *The obturator nerve (L2/L4)* leaves the plexus medial to the psoas muscle and passes through the obturator canal together with the obturator vein and artery to the inside of the thigh. An accessory obturator nerve, which innervates the capsule of the hip joint, is found in 9% of people. The *obturator nerve* has a very variable sensory area of innervation in the medial thigh and provides motor innervation to the adductors.
- The *femoral nerve (L2/L4)* is the largest nerve of the lumbar plexus and provides the sensory innervation of the front of the thigh, while its sensory terminal branch, the saphenous nerve, innervates the inside of the lower leg as far as the ankle. The femoral nerve passes anterior to the psoas muscle under the inguinal ligament through the muscular lacuna and is the motor nerve for the quadriceps femoris, sartorius, and pectineus muscles.

Sacral Plexus

The sacral plexus constitutes the lower part of the lumbosacral plexus and is the biggest nerve plexus in the human body. The plexus is formed by the junction of the anterior rami of the five sacral nerves and the coccygeal nerve and also receives a substantial trunk, the lumbosacral trunk, from the lumbar nerves, which is composed of the entire anterior ramus of the 5th lumbar nerve and fibres from the 4th lumbar nerve (Fig. 7.**5**). The sacral plexus provides the nerves for the parts of the lower limb that are not supplied by the lumbar plexus, that is, for some of the hip muscles, for the flexor side of the thigh, and for all the muscles of the lower leg and foot. It also innervates the skin in part of the buttock area, the posterior side of the thigh, and the posterior, fibular and anterior side of the lower leg and foot (Fig. 7.**7**).
For anesthesia of the lower extremity, only the so-called sciatic plexus is of importance. It derives its roots from part of the anterior ramus of the 4th lumbar nerve and from the entire anterior ramus of the 5th lumbar nerve, which together form the lumbosacral trunk, and from the anterior rami of the 1st and 2nd and part of the 3rd sacral nerve. The anterior ramus of the 1st sacral nerve is

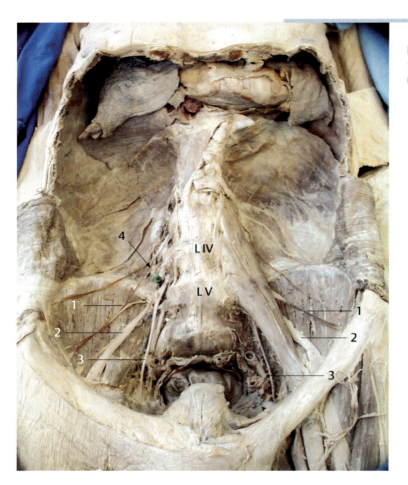

Fig. 7.**4**   Lumbar plexus, anterior view via the abdominal cavity: the psoas major muscle has been removed on the right side.

1   Lateral cutaneous nerve of the thigh
2   Femoral nerve
3   Obturator nerve
4   Destination of needle tips in psoas compartment block

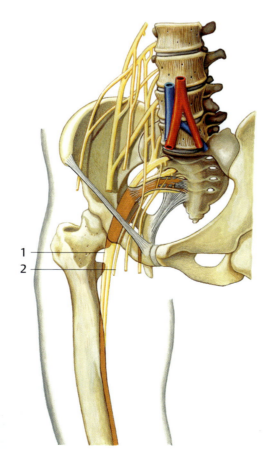

Fig. 7.**5**   Course of the sciatic nerve, the main nerve from the sacral plexus.

1   Sciatic nerve
2   Posterior cutaneous nerve of the thigh

Fig. 7.**6**   Sciatic nerve, posterior view.

1   Sciatic nerve
2   Piriformis
3   Biceps femoris
4   Semitendinosus

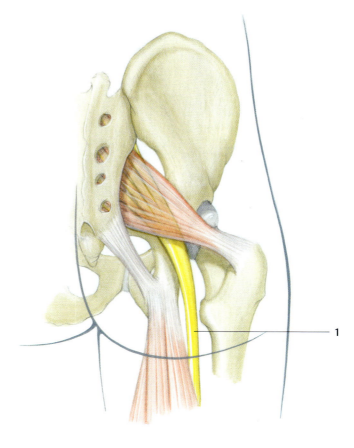

not only the biggest branch of the lumbosacral plexus, but the biggest anterior
ramus overall. All roots of the plexus converge from their exit sites toward the greater
sciatic foramen, so that the plexus forms a
triangular sheet, the tip of which points
toward the infrapiriform foramen where the
sciatic nerve emerges. The nerve plexus lies
largely on the piriformis muscle and is ven-
trally covered by the parietal peritoneum or
the tissues and branches of the iliac artery
that lie beneath it. Both the superior and
inferior gluteal arteries are related to the
plexus in that the former passes between
the lumbosacral trunk and the root of the
1st sacral nerve, the latter between the 2nd
and 3rd sacral nerves.

The articular rami, which supply parts of the
hip capsule, and the periosteal branches,
which innervate the periosteum of the
ischial tuberosity, the greater trochanter, and
the lesser trochanter, are derived from the
sciatic plexus.

The following are the nerves relevant for
anesthesia of the lower limb (Meier 2003):

- The *posterior cutaneous nerve* of the thigh
  (S1–S2), a purely sensory nerve, leaves the
  pelvis minor through the infrapiriform
  foramen and passes downward on the

back of the thigh toward the back of the
knee.

- The *sciatic nerve* (L4–L3) is the biggest
  nerve in the body (Fig. 7.6). It derives its
  fibres from all the roots of the sacral
  plexus and innervates the entire lower leg
  and foot, the ischiocrural muscles of the
  thigh, and the small external rotators of
  the hip. It leaves the pelvis through the
  infrapiriform foramen and then passes
  downward between the ischial tuberosity
  and the greater trochanter. In the proximal part of the popliteal fossa at the
  latest, it divides into its two terminal
  branches, the *tibial nerve* for the flexor
  muscles of the ankle and sole of the foot
  and the common *fibular nerve* (also
  known as the common peroneal nerve)
  for the extensor side of the ankle and the
  dorsum of the foot.

- The *tibial nerve* supplies the motor innervation to the flexor muscles of the ankle
  and is responsible for the flexors of the
  toes and foot. It provides sensory innervation to the skin of the lateral lower leg
  and the sole of the foot, and after joining
  the communicating branch of the *fibular
  nerve* it innervates the lateral margin of
  the heel and foot as the *sural nerve* (Fig.

7.**7**). Complete anesthesia of the tibial
nerve makes plantar flexion of the foot
and toes and spreading and closing of the
toes impossible.

- The *common fibular nerve* (L4–S2) runs in
  the popliteal fossa lateral to the tibial
  nerve and medial to the biceps femoris
  muscle as far as its attachment to the
  head of the fibula, around which the
  nerve winds to reach the front of the
  lower leg. Here it enters the gap between
  the origins of the fibularis longus muscle
  (also known as the peroneus longus) and
  immediately divides into its two
  branches. One of them is predominantly
  sensory (superficial fibular nerve) and the
  other is mainly motor (deep fibular
  nerve). The superficial fibular nerve supplies "little muscle and a lot of skin,"
  which means the motor supply only to
  the fibular muscles and the sensory
  supply to the skin of the lower leg, the
  dorsum of the foot, and the toes. The
  deep fibular nerve in contrast supplies "a
  lot of muscles and little skin," namely, the
  tibialis anterior and extensor muscles,
  with sensory supply only to the adjacent
  sides of the 1st and 2nd toes.

7.2   Sensory Innervation of the Leg

The *sensory innervation of the leg* (Fig. 7.**7**) can be variable. There are regions where two nerves can overlap to provide the sensory innervation. In particular, the division of the sensory innervation of the anterior and medial parts of the thigh is very variable. In most cases, a femoral nerve block in conjunction with a sciatic nerve block is adequate for complete block of the leg. The obturator nerve does not appear to be consistently involved in the sensory innervation of the knee. In some cases, an additional block of the obturator nerve is required. A psoas compartment block as an *alternative* to femoral nerve block includes the blockade of the obturator nerve in contrast to the femoral nerve block. The question of which area of skin receives its sensory innervation from the obturator nerve cannot be answered clearly, and occasionally the obturator nerve does not appear to have any "area" of its own.

Clinical experience in individual cases also contradicts the periostal *innervation of the*

lower limb accepted today (Fig. 7.**8**). The head of the tibia is considered to be innervated essentially by parts of the sciatic nerve (Fig. 7.**8**); however, in clear contradiction to this, a selective femoral nerve block is extremely effective for pain management of the often very painful fracture of the head of the tibia, especially after surgical treatment. The bony innervation of the femur close to the hip is also inconsistent with the usually successful pain therapy by means of femoral nerve block after hip fractures. One explanation might be that the soft tissues (innervated by the femoral nerve) are essentially responsible for the pain.

Innervation of the Bones (Innervation of Periosteum)

(Fig. 7.**8**)
Relevant anatomical relations (periosteal innervation) for anesthesia and pain therapy:
The *periosteum of the femur* is innervated

from behind and in front by the sciatic nerve in the upper third, by the obturator nerve in the middle third, and in the distal third laterally by the sciatic nerve and medially by the femoral and obturator nerves.
The *knee joint is innervated* by branches of the femoral and sciatic nerves anteriorly, and posteriorly by branches of the sciatic, obturator, and saphenous nerves.
The *periosteum of the tibia and fibula* is supplied by the tibial nerve, apart from the lateral head of the tibia and the head of the fibula (common fibular nerve) (important for lower leg amputations, fractures).
The *ankle* receives its sensory supply from the tibial and sural nerves.
The *periosteum of the tarsal bones* is innervated by the sural nerve and parts of the tibial nerve, and the metatarsals and the phalanges are innervated by the deep fibular nerve and terminal branches of the tibial nerve (Wagner 1994).

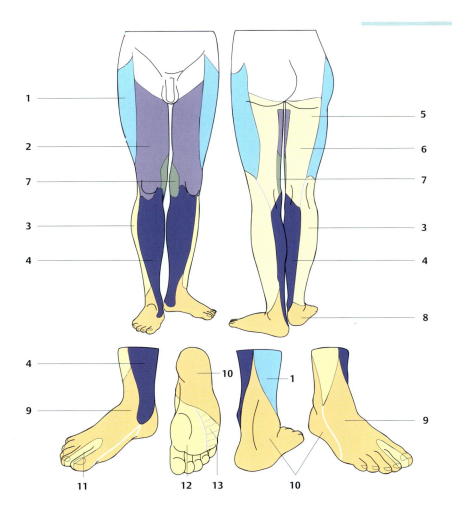

Fig. 7.**7**   Sensory innervation of the lower limb. *Blue:* area of the femoral nerve and its branches. *Yellow:* area of the sciatic nerve and its branches. *Light blue:* area of the lateral cutaneous nerve of the thigh. *Green:* area of the obturator nerve.

1   Lateral cutaneous nerve of the thigh
2   Femoral nerve
3   Fibular nerve
4   Saphenous nerve
5   Sciatic nerve
6   Posterior cutaneous nerve of the thigh
7   Obturator nerve
8   Posterior tibial nerve
9   Superficial fibular nerve
10   Sural nerve
11   Deep fibular nerve
12   Medial plantar nerve
13   Lateral plantar nerve (tibial nerve)

Fig. 7.**8**   Bony sensory innervation of the lower limb. *Blue:* area of the femoral nerve and its branches. *Yellow:* area of the sciatic nerve and its branches. *Green:* area of obturator nerve (innervation varies).

1   Sciatic nerve
2   Obturator nerve
3   Tibial nerve
4   Femoral nerve
5   Common fibular nerve

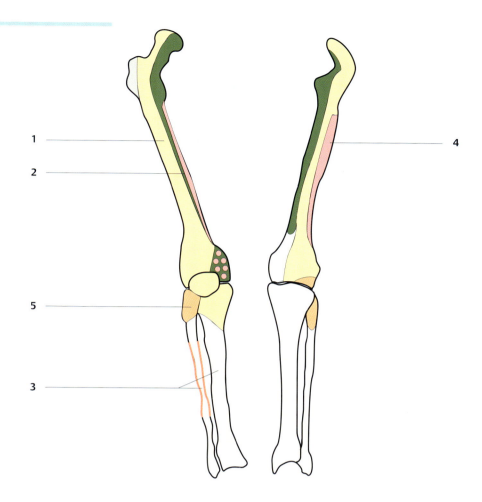

References

Gligorijevic S. Lower extremity blocks for day surgery. Techniques in Regional Anesthesia and Pain Management 2000;4:30-7.

Meier G. Nervenblockaden an den unteren Extremitäten. In: Niesel HC, Van Aken H, eds. Lokalanästhesie, Regionalanästhesie, Regionale Schmerztherapie. 2nd ed. Stuttgart: Thieme; 2003:306-93.

Wagner F. Beinnervenblockaden. In: Niesel HC, ed. Regionalanästhesie, Lokalanästhesie, Regionale Schmerztherapie. Stuttgart: Thieme; 1994;417-521.

8   Psoas Compartment Block

8.1   Anatomical Overview

The anterior rami of the first four lumbar nerves lie between the deep and the superficial parts of the psoas muscle and form the lumbar plexus. The ramus of the 4th lumbar nerve divides into a cranial and a caudal branch. The caudal branch combines with the anterior ramus of the 5th lumbar nerve to form the lumbosacral trunk, which is involved in forming the sacral plexus (Figs. 8.**1**, 8.**2**).

The first branch from the lumbar plexus, the iliohypogastric nerve, lies at the lateral border of the psoas major muscle. It is usually followed by the ilioinguinal nerve, passing through the psoas muscle and running almost parallel. The next nerve passing through psoas major is the genitofemoral nerve, which divides at a variable level into the genital branch and the femoral branch. A further branch of the lumbar plexus lying at the lateral border of the psoas major muscle is the lateral cutaneous nerve of the thigh, which reaches the muscular lacuna far laterally close to the anterior superior iliac spine. The biggest branch, the femoral nerve, runs in the groove between the iliacus and psoas major muscles and passes through the muscular lacuna to the thigh. The last branch, the obturator nerve, is the only one to run medial to the psoas major muscle and reaches the obturator canal after passing beneath the external iliac artery and vein (Figs. 8.**2**, 8.**3**).

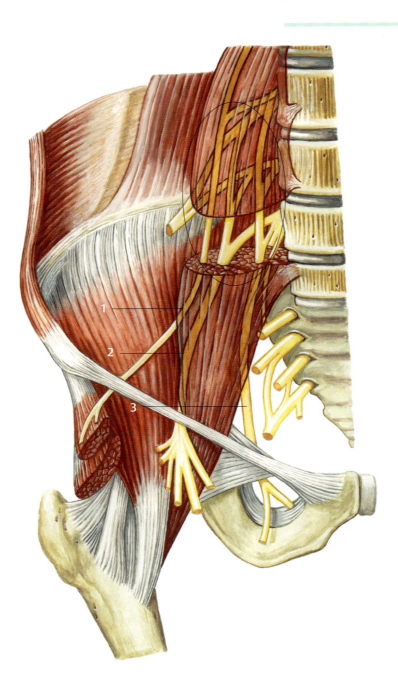

Fig. 8.**1**   The lumbar plexus penetrates the psoas major muscle. The compartment where psoas major is located with the lumbar plexus is found so that the local anesthetic can be injected here.

1   Lateral cutaneous nerve of the thigh
2   Femoral nerve
3   Obturator nerve
◯   Region included by psoas compartment block

Fig. 8.**2**   Anatomy of the lumbar plexus. The lumbar plexus is formed from the anterior rami of the nerve roots of T12 and L1–4. It gives branches to the sacral plexus (nervus furcalis). The psoas compartment block acts very proximally so that block of the obturator nerve can be expected.

1   Iliohypogastric nerve
2   Ilioinguinal nerve
3   Genitofemoral nerve
4   Lateral cutaneous nerve of the thigh
5   Femoral nerve
6   Obturator nerve
7   Root of L4
8   Nervus furcalis (connecting L4/L5)
9   Root of L5, going to the sacral plexus
◯ Region included in psoas compartment block

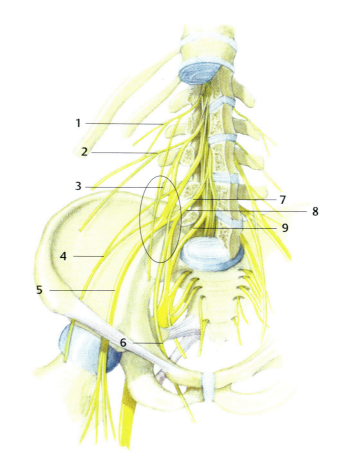

Fig. 8.**3**   Lumbar plexus, anterior view through the abdominal cavity: the psoas major muscle has been removed on the right. The site where the needle meets the lumbar plexus from behind is marked with a green cap on the tip of the needle.

1   Lateral cutaneous nerve of the thigh
2   Femoral nerve
3   Obturator nerve
4   Destination of the needle point in psoas compartment block

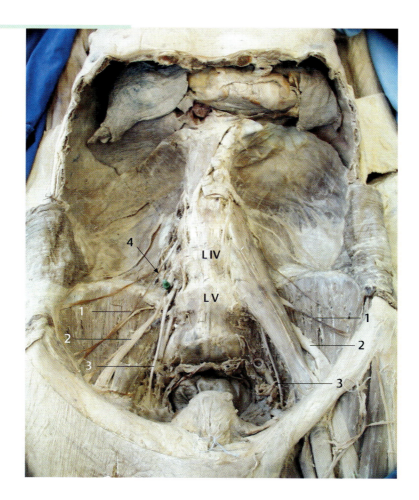

8.2 Technique of Psoas Compartment Block

Classical Technique (according to Chayen)

The position of the lumbar plexus between the fasciae of the psoas muscle, quadratus lumborum, and the vertebral bodies (psoas compartment) allows a cranial block of the lumbar plexus (Platzer 1999) (Fig. 8.4).

Position of the Patient

The patient is positioned on his or her side with the legs drawn up and the spine flexed with the side to be anesthetized uppermost (Fig. 8.6). Alternatively: patient in sitting position, similar to neuraxial anesthesia (Fig. 8.7).

Landmarks

A dorsal line between the iliac crests marks the spinous process of the 4th lumbar vertebra. From the spinous process of LIV a 3 cm line is drawn caudally at the midline. From the caudal end of this line a 5 cm line is drawn laterally at a right angle toward the side to be blocked. This second line ends a little before the medial border of the iliac crest, cranial to the posterior superior iliac spine, and corresponds to the puncture site (Fig. 8.5).

Method

Using continuous stimulation with a current of 0.5-1.0 mA, a 22G 10-12 cm insulated needle is advanced at a right angle to the skin in a strictly sagittal direction (Figs. 8.6-8.8). Contact between the needle tip and the transverse process of the 5th lumbar vertebra is first sought at a depth of 5 cm to a maximum of 8 cm (Figs. 8.7, 8.8). After making bone contact and withdrawing the needle about 4 cm, the needle is changed to a more cranial direction and advanced again. The needle should on no account be advanced more than 2.5 cm beyond the first

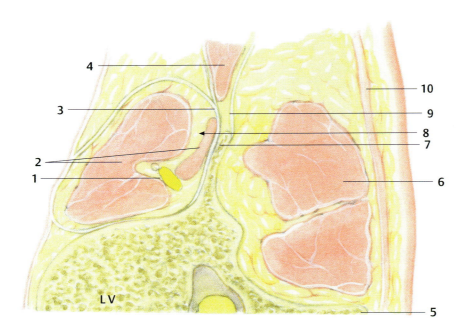

Fig. 8.4 Anatomy at the level of the puncture site for psoas compartment block (transverse section).

1. Lumbar plexus, nerve roots
2. Psoas major
3. Psoas fascia
4. Quadratus lumborum
5. Spinous process of L5
6. Erector spinae muscle
7. Transverse process of L5
8. Direction of needle
9. Transversalis fascia
10. Thoracolumbar fascia

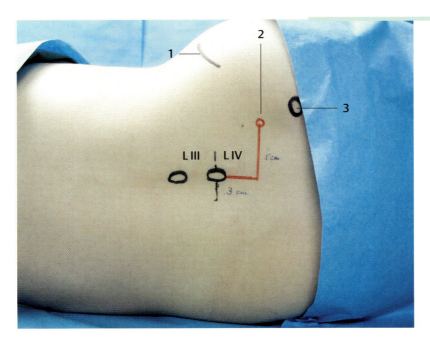

Fig. 8.5 Psoas compartment block can be performed in the lateral decubitus or sitting position. The injection site is 3 cm below the spinous process of LIV and 5 cm lateral to the interspinous line. A distance of 4-4.5 cm should be selected in slim patients.

1. Iliac crest
2. Injection site
3. Posterior superior iliac spine

Fig. 8.**6** The needle must be directed strictly sagittally in psoas compartment block, i.e., perpendicular to the lumbosacral/dorsal plane.

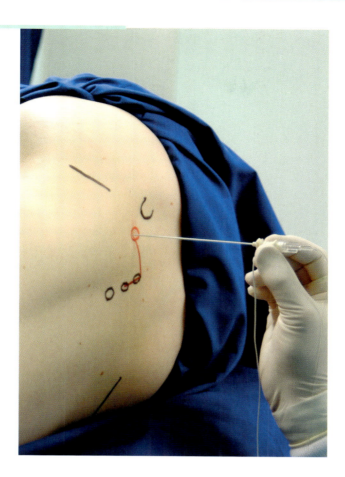

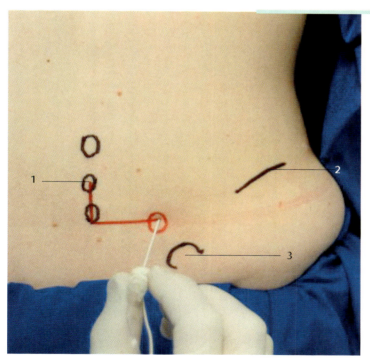

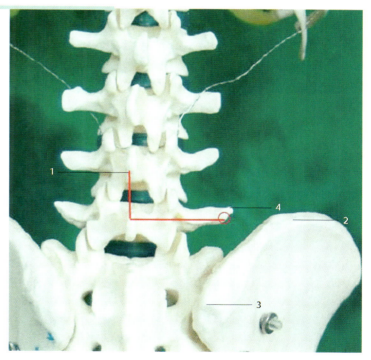

Fig. 8.**7** Psoas compartment block can be performed in the lateral decubitus or sitting position. The injection site is 3 cm below the spinous process of LIV and 5 cm lateral to the interspinous line. The 5 cm distance occasionally proves to be too far laterally, so that a distance of 4–4.5 cm should be selected in slim patients. The needle must be directed strictly sagittally in psoas compartment block, i.e., perpendicular to the dorsal plane. After about 5–8 cm the costal (transverse) process of L5 is usually encountered. After withdrawing it slightly, the needle is advanced further cranial to the process. A further 2 cm (up to 2.5 cm) deeper than the transverse process a loss of resistance is felt when the transversalis fascia or quadratus lumborum is penetrated (especially with a short-bevel needle). The nerve stimulator shows a response in the quadriceps muscle when the lumbar plexus is reached. A response in the region of the foot can occasionally be observed; in this case parts of the L4 root passing to the sacral plexus have been stimulated, and this indicates that the needle direction is too medial.

1 Spinous process of LIV
2 Iliac crest
3 Posterior superior iliac spine
4 Transverse process of LV

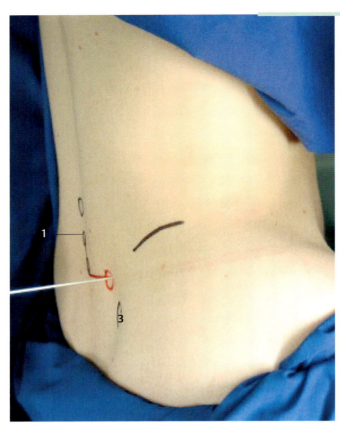 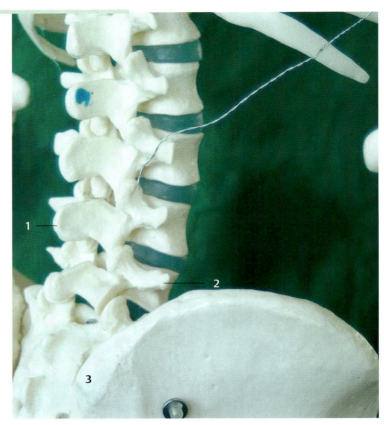

Fig. 8.**8**   The needle must be directed strictly sagittally in psoas compartment block, i.e., perpendicular to the dorsal plane. The transverse process of L5 is usually encountered after about 5–8 cm. After withdrawing it slightly, the needle is advanced just cranial to the process. Contact with the transverse process is helpful for depth orientation and the needle should not be advanced more than 2–2.5 cm after bone contact, in general never deeper than 11 cm.

1   Spinous process of LIV
2   Transverse process of LV
3   Posterior superior iliac spine

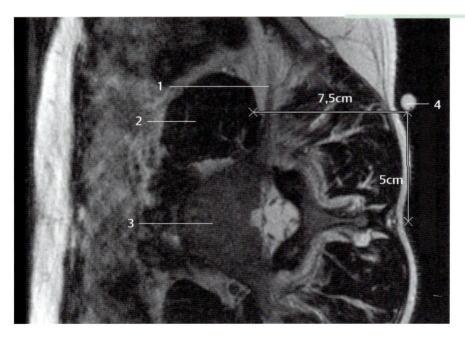

Fig. 8.**9**   MRI scan at the level of the injection site for psoas compartment block. Note the depth of 7.5 cm at which the psoas major muscle is reached (average male, 75 kg, 185 cm).

1   Transverse process of LV
2   Psoas major
3   LV
4   Puncture site, marked

Fig. 8.**10** Schematic description of anatomy corresponding to the plane of the MR image in Fig. 8.**9**.

1 Lumbar plexus
2 Psoas major
3 LV
4 Psoas fascia
5 Transversalis fascia
6 Erector spinae

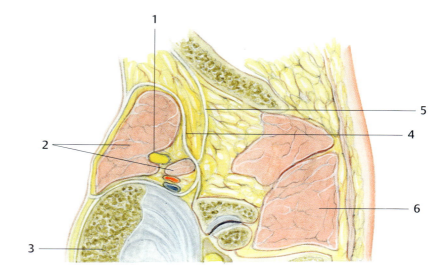

Fig. 8.**11** Cross section through a torso at the level of LV, view from above. The lumbar plexus lies embedded with its nerve roots in psoas major muscle. On passing through the quadratus lumborum muscle with the transversalis fascia, a "loss of resistance" is felt. However, the block should generally be performed with the nerve stimulator.

1 Lumbar plexus
2 Psoas major (muscle layers divided to show the lumbar plexus)
3 Quadratus lumborum
4 Transversalis fascia
5 Erector spinae
6 Thoracolumbar fascia
7 Needle tip
8 Vertebral body (L5)

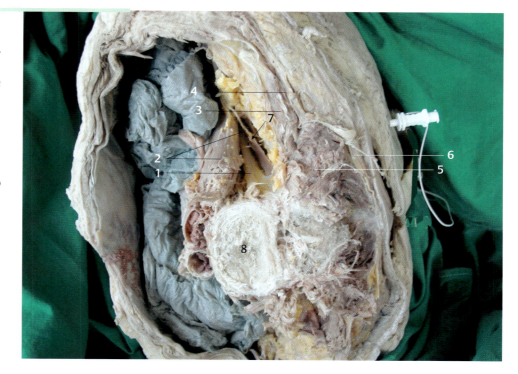

bone contact, and usually never more than 11 cm overall (Fig. 8.**8**). When the needle has passed the transverse process of the 5th lumbar vertebra, the loss of resistance after passing through the quadratus lumborum muscle and transversalis and psoas fascia indicates that the psoas compartment has been reached (Figs. 8.**9**-8.**13**). Muscle contractions of the quadriceps (anterior thigh) at a current of 0.3 mA and pulse duration of 0.1 ms indicate that the tip of the needle is in the correct position close to the femoral nerve (Fig. 8.**14**). The desired response corresponds to the motor block obtained by femoral nerve block.

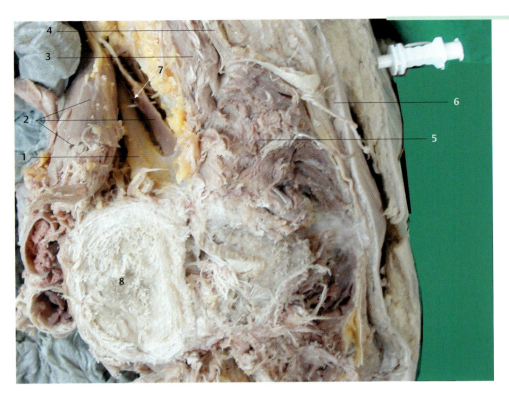

Fig. 8.**12**   Cross section through a torso at the level of LV, view from above. Section of Fig. 8.**11** enlarged.

1   Lumbar plexus
2   Psoas major (muscle layers divided to show the lumbar plexus)
3   Quadratus lumborum
4   Transversalis fascia
5   Erector spinae
6   Thoracolumbar fascia
7   Needle tip
8   Vertebral body (L5)

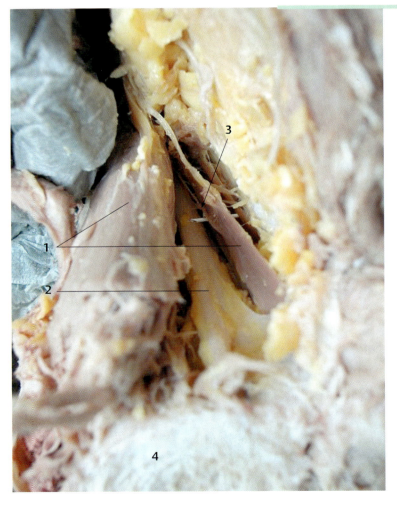

Fig. 8.**13**   Section of Fig. 8.**11** enlarged.

1   Psoas major (muscle layers divided to show the lumbar plexus)
2   Nerve roots of the lumbar plexus
3   Needle tip
4   Vertebral body (L5)

Fig. 8.**14**   The response is expected in the quadriceps muscle (see assistant's left hand). Aspiration before injection of the LA. Both before injecting through the needle and before injecting through the catheter, as in epidural anesthesia a test dose (3 ml of a medium-acting LA) must be given to exclude an intrathecal position.

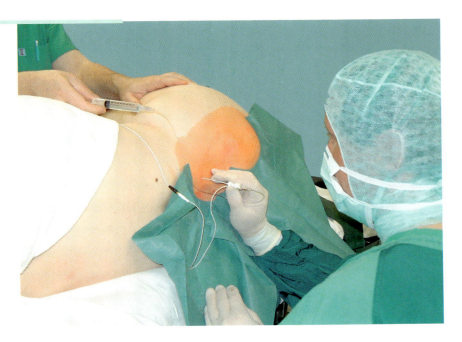

Fig. 8.**15**   Initially (following the test dose) 40–50 ml of LA is given. This can be divided when a catheter is being placed (e.g., 20 ml through the needle, 20–30 ml through the catheter).

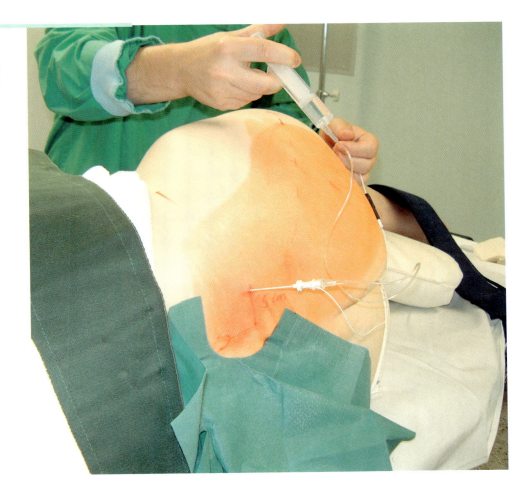

After careful aspiration, a test dose of 3 ml of local anesthetic (LA) is injected to exclude an incorrect intrathecal position. This is followed by injection of 30–50 ml of a medium-acting or long-acting LA (Fig. 8.**15**). After each 10 ml, further aspiration should be performed to exclude an accidental intravascular position. Initially, e.g., 40–50 ml of mepivacaine 1% or lidocaine 1% (10 mg/ml) or 30 ml of mepivacaine 1% (10 mg/ml) in combination with 10 ml of ropivacaine 0.75% (7.5 mg/ml) can be injected (Büttner and Meier 1999; Geiger 1999; Meier and Büttner 2001).

Continuous Psoas Compartment Block (according to Mehrkens and Geiger)

The anatomical orientation corresponds to the landmarks given by Chayen (see above). The puncture is made with a 19.5G 12 cm insulated needle, which allows a catheter to

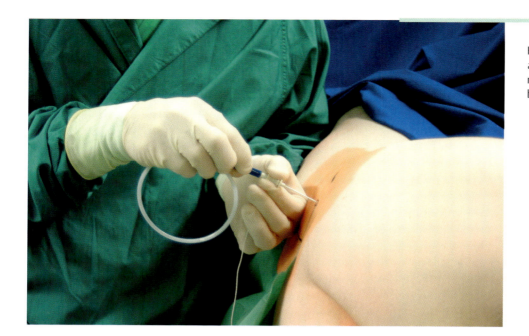

Fig. 8.**16**   Psoas compartment block can also be performed as a continuous technique. The catheter is advanced about 5 cm beyond the tip of the needle.

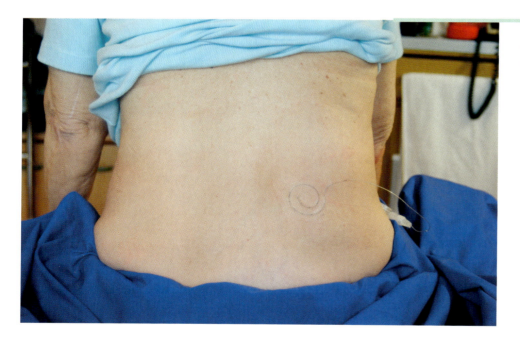

Fig. 8.**17**   Psoas compartment catheter in situ.

be introduced (e.g., Plexolong B according to Meier, 12 cm, Pajunk). When advancing the needle, the transverse process of the 5 th lumbar vertebra does not absolutely have to be contacted. Contractions of the quadriceps demonstrate the immediate vicinity of the femoral nerve. After correct stimulation at 0.3 mA/0.1 ms, negative aspiration, and a *test dose of a local anesthetic* (3 ml of a medium-acting LA to exclude an intrathecal position), 50 ml of LA is fractionally injected. The

catheter is advanced caudally into the psoas compartment (Fig. 8.**16**). Slight resistance at the end of the needle during advancement is normal and is caused by the transition of the needle tip to the tissue. Usually this slight resistance is easily overcome (Geiger 1999). A trial aspiration is performed again to exclude an intravascular position, and another test dose is given through the catheter to exclude an intrathecal position. *Initially*, e.g., 40 ml of mepivacaine 1 %

(10 mg/ml) mixed with 10 ml of ropivacaine 0.5 % (5 mg/ml); for *continuous administration*, 5-15 ml/h of ropivacaine 0.2 % (2 mg/ml); or *bolus injections* of 20 ml of ropivacaine 0.2-0.375 % (2-3.75 mg/ml) can be injected. We recommend a maximum ropivacaine dose of 37.5 mg/h (Büttner and Meier 1999; Meier 2001; Meier and Büttner 2001) (Figs. 8.**17**-8.**19**).

Fig. 8.**18**   After advancing the catheter, further injection of a test dose to exclude an intrathecal position.

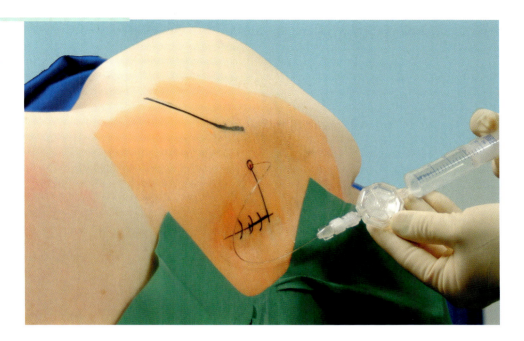

Fig. 8.**19**   Spread of contrast with correct psoas compartment block. Note the shadow of the psoas edge.
Arrows: Psoas edge shadow

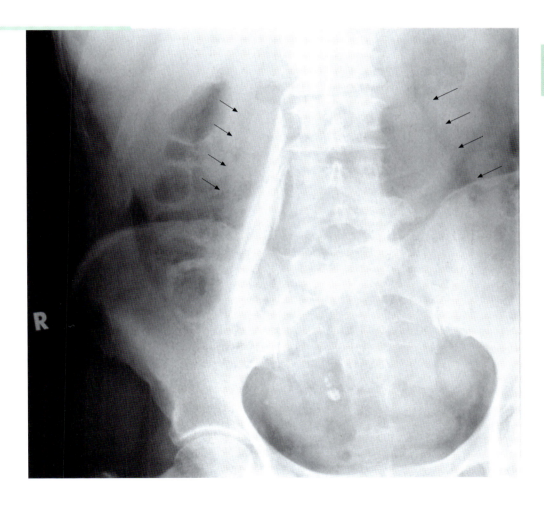

8.3   Sensory and Motor Effects

While the iliohypogastric, ilioinguinal, and genitofemoral nerves are not important for leg innervation, the following nerves are usually fully anesthetized by psoas compartment block:

- The *lateral cutaneous nerve of the thigh (L2/3)* passes over the iliacus muscle medial to the anterior superior iliac spine under the inguinal ligament and is a purely sensory nerve innervating the skin of the lateral side of the thigh.

- The *obturator nerve (L2/L4)* leaves the plexus medial to the psoas muscle and passes together with the obturator artery and nerve through the obturator canal to the inside of the thigh. In 9% of people an accessory obturator nerve is found, which innervates the capsule of the hip joint. The obturator nerve has a very variable sensory area of innervation on the medial thigh and provides motor innervation to the adductors.

- The *femoral nerve (L2/L4)* is the biggest nerve of the lumbar plexus and provides the sensory innervation of the front of the thigh and the inside of the lower leg as far as the ankle. It passes anterior to the psoas muscle below the inguinal ligament through the muscular lacuna and is responsible for the motor innervation of the quadriceps femoris, sartorius, and pectineus muscles.

8.4   Indications and Contraindications

Indications
- All operations on the lower limb (including hip, knee, and ankle joint replacement) can be performed under lumbar plexus block in combination with a sciatic nerve block (sacral plexus).
- Pain therapy after operations on the knee or hip (e.g., after cruciate ligament surgery, synovectomy, total joint replacement).

- Wound management, skin grafting in the anterior and lateral thigh.
- Need for early mobilization after operation and painless physiotherapy.

Contraindications
- General contraindications (see Chapter 15).
- Coagulation disorders: in contrast to all other peripheral blocks, the same rules

apply with regard to coagulation as for neuraxial blocks (Gogarten et al. 2003; Horlocker 2003).
- Peritoneal infection.
- Relative: major alterations of the spine (e.g., kyphoscoliosis).

8.5   Complications, Side Effects, Method-Specific Problems

Complications
- Bilateral anesthesia (epidural-like spread).
- Total spinal anesthesia (Auroy et al. 2002; Morisot 1979) or epidural anesthesia (Figs. 8.20-8.22).
- Peritoneal injection (Farny et al. 1994a) (Fig. 8.23).

- Subcapsular hematoma of the kidney (rare), (Aida et al. 1996) (Fig. 8.24).
- Infection (psoas abscess with continuous technique) (Fig. 8.25).
- Systemic toxicity due to the local anesthetic in the event of accidental intravascular injection (Auroy et al. 2002).

Practical Notes
- Because of the risk of renal puncture, the orientation lines should start from LIV, not from LIII.
- Contact with the transverse process of LV is helpful for orientation. The needle should be advanced a maximum of 2.5 cm beyond this distance.

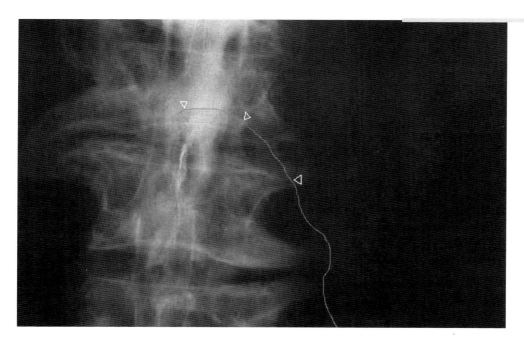

Fig. 8.20   Advancing the catheter too far can lead to an epidural position with corresponding spread and effect of the LA (see contrast). For this reason the patient requires adequate monitoring after injection of the LA, as a test dose does not exclude an epidural position. By withdrawing the catheter 7.5 cm, a correct catheter position was obtained in this case. (The radiograph was kindly provided by H. Kaiser.)

Fig. 8.**21** Note the close vicinity of the spinal cord: bilateral anesthesia, disorders of bladder function, and even high spinal anesthesia with cardiocirculatory arrest have been described. The tight vascularization may lead to hematoma with temporary neurological impairment. With regard to coagulation, the rules applying to neuraxial blocks should be followed in psoas compartment block. These rules can be followed more liberally with other peripheral blocks.

1 Dura mater
2 Nerve roots
3 Lumbar plexus in psoas major
4 Iliac crest
5 Spinous process of LIV

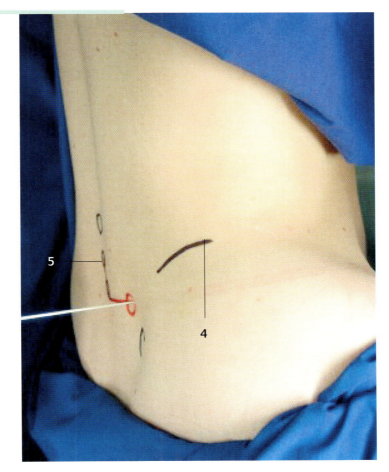

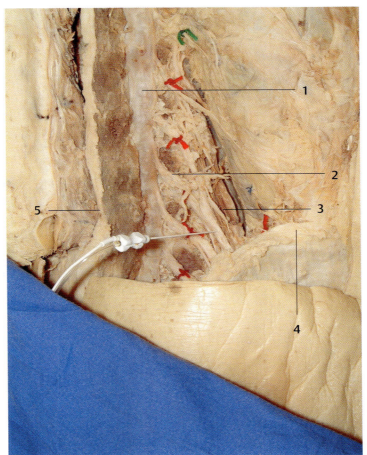

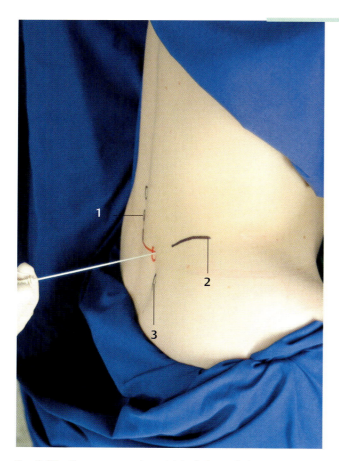
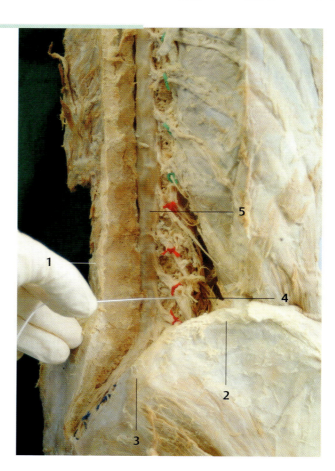

Fig. 8.**22**   Psoas compartment block, lateral view.

1   Spinous process of LIV   3   Posterior superior iliac spine   5   Dura mater
2   Iliac crest   4   Psoas major

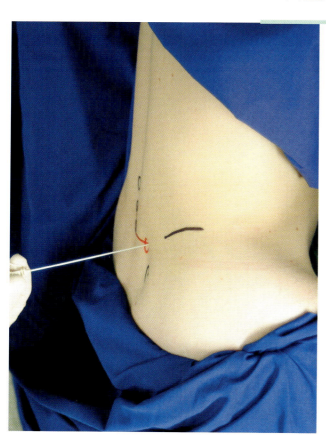
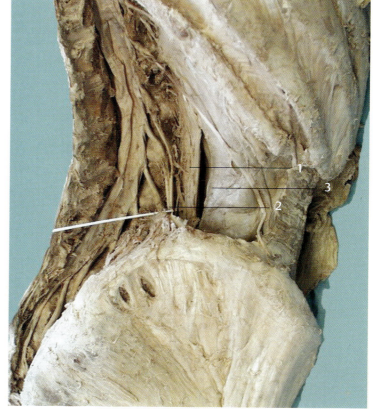

Fig. 8.**23**   Psoas compartment block, lateral view. Because of the risk of penetrating the peritoneal cavity, the depth of needle penetration should not exceed 11 cm.

1   Psoas major   2   Lumbar plexus   3   Peritoneum

Fig. 8.**24**   Psoas compartment block, anterior view. Note the safe distance from the lower pole of the kidney when LIV is the reference level for determining the puncture site.

  1 Psoas major
  2 Lumbar plexus
  3 Needle tip

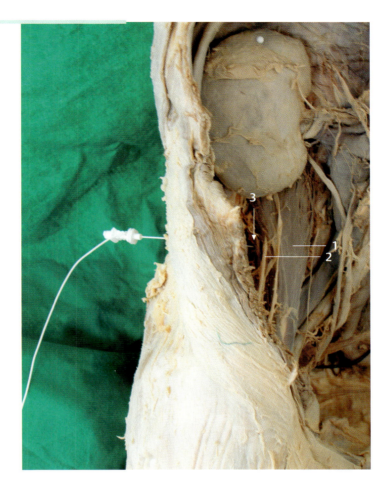

Fig. 8.**25**   Psoas abscess on the left: in rare cases a psoas abscess due to infection via a psoas compartment catheter can occur. In this case the abscess healed without surgical intervention and without sequelae.

  1 Psoas abscess on the left after psoas compartment catheter

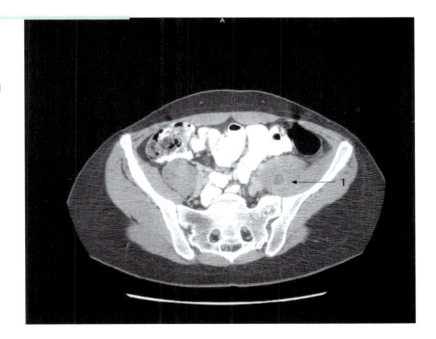

- Use nerve stimulation. Combination with a loss of resistance technique can simplify the procedure.
- Excessively deep injection (over 11 cm) should be avoided (see below).
- A test dose is indispensable (exclusion of an intrathecal position).

- A volume of 30-50 ml of the LA is required for sufficient anesthesia.
- If the lateral cutaneous nerve of the thigh has a very high origin from the plexus, incomplete anesthesia of the outside of the thigh is possible (rare compared to inguinal lumbar plexus block) (Bruelle et al. 1998).

- An intrathecal or epidural position can be excluded by a radiological check of the catheter's position.

8.6   Remarks on the Technique

In anatomical investigations, Farny et al. (1994a) found that the average distance between the skin and the femoral nerve is 9.0 cm (± 1.4 cm) in women and 9.9 cm (± 2.1 cm) in men. Farny therefore regards peritoneal injection as possible with a needle length of 11 cm or more. For this reason, the needle should not be longer than 10-12 cm.

Peripheral nerve stimulation (PNS) facilitates performance and improves the success rate with this technique (Ayers and Kayser 1999; Kaiser et al. 1990; Mehrkens et al. 1987; Parkinson et al. 1989; Vaghadia et al. 1992). The combination of PNS and loss of resistance technique is recommended. Insulated needles with a short-bevel or pencil-point tip have therefore also proved to be suitable for this technique. Contraction of the vastus muscles of the adductors should be obtained. Contact of the needle with the transverse process of the 5th lumbar vertebra is helpful for anatomical orientation (Chayen et al. 1976; Parkinson and Mueller 1989; Parkinson et al. 1989). In cases where the direction of the needle is corrected, this should only be in the cranial direction over the transverse process and not in the medial direction. The transverse process of the 5th lumbar vertebra is very short, so if the needle is directed medially there can be a response from parts of the sacral plexus (sciatic nerve) (Fig. 8.**7**), as the lumbosacral trunk lies furthest medially and paravertebrally while the femoral nerve lies in the middle of the lumbosacral plexus. This often leads to an unwanted paravertebral, epidural-like spread of anesthesia with the corresponding side effects, but without achieving complete lumbosacral plexus anesthesia (Ayers and Kayser 1999; Gligorijevic 2000). However, even when performed correctly, bilateral spread of the block must be anticipated. The incidence is between 8% and 88% (Geiger 1999; Parkinson et al. 1989; Rogers and Ramamurthy 1996; Vaghadia et al. 1992). The bilateral effects can probably be attributed to diffusion of the local anesthetic into the epidural space (Farny et al. 1994b; Geiger 1999; Hahn et al. 1996).

Occasionally the 5 cm distance from the interspinous line proves to be too great and a distance of 4-4.5 cm can be selected in slim patients, although here too directing the needle medially must be strictly avoided. A variant using a distance of 3 cm from the interspinous line has also been described with good results (3 cm caudally from LIV and 3 cm on the side to be blocked) (Pandin et al. 2002).

The monitoring of the patients must be similar to that in neuraxial anesthesia as an incorrect intrathecal or epidural position cannot absolutely be excluded. Accidental spinal anesthesia and high epidural anesthesia have been described (Gentili et al. 1998). In a review article involving a total of 394 psoas compartment blocks, Auroy reports one cardiocirculatory arrest with fatal outcome, two cases of acute respiratory insufficiency (complete respiratory paralysis) as a result of accidental intrathecal injection of the local anesthetic, and one seizure due to intravascular injection of the local anesthetic (Auroy et al. 2002). This represents a major complication rate of 0.8% associated with this technique. An intrathecal or epidural catheter position can also be excluded by a subsequent radiograph (Douglas and Bush 1999). Studies suggest that the use of ultrasound may improve and facilitate orientation and checking of the catheter position in psoas compartment block (Kirchmair et al. 2000a, 2000b).

The lateral cutaneous nerve of the thigh often leaves the lumbar plexus very far cranially, so incomplete anesthesia in the area supplied by this nerve is possible even when the psoas compartment block is performed correctly (Bruelle et al. 1998). Puncture using LIII for orientation instead of LIV confers no advantages (Bartmann et al. 1993), and the risk of a subcapsular hematoma of the kidney is increased (Aida et al. 1996). In discussions of the side effects or complications of the technique, there are few reports on its use in the case of coagulation disorders. Theoretically, psoas compartment block has a better risk-benefit ratio in patients on anticoagulant therapy compared to epidural anesthesia (Ayers and Kayser 1999). However, in the case of coagulation disorders, psoas compartment block should be avoided. Case descriptions report extensive retroperitoneal hematomas after psoas compartment blocks (Klein et al. 1997; Weller et al. 2003). In one case, the block was performed under prophylactic administration of enoxaparin; reversible plexus injury occurred (Klein et al. 1997). In another case, the anticoagulation was given after performing the continuous psoas compartment block but before withdrawing the catheter. There were no neurological deficits but there was a drop in hemoglobin necessitating a transfusion and causing renal failure and ileus. In a third case with normal coagulation status, a hematoma requiring transfusion occurred despite perioperative discontinuation of continuous adminis-

tration of unfractionated heparin (Weller et al. 2003).

- As far as coagulation is concerned, in contrast to all other peripheral blocks the rules that apply to neuraxial blocks also apply to the psoas compartment block (Gogarten et al. 2003; Horlocker 2003). Compared to general anesthesia or neuraxial anesthesia, patients have better circulatory stability with the psoas compartment block.

For most operations on the leg, particularly when they are performed with a tourniquet at the thigh, the *combination of psoas compartment and sciatic nerve block is necessary for anesthesia.* For this combination, relatively large volumes of LA are required. The sciatic nerve is adequately blocked with 20-25 ml of LA, while volumes of 40-50 ml are required for block of the lumbar plexus in the psoas compartment (Fig. 8.**26**).

- A combination of 40 ml of a medium-acting LA with 20 ml of ropivacaine 0.75% (7.5 mg/ml) or 40 ml of ropivacaine 0.375% (3.75 mg/ml) is possible for combined psoas compartment and sciatic nerve block.

The advantage of a psoas compartment-sciatic nerve block compared to an inguinal femoral nerve-sciatic nerve block in knee operations is based on the more complete lumbar plexus anesthesia, which also includes obturator nerve block (Luber et al. 2001; Uckunkaya et al. 2000). The hip is innervated by branches of the lumbar plexus and the sacral plexus (Birnbaum et al. 1997). Cranial anesthesia of the lumbar plexus can also be used successfully in combination with a sciatic nerve block and sedation of the patient for anesthesia for operations on the hip (total hip replacement) (Bruckenmeier et al. 2001; Chudinov et al. 1999; Geiger et al. 1994; Mitchell 1999; Türker et al. 2000; de Visme et al. 2000). Further studies indicate a beneficial effect with regard to diminished blood loss in hip operations (Stevens et al. 2000; Twyman et al. 1990). Beyond the positive results with regard to good intraoperative anesthesia with comparatively less impairment of the hemodynamic parameters, the continuous technique also offers the possibility of postoperative pain therapy (Fig. 8.**27**).

Fig. 8.**26** Spread of contrast in combined psoas compartment and sciatic nerve block. Initially, e.g., about 30 ml of a 1 % (10 mg/ml) medium-acting local anesthetic (prilocaine/mepivacaine) in combination with 15(–20) ml of 0.375 % (3.75 mg/ml) ropivacaine or 10 ml of ropivacaine 0.75 % (7.5 mg/ml) can be given in each catheter.

1 Spread of contrast in psoas compartment block
2 Spread of contrast in sciatic nerve block

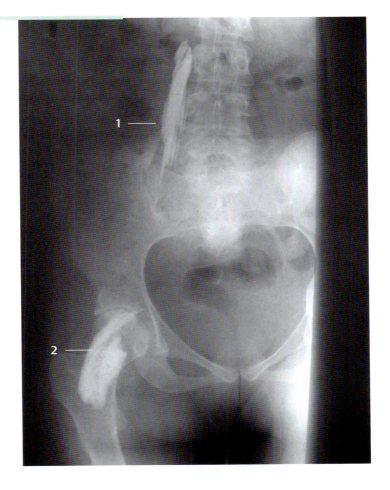

Fig. 8.**27** Psoas compartment block can be used in conjunction with posterior proximal sciatic nerve block for complete anesthesia of the entire leg (also as a continuous technique). In the continuous technique both catheters can, for example, each be infused with 6 ml of 0.33 % (3.3 mg/ml) ropivacaine per hour

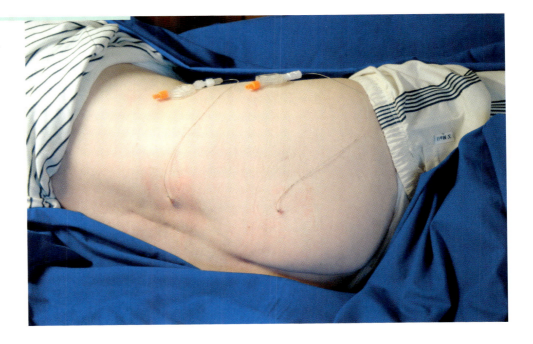

8.7   Summary

Psoas compartment block can be performed in sitting position or with the patient lying on his or her side. It consists of a cranial approach to the lumbar plexus with a high success rate. The procedure requires sterile conditions. Full supervision and monitoring of the patient must be ensured. During this monitoring, the possibility of the development of epidural-like spread or spinal anesthesia must be borne in mind. Peritoneal infections, coagulation disorders, and major abnormalities of the spine must be regarded as contraindications. In combination with sacral plexus block, the technique leads to sufficient anesthesia in operations on the leg and is well suited for pain therapy and mobilization with operations on the hip and knee.

References

Aida S, Takahashi H, Shimoji K. Renal sub-capsular hematoma after lumbar plexus block. Anesthesiology. 1996;84:452-5.

Auroy Y, Benhamou D, Bargues L. Major complications of regional anesthesia in France. Anesthesiology. 2002;97:1274-80.

Ayers J, Kayser EF. Continuous lower extremity techniques. Techniques in Regional Anesthesia and Pain Management 1999;3:47-57.

Bartmann E, Mehrkens HH, Geiger P, Herrmann M. Anatomic examinations to optimize the paravertebral approach to the psoas compartment. Surgical and radiologic anatomy. J Clin Anat. 1993;15:3.

Birnbaum K, Prescher A, Hepler S, Heller KD. The sensory innervation of the hip joint—An anatomical study. Surg Radiol Anat. 1997;19:371-5.

Bruckenmeier CC, Xenos JS, Nilsen SM. Lumbar plexus block with perineural catheter and sciatic nerve block for total hip arthroplasty. Int Monitor Reg Anesth. 2001;(A)53.

Bruelle P, Cuvillon P, Ripart J, Eledjam JJ. Sciatic nerve block: Parasacral approach. Reg Anesth. 1998;(S)23:78.

Büttner J, Meier G. Kontinuierliche periphere Techniken zur Regionalanästhesie und Schmerztherapie - Obere und untere Extremität. Bremen: Uni-Med-Verlag; 1999.

Chayen D, Nathan H, Cayen M. The psoas compartment block. Anesthesiology. 1976;45:95-9.

Chudinov A, Berkenstadt H, Salai M, Cahana A, Perel A. Continuous psoas compartment block for anesthesia and perioperative analgesia in patients with hip fractures. Reg Anesth Pain Med. 1999;24:563-8.

Douglas I, Bush D. The use of patient-controlled bolus of local anesthetic via a psoas sheath catheter in the management of malignant pain. Pain. 1999;82:105-7.

Farny J, Drolet P, Girad M. Anatomy of the posterior approach to the lumbar plexus block. Can J Anaesth. 1994 a;41:480-5.

Farny J, Girard M, Drolet P. Posterior approach to the lumbar plexus combined with a sciatic nerve block using lidocaine. Can J Anaesth. 1994 b;41:486-91.

Geiger P. Der Psoas-Kompartment-Block. In: Mehrkens HH, Büttner J, eds. Kontinuierliche periphere Leitungsblockn zur postoperativen Analgesie. München: Arcis-Verlag; 1999:29-42.

Geiger P, Bartmann E, Gelowicz-Maurer M, Mehrkens HH. Combined sciatic nerve plus continuous paravertebral lumbar plexus block in orthopaedic knee surgery. XIII Annual ASRA-Congress, Barcelona (special abstract issue); 1994:57.

Gentili M, Aveline C, Bonnet F. Total spinal anesthesia after posterior lumbar plexus block. Ann Fr Anesth Reanim. 1998;17:740-2.

Gligorijevic S. Lower extremity blocks for day surgery. Techniques in Regional Anesthesia and Pain Management 2000;4:30-7.

Gogarten W, van Aken H, Büttner J. Rückenmarksnahe Regionalanästhesien und Thromboembolieprophylaxe/antithrombotische Medikation. Anästh Intensivmed. 2003;44:218-30.

Hahn MB, McQuillan PM, Sheplock GJ. Regional anesthesia: an atlas of anatomy and techniques. St. Louis: Mosby; 1996.

Horlocker TT. Regional anesthesia in the anticoagulated patient: Defining the risks (The second ASRA consensus conference on neuraxial anesthesia and anticoagulation). Reg Anesth Pain Med 2003;28:172-97

Kaiser H, Niesel HCh, Klimpel L. Grundlagen und Anforderungen der peripheren elektrischen Nervenstimulation. Ein Beitrag zur Erhöhung des Sicherheitsstandards in der Regionalanästhesie. Reg Anaesth. 1990;13:143-4.

Kirchmair L, Entner T, Burger R, Künzel KH, Maurer, H, Mitterschiffthaler G. Ultrasound (US) guided psoas compartment block (PCB): Verification of a new technique with CT. Int Monitor Reg Anesth. 2000 a;(A) 12:199.

Kirchmair L, Entner T, Burger R, et al. Ultrasound (US) guided psoas compartment block (PCB): Anatomical fundamentals. Int Monitor Reg Anesth. 2000;(A) 12:197.

Klein SM, D'Ercole F, Greengrass R. Enoxaparin associated with psoas hematoma and lumbar plexopathy after lumbar plexus block. Anesthesiology. 1997;87:1576-9.

Luber MJ, Greengrass R, Vail TP. Patient satisfaction and effectiveness of lumbar plexus and sciatic nerve block for total knee arthroplasty. J Arthroplasty. 2001;16:17-21.

Mehrkens HH, Schleinzer W, Geiger P. Successful peripheral regional anesthesia by aid of an improved nerve stimulator. (Abstract) 6. Annual Meeting, ESRA, Paris 1987.

Meier G. Periphere Blockaden der unteren Extremität. Anesthesist. 2001;50:536-59.

Meier G, Büttner J. Regionalanästhesie - Kompendium der peripheren Blockaden. München: Arcis Verlag; 2001.

Mitchell ME. Regional anesthesia for hip surgery. Techniques in Regional Anesthesia and Pain Management 1999;3:94-106.

Morisot P. Les blocs du membre inférieur. Encyclop Med-chir Anesthesie. 1979;363:23.

Pandin PC, Vandesteene A, d'Hollander A. A catheter placement description using electrical nerve stimulation. Anesth Analg. 2002:95:1428-31.

Parkinson S, Mueller JB. A simple technique for continuous lumbar sympathic block. Anesth Analg. 1989;68:218.

Parkinson S, Mueller WL, Little S, Bailey L. Extent of block with various approaches to the lumbar plexus. Anesth Analg. 1989;68:243-8.

Platzer W. Taschenatlas der Anatomie - Bewegungsapparat. 7th ed. Stuttgart: Thieme; 1999.

Rogers NR, Ramamurthy S. Lower extremity blocks. In: Brown, DL, eds. Regional anesthesia and analgesia. Philadelphia: Saunders; 1996:284-5.

Stevens RD, van Gessel E, Flory N, Fournier R, Gamulin Z. Lumbar plexus block reduces pain and blood loss associated with total hip arthroplasty. Anesthesiology. 2000;93:115-21.

Türker G, Uckunkaya N, Yilmazlar A. Postoperative analgesia with psoas compartment block after prosthetic hip surgery. Int Monitor Reg Anesth. 2000;(A) 12:246.

Twyman R, Kirwan T, Fenelly M. Blood loss reduced during hip arthroplasty by lumbar plexus block. J Bone Joint Surg Br. 1990;72:770-1.

Uckunkaya N, Türker G, Yilmazlar A, Sahin S. Combined psoas compartment and sciatic nerve blocks for lower limb surgery. Int Monitor Reg Anesth. 2000;(A) 12:196.

Vaghadia H, Kapnoughis P, Jenkins L, Taylor D. Continuous lumbosacral block using a Tuohy needle and catheter technique. Can J Anaesth. 1992;39:75-8.

Visme V de, Picart F, Jouan R le, Legrand A, Savry Ch, Morin V. Combined lumbar and sacral plexus block compared with plain bupivacaine spinal anesthesia for hip fractures in the elderly. Reg Anesth Pain Med. 2000;25:158-62.

Weller RS, Gerancher JC, Crews JC. Extensive retroperitoneal hematoma without neurologic deficit in two patients who underwent lumbar plexus block and were later anticoagulated. Anesthesiology. 2003;98:31-7.

9   Inguinal Paravascular Lumbar Plexus Anesthesia
("3-in-1 Technique" according to Winnie, Femoral Nerve Block)

9.1   Anatomical Overview

The femoral nerve arises within the psoas muscle, usually from the anterior divisions of the four large roots L1-L4 but sometimes only from L2-L4, and is the largest nerve of the lumbar plexus (Fig. 9.**1**). It passes to the thigh in the fascial space between psoas major and iliacus through the muscular lacuna (Fig. 9.**2**). The iliopectineal fascia separates the muscular lacuna and thus the femoral nerve from the vascular lacuna through which the lymphatic vessels and the femoral artery and vein run. After giving off a few superficial cutaneous branches (anterior cutaneous branches) it lies under the fascia lata and the iliac fascia in the femoral trigone (Hahn et al. 1996; Platzer 1999; Woodburne 1983), (Figs. 9.**3**, 9.**4**). In the region of the inguinal ligament, the femoral nerve is ca. 1 cm lateral to the artery, where it soon branches (Figs. 9.**5**, 9.**6**).

The femoral nerve provides the *sensory* innervation of the anterior thigh and is involved in the innervation of the hip and knee and of the femur. It is the *motor* supply to the knee extensors and hip flexors (see Fig. 7.**7**).

Fig. 9.**1**   Anatomical overview of the lumbar plexus and the femoral nerve.

1   Obturator nerve
2   Femoral nerve
3   Lateral cutaneous nerve of the thigh
4   Inguinal ligament

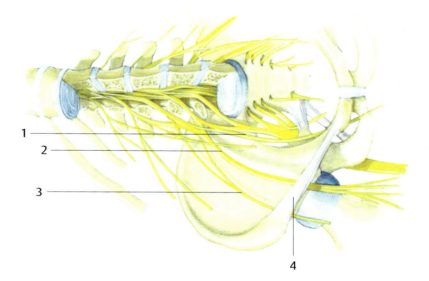

Fig. 9.**2**   Lumbar plexus with femoral nerve and obturator nerve. Note the arcus ileopectineus, a sheet of connective tissue that separates the vascular lacuna from the muscular lacuna. In femoral nerve block, the psoas muscle may prevent spread of the local anesthetic to the obturator nerve proximal to the inguinal ligament. Distal to the inguinal ligament, the spatial distance and separation by the iliac fascia make inclusion of the obturator nerve by a femoral nerve block almost impossible.

1   Psoas
2   Femoral nerve
3   Arcus ileopectineus
4   Obturator nerve
5   Femoral artery
6   Inguinal ligament

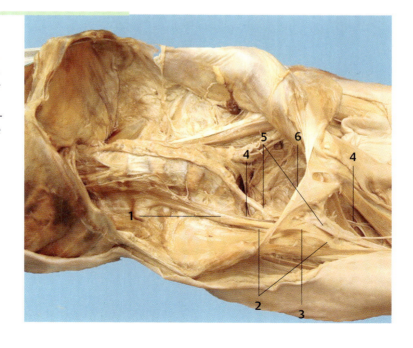

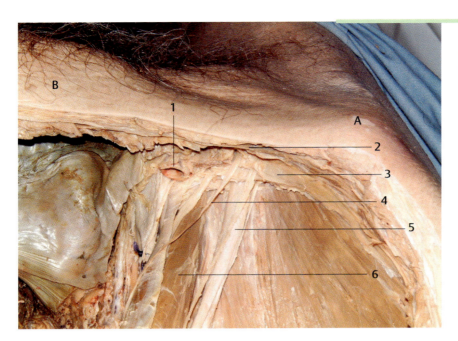

Fig. 9.**3** Cranial view of the right inguinal region. Note that the fascia lata and the iliac fascia have to be penetrated to block the femoral nerve ("double-click").

1 Femoral artery
2 Fascia lata
3 Iliac fascia with arcus iliopectineus
4 Genitofemoral nerve
5 Femoral nerve
6 Psoas major
A Anterior superior iliac spine
B Symphysis

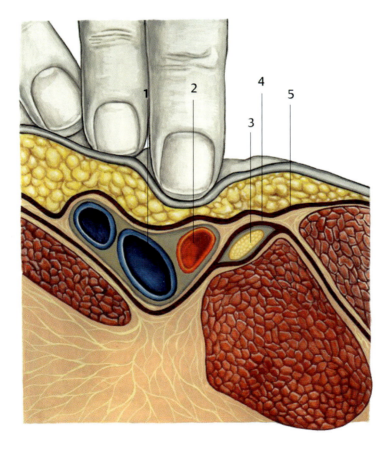

Fig. 9.**4** Cranial view of the right inguinal region. Note that the fascia lata and the iliac fascia have to be penetrated to block the femoral nerve ("double-click," see also Fig. 9.**3**).

1 Femoral vein
2 Femoral artery
3 Femoral nerve
4 Iliac fascia
5 Fascia lata

Fig. 9.**5**   Anatomical overview of the inguinal region: note IVAN (Inside Vein, Artery, Nerve).

1   Lateral cutaneous nerve of the thigh
2   Femoral nerve
3   Femoral artery
4   Femoral vein
5   Obturator nerve

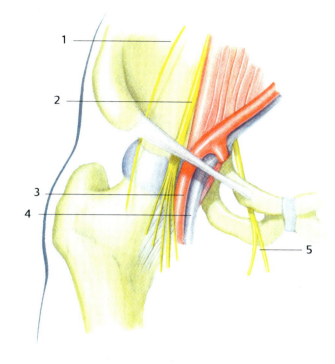

Fig. 9.**6**   Anatomical overview of the inguinal region: note IVAN (Inside Vein, Artery, Nerve). The femoral nerve has a cauda equina-like division after passing through the inguinal ligament.

1   Sartorius
2   Femoral nerve (looped)
3   Femoral artery
4   Femoral vein
5   Branch of the obturator nerve

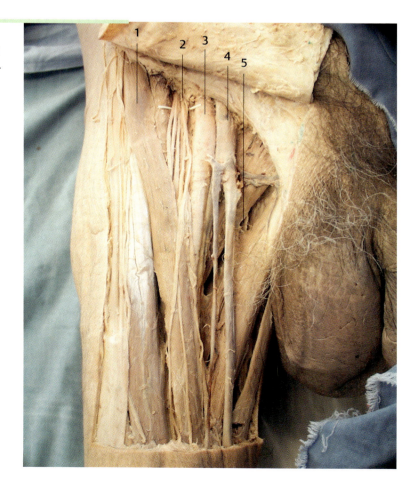

9.2   Femoral Nerve Block ("3-in-1 Technique")

Landmarks
Anterior superior iliac spine, pubic tubercle. The anterior superior iliac spine and the pubic tubercle are marked and joined by a line. This connecting line corresponds to the

inguinal ligament. The classically described puncture site is 1 cm below the inguinal ligament and ca. 1.5 cm lateral to the femoral artery (note: IVAN = **I**nside **V**ein, **A**rtery, **N**erve) (Figs. 9.**7**, 9.**8**).

Divergence from the original technique is recommended, selecting the injection site ca. 1 cm below the inguinal *crease*, that is, markedly further distally (Figs. 9.**9**-9.**12**).

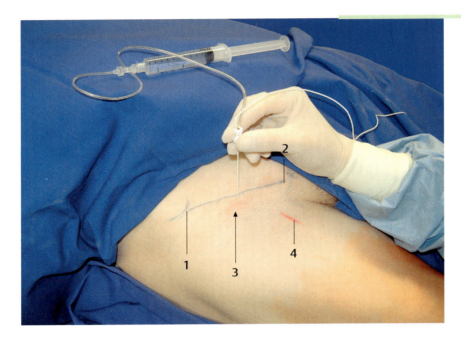

Fig. 9.**7**   Classical injection site according to Winnie and Labat just below the inguinal ligament. The nerve is here at a greater distance from the skin and is encountered at an angle of almost 90° (see Fig. 9.**8**). It is advisable to seek orientation further distally just below the inguinal crease (see Fig. 9.**9**).

1   Anterior superior iliac spine
2   Pubic tubercle
3   Injection site according to Winnie and Labat
4   Femoral artery

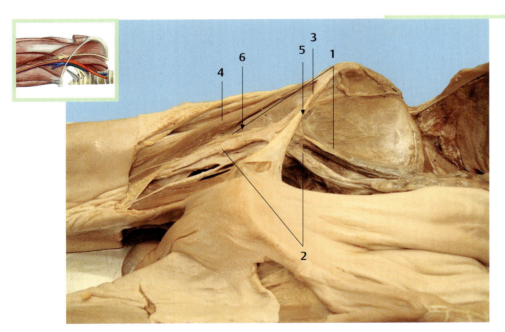

Fig. 9.**8**   **The** femoral nerve emerges from beneath anteriorly, crosses the iliopubic eminence, and then divides into the individual branches. The shortest skin–nerve distance is at about the level of the inguinal crease. If puncture is performed in the region of the inguinal ligament, a greater skin–nerve distance must be anticipated.

1   Femoral nerve
2   Femoral artery
3   Inguinal ligament
4   Sartorius
5   Note the skin–femoral nerve distance at the level of the inguinal ligament
6   The femoral nerve crosses the iliopubic eminence

Fig. 9.**9**   Recommended technique for femoral nerve block: puncture site about 1.5 cm lateral to the femoral artery, which can be palpated, and ca. 1 cm below the inguinal crease. Note that the needle is directed tangentially and proximally.

1   Inguinal ligament
2   Inguinal crease
3   Femoral artery
4   Puncture site
A   Anterior superior iliac spine
B   Greater trochanter

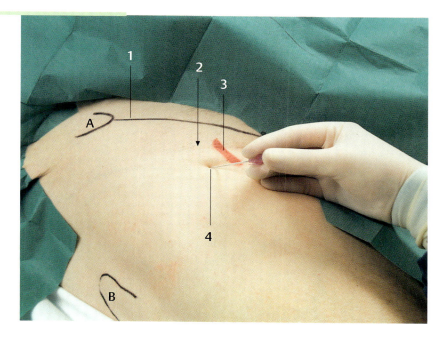

Fig. 9.**10**   See Fig. 9.**9**; here, medial view. Right thigh

1   Inguinal ligament
2   Inguinal crease
3   Femoral artery

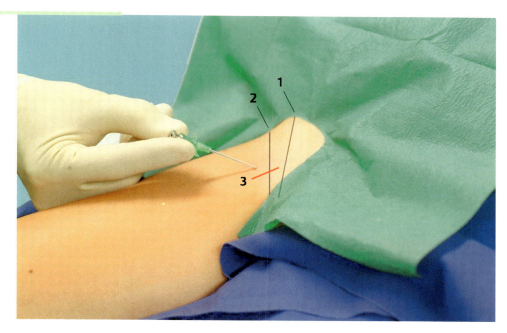

Position

The patient lies supine and the leg is slightly abducted and externally rotated. In difficult anatomical situations, a flat pad can be placed under the patient's buttocks in order to show the topography of the inguinal region better.

Method

The landmarks are marked and the femoral artery is palpated. If the artery is impalpable, a Doppler probe can be used for orientation (Fig. 9.**13**).

After skin disinfection and intracutaneous or superficial subcutaneous local anesthesia ca. 3 cm (Härtel 1916; Moore 1969) below the inguinal ligament (or 1 cm below the inguinal crease) and ca. 1.5 cm lateral to the artery, the skin is incised with a small lancet. An 18G, 45° short-bevel needle with a surrounding plastic cannula is advanced cranially and dorsally at an angle of 30° to the skin and parallel to the artery until the tough resistance of the fascia lata is felt. The

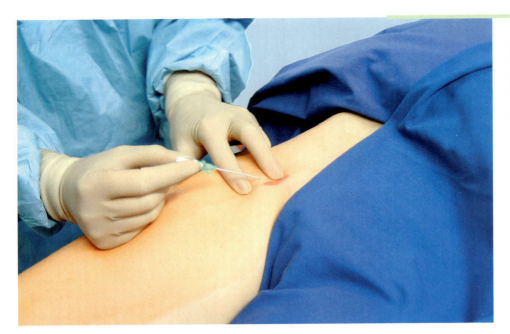

Fig. 9.**11**   When the index and middle fingers are on the femoral artery, the injection site is laterally located at the level of the distal interphalangeal joints.

Right thigh

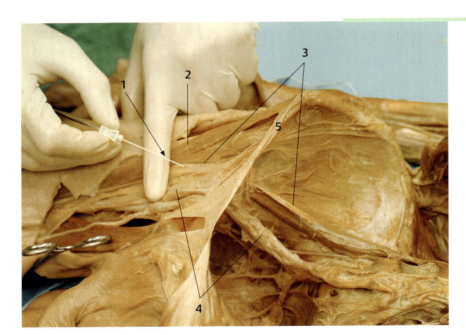

Fig. 9.**12**   Recommended puncture site for femoral nerve block. The nerve is relatively superficial just below the inguinal crease. Note the tangential needle direction. When the finger palpates the femoral artery from the lateral aspect, the injection site is at the level of the distal interphalangeal joint.

Right inguinal region
  1 Puncture site
  2 Sartorius
  3 Femoral nerve
  4 Femoral artery
  5 Inguinal ligament

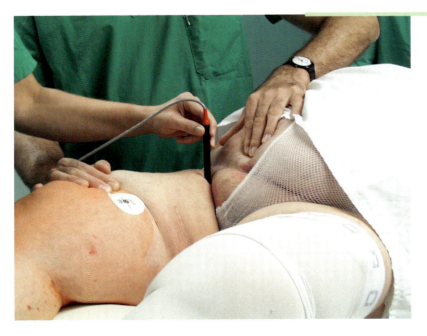

Fig. 9.**13**   In difficult anatomical situations, use of a Doppler probe can facilitate finding the femoral artery.

resistance is overcome by slightly increasing pressure (Figs. 9.**14**, 9.**15**).

While cautiously advancing the needle further, there is often a second "loss of resistance" when the tip of the needle passes through the iliac fascia (so-called "double-click"). The end of the needle should then be lowered, and it is advanced further proximally parallel to the artery under stimulation (PNS) (Figs. 9.**16**, 9.**17**).

Contractions in the quadriceps femoris and "dancing" of the patella at 0.3 mA with a pulse duration of 0.1 ms indicate that the tip of the needle is in the correct position in the immediate vicinity of the femoral nerve. Following negative aspiration, 20-40 ml of a medium-acting or long-acting local anesthetic (LA) is injected. Digital pressure distal to the needle can promote distribution of the LA in a cranial direction (Figs. 9.**18**-9.**20**). If a continuous technique is planned, a flexible 20G catheter is advanced 5 cm beyond the end of the cannula after injection of the LA (Figs. 9.**21**, 9.**22**). Before connecting the catheter to a bacterial filter, the catheter should be aspirated again to exclude an intravascular position (Fig. 9.**23**).

Local Anesthetic, Dosages

Initially: 30-50 ml of a medium-acting LA (e.g., 1% [10 mg/ml] mepivacaine, lidocaine) or a long-acting LA (e.g., ropivacaine 0.75% [7.5 mg/ml]).

Continuous: 8-10 ml/h ropivacaine 0.2-0.375% (2-3.75 mg/ml)

Combination block with the sciatic nerve: see below.

Fig. 9.**14**   Puncture of the femoral nerve. The fascia lata and iliac fascia have to be penetrated.

Right inguinal region
  1   Fascia lata
  2   Iliac fascia with iliopectineal fascia

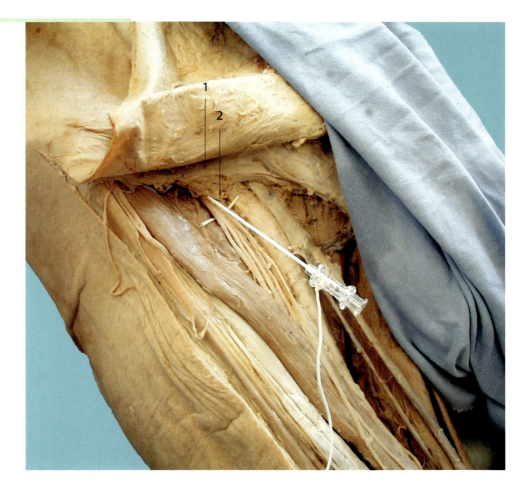

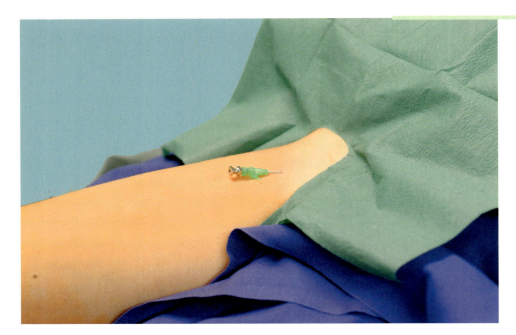

Fig. 9.**15** Puncture for femoral nerve block. The needle is advanced proximally in the surrounding sheath using electrostimulation. It must not be forced against resistance. If the response is lost, it can be useful to direct the needle tip somewhat anteriorly by lowering the hub of the needle.

Right thigh

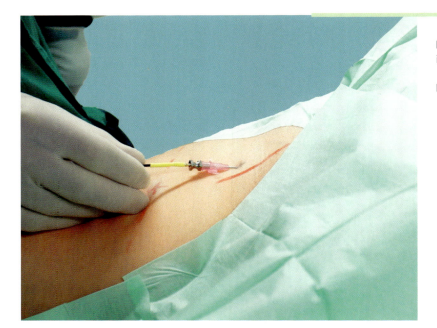

Fig. 9.**16** Advancing proximally beneath the iliac fascia using nerve stimulation.

Right inguinal region

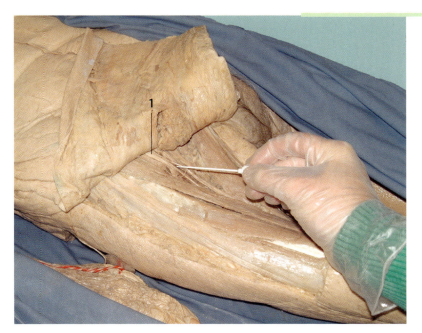

Fig. 9.**17** After crossing the iliopubic eminence as the highest point, the femoral nerve goes deeper again further peripherally. With a more peripheral puncture below the inguinal ligament, advancing the needle in the cranial direction (under nerve stimulation) within the surrounding sheath may necessitate lowering the hub of the needle in order to advance it virtually "uphill."

1 Femoral nerve

Fig. 9.**18**   After aspiration, 30–40 ml of LA is injected slowly and with repeated aspiration. Digital compression distal to the needle can be helpful.

Right inguinal region

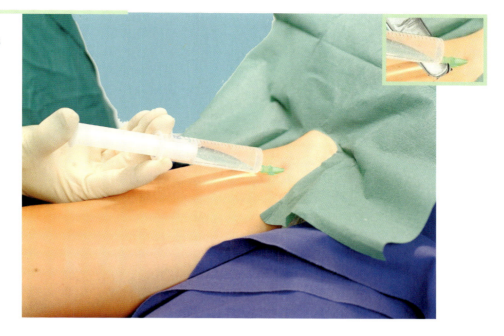

Fig. 9.**19**   Backflow of drops of the LA after injection of 30–40 ml indicates correct injection into the nerve compartment.

Right inguinal region

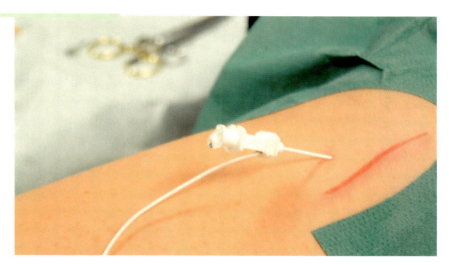

Fig. 9.**20**   Spread of the LA, shown radiologically using contrast. Note the spread laterally; contrary to what is imagined of a "3-in-1 block" there is not always central spread toward the lumbar plexus.

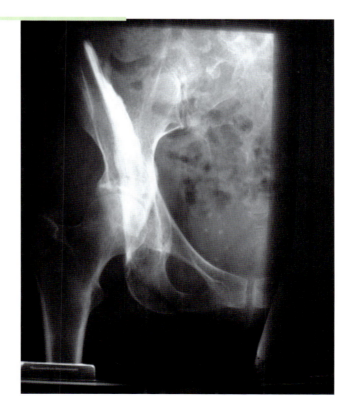

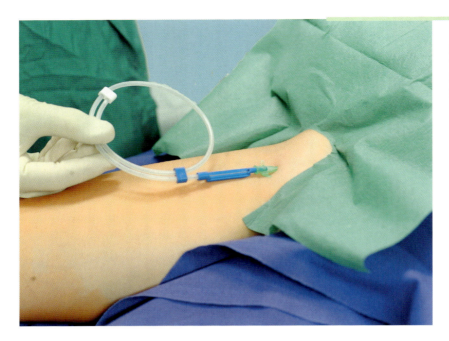

Fig. 9.**21**   Introduction of a flexible catheter through the needle. The catheter should not be advanced more than 3–4 cm beyond the needle tip.

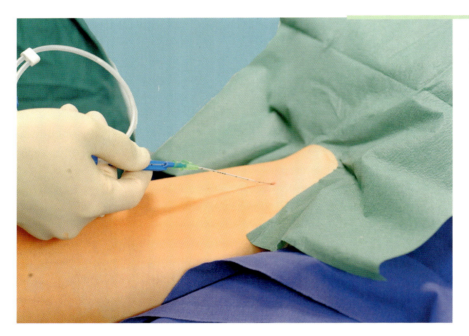

Fig. 9.**22**   Removal of the cannula after advancing the catheter.

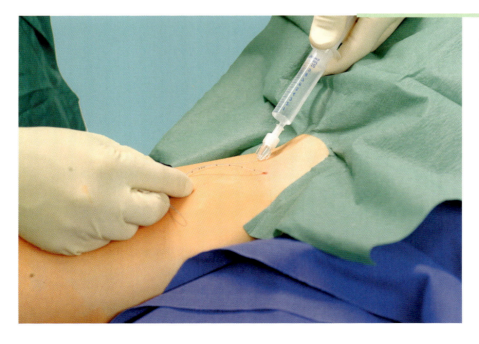

Fig. 9.**23**   Aspiration through the catheter before connecting a bacterial filter.

9.3   Sensory and Motor Effects

The femoral nerve provides the *sensory* innervation of the front of the thigh and is involved in the innervation of the hip, knee, and femur. It is the *motor* supply to the knee extensors and hip flexors. The saphenous nerve is the sensory terminal branch of the femoral nerve and supplies the inside of the lower leg. The anesthesia can include the great toe in a few cases (Clara 1959).

9.4   Indications and Contraindications

Indications
- In combination with a block of the sciatic nerve (sacral plexus), all operations on the leg (including total joint replacement of the knee and ankle) can be performed.
- Wound management and skin grafts on the anterior and lateral thigh and on the inside of the lower leg.
- Pain therapy after operations on the knee (e.g., arthroscopic operations, anterior cruciate ligament repair, knee replacement, etc.) and pain reduction after hip operations or thigh amputation.
- Pain therapy (e.g., in femoral shaft fracture [Tobias 1994]; patellar fracture; positioning for spinal anesthesia, e.g., before surgery of femoral neck fractures; mobilization; physiotherapy).

Contraindications
- General contraindications (see Chapter 15).
- Tumor in the groin (relative: painful lymph nodes in the groin).
- Previous inguinal vascular surgery (relative).

9.5   Complications, Side Effects, Method-Specific Problems

Vascular puncture with subsequent hematoma is possible. Femoral nerve lesions have been described in case reports.

Practical Notes
- Identification of the perineural space is possible in principle without a nerve stimulator and with the loss-of-resistance technique only. However, the nerve stimulator should not be omitted as the femoral nerve is primarily a motor nerve and therefore paresthesia is not produced in every case in the event of (unintentional) puncture of the nerve (Urmey 1997).
- The femoral nerve is separated from the artery by the iliac fascia (Figs. 9.2-9.4). A transarterial technique, such as that described for the brachial plexus, is therefore not possible (Rosenquist and Lederhaas 1999; Urmey 1997).
- Misinterpretation due to muscle contractions on direct intramuscular stimulation of the sartorius muscle or stimulation of superficially situated motor branches innervating sartorius muscle can lead to failures (Fig. 9.**24**). So-called "dancing" of the patella should therefore always be achieved.
- The classical technique was described in 1924 by Labat. In this technique the puncture site was 1 cm below the inguinal

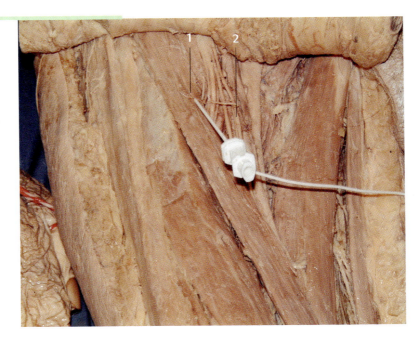

Fig. 9.**24**   A motor response in the region of the sartorius muscle can be caused by direct stimulation of the muscle or by stimulation of the motor branch of the femoral nerve, which supplies the sartorius. In both cases, the needle position must be corrected, medially in the first case and slightly laterally and a little deeper in the second case. Only a "dancing patella" or response from the different quadriceps muscles produced by slight "wobbling" movements of the needle is secure evidence that the needle is in the correct position (at appropriate stimulation intensity).

1   Sartorius
2   Motor branch to sartorius

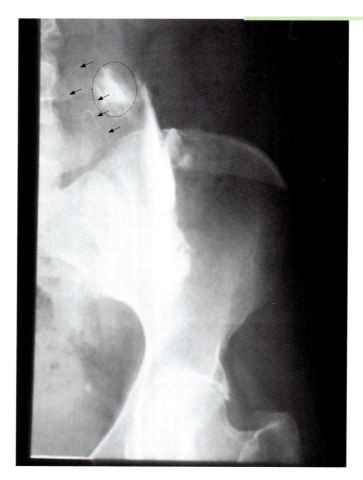

Fig. 9.**25** Advancing the catheter too far may lead to looping and an incorrect catheter position.

———▶ Catheter

 Diffuse spread of contrast injected through the catheter

ligament. Compared to a puncture site in the region of the inguinal ligament, the femoral nerve 1 cm below the inguinal crease is wider and markedly closer under the fascia lata (Figs. 9.**8**, 9.**12**). Puncture somewhat *distal to the inguinal crease* is therefore recommended and not, as in the classical technique of femoral

nerve block, at the level of the inguinal ligament.
● The quality of anesthesia is not improved by advancing the catheter further forwardand/or using greater injection volume than stated (Singelyn et al. 1996) (Fig. 9.**25**).
● The anesthesia may, in a few cases, include the great toe through the

saphenous nerve (sensory terminal branch of the femoral nerve) (Clara 1959).
● Persistent pain in the region of the knee with otherwise complete anesthesia on the front of the thigh and a good motor block of the hip flexors and knee extensors can indicate insufficient obturator nerve block (Paul 1999).

9.6   Remarks on the Technique

Cranial to the inguinal ligament, the femoral nerve passes in a fascial sheath that is formed posterolaterally by the iliac fascia, medially by the psoas fascia, and anteriorly by the transversalis fascia. When it passes under the inguinal ligament, the nerve begins to split underneath and soon comes closer to the surface, dividing into its terminal branches. Immediately below the inguinal ligament, the femoral nerve is separated from the artery by the iliopectineal fascia, which now forms the fascial sheath that

continues to surround the medial part of the nerve, which is composed posterolaterally of the merged iliopsoas fascia and anteriorly of the fascia lata.
Alon Winnie postulated in 1973 that this fascial sheath should be understood as a sheath surrounding the nerve plexus throughout from the proximal psoas compartment to its distal branching. According to Winnie, this fascial tube can be "filled" with local anesthetic by an appropriate injection technique not only from above as a psoas compartment

block but also from the groin. According to Winnie, the femoral, obturator, and lateral cutaneous nerves of the lumbar plexus should be reached with 20 ml of local anesthetic. This technique is also described as the anterior approach to the psoas compartment (Hahn et al. 1996). Winnie called the method the "3-in-1 technique" (Winnie et al. 1973, 1974). Winnie's classic concept is currently under discussion on the basis of recent information. The shared and continuous fascial sheath he described was not always

Fig. 9.**26**   Lumbar plexus with femoral nerve and obturator nerve. In femoral nerve block, the psoas major muscle (largely removed on the right) usually prevents spread of the LA to the obturator nerve in femoral nerve block.

1   Ilioinguinal nerve
2   Lateral cutaneous nerve of the thigh
3   Obturator nerve
4   Femoral nerve
5   Psoas major (largely removed on the right)
6   Femoral artery
7   Femoral vein

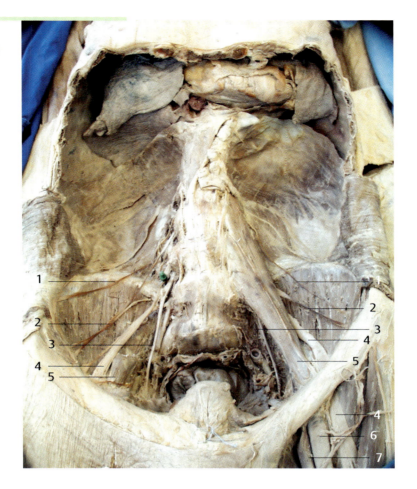

Fig. 9.**27**   Cranial view of the retroperitoneal region. The psoas major muscle prevents spread of the LA to the obturator nerve in femoral nerve block.

1   Lateral cutaneous nerve of the thigh
2   Femoral nerve
3   Psoas major
4   Obturator nerve

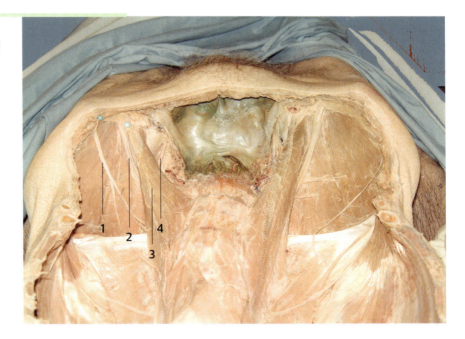

found in anatomical studies. In particular, it is doubted whether the obturator nerve is reached at all with this block (Capdevila et al. 1998; Cauhepe et al. 1989; Dupré 1996; Kozlov et al. 1991; Ritter 1996) (Figs. 9.**26**-9.**28**).

Lang found in a prospective study that when the Winnie technique was used, the femoral nerve was anesthetized in 81% and the lateral cutaneous nerve of the thigh in 96%, but that the obturator nerve was blocked in only 4% (Lang et al. 1993). The area of

sensory innervation of this nerve on the inside of the thigh is very inconstant and is not suitable for investigation (Bergmann 1994). Demonstration of the degree to which the obturator nerve is involved in the block is therefore very difficult. Paul and Drechsler

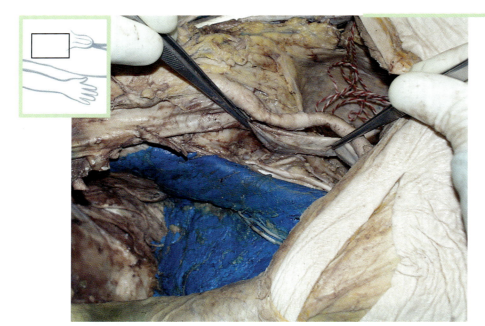

Fig. 9.**28**   Dye introduced through a correct access to the femoral nerve block (before dissection) does not reach the obturator nerve.

Right lower abdomen
   1   Femoral artery
   2   Femoral vein
   3   Obturator nerve
   4   Psoas
   5   Femoral nerve

(1993) found a completely anesthetized area of skin in only 5 % of cases in isolated obturator nerve blocks despite the fact that there was obvious motor block of the adductors. On the basis of these observations, the obturator nerve appears to be of subordinate importance for the innervation of the knee in most cases. That would explain the very effective use of the so-called "3-in-1 technique," even if this probably leads only to a "2-in-1 block" (Rosenquist and Lederhaas 1999). The extent and significance of block of the lateral cutaneous nerve of the thigh have not yet been conclusively elucidated. In the technique described by Winnie, the puncture site selected was 1 cm below the inguinal ligament with the needle directed vertically toward the nerve. At this point, the femoral nerve is still relatively deep. Löfström mentions a depth of 3.5-4 cm (Löfström 1980) (Fig. 9.**8**). For this reason, Härtel (1916) and later Moore (1976) recommended a puncture site 2-3 cm further distal. In its further course, the nerve very quickly becomes more superficial and divides. Vloka et al. (1999) found that a puncture site at the level of the inguinal crease and directly lateral to the artery led most frequently (in 71 %) to contact between the needle and the nerve. The nerve was significantly wider at this point (1.4 cm vs. 0.98 cm) and was closer to the fascia lata (0.68 cm vs. 2.64 cm) than at the level of the inguinal ligament (Vloka et al. 1999) (Fig. 9.**12**). Because of the branching of the nerve, however, a puncture site even further distally might be problematic and might also make placement of a catheter more difficult (Urmey 1997).

Good anatomical orientation is possible even without producing paresthesia. The "double-click," a loss of resistance that can be felt on penetrating the fascia lata and the iliac fascia, especially when short-bevel needles are used, is a very reliable indication that the tip of the needle is in the correct position. Whether the success rate can be improved by peripheral nerve stimulation during femoral nerve block is controversial. However, as the femoral nerve in the majority of cases has motor fibers, an intraneural injection might remain unnoticed on the basis of absent paresthesia if the nerve is approached too closely. With pure motor neurons, an overproportionate incidence of intraneural injection can be anticipated (Gentili and Wargnier 1993; Graf and Martin 2001; Urmey 1997). For safety reasons, the use of peripheral nerve stimulation is strongly recommended.

The *indications* for inguinal paravascular femoral nerve block for intraoperative anesthesia are very limited.

Femoral nerve block, when performed on admission to hospital in the case of femoral neck or femoral shaft fractures, can allow pain-free examination and also administration of spinal anesthesia for surgery. Complete analgesia in the hip cannot be achieved as the hip is also supplied by the sacral plexus, but a clear reduction in pain is obtained (Esteve et al. 1990; Fournier et al. 1998).

A combination of spinal anesthesia and the "3-in-1 block" in transurethral operations on the bladder wall to eliminate the obturator reflex seldom leads to the desired effect. By blocking the obturator nerve, contractions of the adductor muscles due to unintentional stimulation by electroresection should be prevented. However, the "3-in-1 block" not only leads to an inadequate obturator nerve block but is also cranial to the site of stimulation. In order to obtain an effective block of the obturator nerve for this purpose, a selective obturator nerve block must be performed distal to the bladder.

Femoral nerve block can be combined very successfully with sciatic nerve block for operations on the leg (Anke-Moller et al. 1990; Elmas and Atanassoff 1993; Geiger et al. 1989, 1995; Kaiser et al. 1986; Mackenzie 1997; Sprotte 1981).

For surgery requiring a thigh tourniquet and operations on the knee, where dorsal parts of the knee are also involved, combination with a proximal sciatic nerve block is always necessary. 20-40 ml of a 1 % (10 mg/ml) medium-acting amide for the femoral nerve block ("3-in-1 block") plus 20-30 ml for the sciatic block is recommended (Büttner and Meier 1999; Meier and Büttner 2001). Sufficient anesthesia of the femoral nerve ("3-in-1 block") can also be obtained with 20 ml of ropivacaine 0.5 % (5 mg/ml)or 20 ml of bupivacaine 0.5 % (5 mg/ml) (Marhofer et al. 2000 a, 2000 b).

The technique of femoral nerve block is easy to learn, simple to perform, and safe. In combination with a proximal sciatic block, it enables operations to be performed on the lower limb. As continuous pain therapy, femoral nerve block provides sufficient analgesia for operations on the femur and patella and reduces pain in operations on the hip or knee. In rehabilitation after knee operations, continuous femoral nerve block provides effective pain relief and leads to shorter hospitalization and better functional results compared to general anesthesia (Capdevila 1999).

References

Anke-Moller E, Dahl JB, Spangsberg NLM, Schultz P, Wernberg M. Inguinal paravascular block (three-in-one block). Ugeskr Laeger. 1990;152:1655-8.

Bergmann RA. Compendium of human anatomic variations. Munich: Urban and. Schwarzenberg; 1994:143-7.

Büttner J, Meier G. Kontinuierliche periphere Techniken zur Regionalanästhesie und Schmerztherapie–Obere und untere Extremität. Bremen: UNI-MED-Verlag; 1999.

Capdevila X, Biboulet P, Bouregba M, Barthelet Y, Rubenovitch J, D'Athis F. Comparison of the three in one and fascia iliaca compartment blocks in adults: Clinical and radiographic analysis. Anesth Analg. 1998;86:1039-44.

Capdevila X, Barthelet Y, Biboulet P. Effects of perioperative analgesic technique on the surgical outcome and duration of rehabilitation after major knee surgery. Anesthesiology. 1999;91:8-15.

Cauhepe C, Oliver M, Colombani R. The "3-in-1" block: myth or reality? Ann Fr Anesth Reanim. 1989;376-8.

Clara M. Das Nervensystem des Menschen. 3rd ed. Leipzig: Barth; 1959.

Dupré LJ. Bloc 3 en 1 ou bloc fémoral. Que faut-il faire et comment le faire? Ann Fr Anesth Réanim. 1996;15:1099-106.

Elmas C, Atanassoff PG. Combined inguinal paravascular (3 in 1) and sciatic nerve blocks for lower limb surgery. Reg Anesth. 1993;2:88-92.

Esteve M, Veillette Y, Ecoffey C, Orhant EE. Continuous block of femoral nerve after surgery of the knee: Pharmacokinetics of bupivacaine. Ann Fr Anesth Reanim. 1990;9:322-5.

Fournier R, Van Gessel E, Gaggero G, Boccovi S, Forster A, Gamulin Z. Postoperative analgesia with "3-in-1" femoral nerve block after prosthetic hip surgery. Can J Anaesth. 1998;45:34-8.

Geiger P, Weindler M, Wollinsky KH, et al. Met-Hb-Spiegel bei kombiniertem Ischiadicus/3 in 1-Block mit alleiniger Verwendung von Prilocain im Vergleich zu einer Prilocain-Bupivacain-Kombination. Zentraleuropäischer Anästhesiekongress, Innsbruck; 1989.

Geiger P, Moßbrucker H, Gelowicz-Maurer M, Mack E, Mehrkens HH. Postoperative analgesia with 3 in 1 or psoas compartment catheter—are there differences in efficiency? XIV Annual ESRA Congress, Prague (special abstract issue); 1995:68.

Gentili ME, Wargnier JP. Peripheral nerve damage and regional anesthesia. Br J Anaesth. 1993;71:324-5.

Graf BM, Martin E. Periphere Nervenblockaden - Eine Übersicht über neue Entwicklungen einer alten Technique. Anaesthesist. 2001;50:312-22.

Hahn MB, McQuillan PM, Sheplock GJ. Regional anesthesia: an atlas of anatomy and techniques. St. Louis: Mosby; 1996.

Härtel F. Die Lokalanästhesie. Stuttgart: Enke; 1916.

Kaiser H., Niesel HC, Klimpel L, Menge M. Technike und Indikationen der kontinuierlichen 3-in-1-Blockade. In: Hempelmann G, Biscoping J, eds. Regionalanästhesiologische Aspekte I. Kontinuierliche Verfahren der Regionalanästhesie. Wedel: Astra; 1986:83-94.

Kozlov SP, Shartrov AI, Svetlov VA. The inguinal paravascular technique of lumbar plexus block—anatomical pretests were unsuccessful. Anesteziol Reanimatol. 1991;5:37-9.

Labat G. Regional anesthesia: Its technique and clinical application. Philadelphia: Saunders; 1924; 45.

Lang SA, Yip RW, Chang PC. The femoral 3-in-1 block revisited. J Clin Anesth. 1993;5:292-6.

Löfström B. Blockaden der peripheren Nerven des Beines. In: Eriksson E, eds. Atlas der Lokalanästhesie. 2nd ed. Berlin: Springer; 1980:101-15.

Mackenzie JW. 3-in-1 block via femoral nerve sheath cannula: a simple method of pain relief for fractured neck of femur. Int Monitor Reg Anesth. 1997;9(3):91.

Marhofer P, Nasel C, Sitzwohl C, Kapral S. Magnetic resonance imaging of the distribution of local anesthetic during the three-in-one block. Anesth Analg. 2000a;90:119-24.

Marhofer P, Oismüller C, Faryniak B, Sitzwohl C, Mayer N, Kapral S. Three-in-one blocks with ropivacaine: evaluation of sensory onset time and quality of sensor block. Anesth Analg. 2000b;90:125-8.

Meier G, Büttner J. Regionalanästhesie - Kompendium der peripheren Blockaden. München: Arcis; 2001.

Moore DC. Lesions of the peripheral nerves. In: Moore DC, ed. Complications of regional anesthesia. Philadelphia: Davis; 1969:112-8.

Moore DC. Regional block: Block of the sciatic and femoral nerves. Springfield: Thomas; 1976;275-99.

Paul W. Die kontinuierliche Blockade des N. femoralis. In: Mehrkens HH, Büttner J, eds. Kontinuierliche periphere Leitungsblockaden. München: Arcis; 1999:49-58.

Paul W, Drechsler HJ. Clinical efficacy and radiological representation of continuous 3-in-1 block placed by the Seldinger technique. Int Monitor Reg Anesth. 1993;531-2.

Platzer W. Taschenatlas der Anatomie - Bewegungsapparat. 7th ed. Stuttgart: Thieme; 1999.

Ritter JW. Femoral sheath for inguinal paravascular lumbar plexus block is not found in human cadavers. J Clin Anesth. 1996;7:470-3.

Rosenquist RW, Lederhaas G. Femoral and lateral femoral cutaneous nerve block. Techniques in Regional Anesthesia and Pain Management 1999;3:33-8.

Singelyn FJ, Gouverneur JMA, Goossens F, van Roy C. During continuous "3-in-1" block a high position of the catheter increases the success rate of the technique. Int Monitor Reg Anesth. 1996;(A)8:105.

Sprotte G. Die inguinale Blockade des Lumbar plexus als Analgesie-Verfahren in der prä- und postoperativen Traumatologie und Orthopädie. Reg Anaesth. 1981;4:39-41.

Tobias JD. Continuous femoral nerve block to provide analgesia following femur fracture in paediatric ICU population. Anaesth Intensive Care. 1994;22:616-8.

Urmey WF. Femoral nerve block for the management of postoperative pain. Techniques in Regional Anesthesia and Pain Management 1997;1:88-92.

Vloka JD, Hadzic A, Drobnik L, Ernest A, Reiss W, Thys DM. Anatomical landmarks for femoral nerve blocks: A comparison of four needle insertion sites. Anesth Analg. 1999;89:1467-70.

Winnie AP, Ramamurthy S, Durrani Z. The inguinal paravascular technique of lumbar plexus anesthesia: The "3-in-1-block". Anesth Analg. 1973;52:989-96.

Winnie AP, Ramamurthy S, Durrani Z, Radonjic R. Plexus blocks for lower extremity surgery. New answers to old problems. Anesth Rev. 1974;11-6.

Woodburne RT. The lower limb. In: Woodburne RT, ed. Essentials of human anatomy. 7th ed. New York: Oxford University Press; 1983:557-71.

10 Proximal Sciatic Nerve Block

10.1 Anatomical Overview

The sacral plexus can be divided into three parts:
- Pudendal plexus
- Coccygeal plexus
- Sciatic plexus

The sacral plexus is not subdivided in all anatomy textbooks. However, as the division is useful from the clinical aspect, it is used as a basis here.

Sciatic Plexus

The sciatic plexus derives its roots from part of the anterior ramus of the 4th lumbar nerve and from the entire anterior ramus of the 5th lumbar nerve, which together form the lumbosacral trunk, along with the anterior rami of the 1st and 2nd and part of the 3rd sacral nerves. The anterior ramus of the 1st sacral nerve is not only the biggest branch of the lumbosacral plexus but the biggest anterior ramus overall. All of the roots of the plexus converge from their exit sites toward the greater sciatic foramen so that the plexus forms a triangular sheet, the apex of which points toward the infrapiriform foramen where the sciatic nerve emerges (Fig. 10.**1**). The nerve plexus lies for the most part just under the piriformis muscle and is covered toward the pelvis by

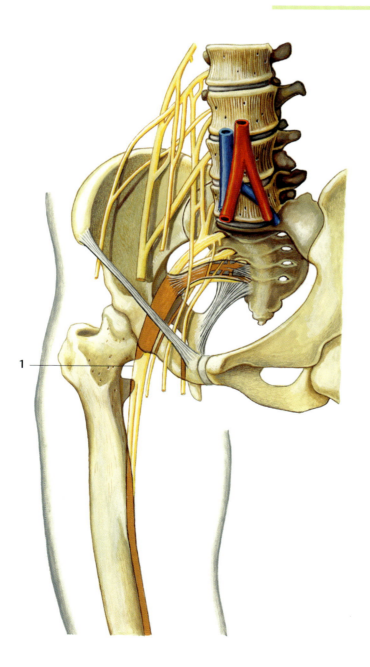

Fig. 10.**1**   Course of the sciatic nerve, main nerve of the sacral plexus.

1   Sciatic nerve

the parietal peritoneum and the tissues and branches of the internal iliac artery lying beneath it. The articular branches that supply parts of the hip joint capsule and the periosteal branches that innervate the periosteum of the ischium, greater trochanter, and lesser trochanter also come from the sciatic plexus.

Sciatic Nerve (L4–S3)

The sciatic nerve derives its fibers from all the roots of the sacral plexus. It is the biggest and longest nerve in the body, it supplies the widest area, and at the same time it has the greatest resistance among all the nerve cords with a tear strength of 91.5 kg (!). Excessive stretching can even tear the nerve trunk from its roots in the spinal cord. The roots of the sciatic nerve unite into the

trunk immediately before the greater sciatic foramen at the lower border of the piriformis (Fig. 10.**2**). It consists of two components, the common fibular nerve (synonym: common peroneal nerve) and the tibial nerve, which are surrounded in the pelvis minor and thigh by a shared connective-tissue sheath and therefore have the appearance of a single nerve trunk. The division into the two branches can occur at a varying level (Figs. 10.**3**, 10.**4**). At dissection,

Fig. 10.**2**   After emerging from the lesser pelvis through the infrapiriform foramen, the sciatic nerve, covered by the gluteal muscles, runs peripherally in the middle between the greater trochanter and the ischial tuberosity behind and medial to the lesser trochanter. The three palpable bony points (posterior superior iliac spine, greater trochanter, and ischial tuberosity) are used for orientation in all dorsal techniques of proximal sciatic nerve block.

  1 Posterior superior iliac spine
  2 Piriformis
  3 Trochanter minor
  4 Sciatic nerve
  5 Ischial tuberosity
  6 Trochanter major

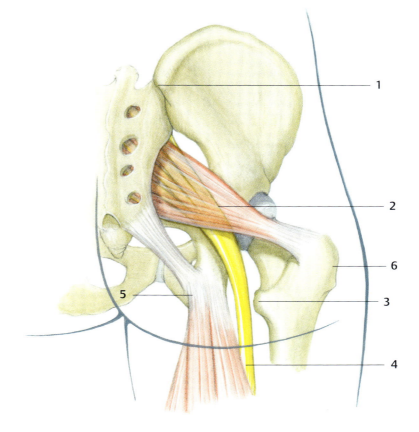

Fig. 10.**3**   The sciatic nerve often divides immediately after passing through the infrapiriform foramen into a fibular and a tibial division. The fibular division is always lateral, the tibial one always medial. However, these two divisions run together until about 10–15 cm above the popliteal crease.

  1 Sciatic nerve, fibular part
  2 Sciatic nerve, tibial part

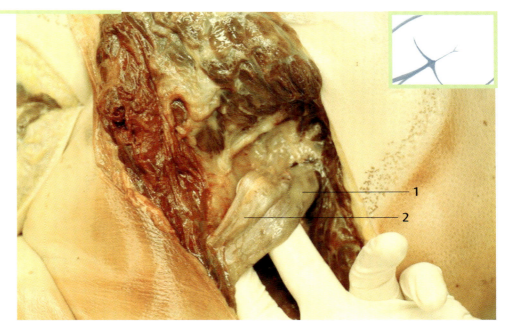

the nerve can almost always be separated into its two divisions as far as the hip region, even if they run in a common sheath (Ericksen et al. 2002).

The sciatic nerve usually leaves the true pelvis (pelvis minor) through the infrapiriform foramen as a 1.4 cm (up to 3 cm) wide and 0.4-05 cm (up to 0.9 cm) thick nerve cord (Figs. 10.**3**, 10.**4**) and enters the gluteal region. It divides into the tibial nerve and the common fibular nerve at the latest when it enters the popliteal fossa. The sciatic nerve provides motor innervation through its tibial division to all of the flexor muscles of the thigh (with the exception of the short head of the biceps femoris) and the lower leg and with its fibular division it supplies the short head of the biceps femoris and the fibular muscles and all the extensors in the lower leg and foot. It provides sensory innervation through both divisions to the skin of the lower leg and foot (see Fig. 7.**7**).

Clinical note: If the trunk of the sciatic nerve is blocked, external rotation of the thigh and knee flexion are greatly impaired. Because of the unopposed extensor action of the quadriceps muscle, the leg behaves like a stilt. The foot is unstable at the ankle and can no longer be dorsiflexed.

Overview of the Nerves of the Sciatic Plexus

The superior gluteal nerve and the inferior gluteal nerve along with the posterior cutaneous nerve of the thigh and the sciatic nerve belong to the sciatic plexus.

Only the *sciatic nerve* (tibial nerve, common fibular nerve) and the *posterior cutaneous nerve* of the thigh have importance for anesthesia and analgesia of the leg.

Posterior Cutaneous Nerve of the Thigh (S1–S3)

The posterior cutaneous nerve of the thigh, which is the sensory supply to the posterior aspect of the thigh, leaves the pelvis together with the sciatic nerve and the inferior gluteal nerve through the infrapiriform foramen. The nerve lies medial and caudal to the sciatic nerve and reaches the posterior surface of the thigh under the gluteus maximus muscle. The distribution of the posterior cutaneous nerve of the thigh is variable and extends from the distal third of the buttocks as far as the distal boundary of the popliteal fossa.

Periosteal Innervation

(see Fig. 7.**8**)

Relevant Facts for Anesthesia and Pain Therapy

The *periosteum of the femur* is supplied from behind by the sciatic nerve in the upper third, by the obturator nerve in the middle third, and in the distal third by the sciatic nerve laterally and by the femoral and obturator nerves medially.

The *innervation of the knee anteriorly* is by branches of the femoral nerve and sciatic nerve and posteriorly by parts of the sciatic nerve, the obturator nerve, and the saphenous nerve.

The *periosteum of the tibia and fibula* is supplied by the tibial nerve, apart from the lateral head of the tibia and the head of the fibula (common fibular nerve) (important for lower leg amputations, fractures).

The *ankle* receives its sensory supply from the tibial nerve and sural nerve.

The *periosteum of the tarsal bones* is innervated by the sural nerve and parts of the tibial nerve, the metatarsals, and the phalanges by the deep fibular nerve and the terminal branches of the tibial nerve (Wagner 1994).

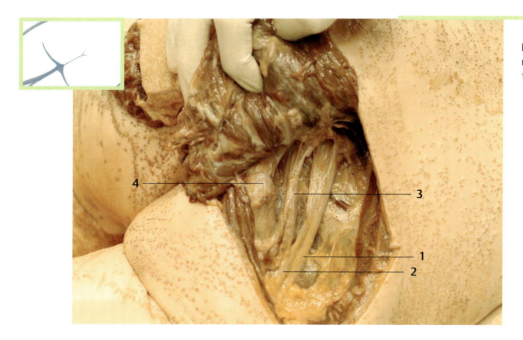

Fig. 10.**4**   As Fig. 10.**3**, here with the posterior cutaneous nerve of the thigh and ischial tuberosity.

1   Sciatic nerve, fibular part
2   Sciatic nerve, tibial part
3   Posterior cutaneous nerve of the thigh
4   Ischial tuberosity

10.2 Anterior Proximal Sciatic Nerve Block (with Patient in Supine Position)

Technique of Anterior (Ventral) Sciatic Nerve Block

Anterior Block of the Sciatic Nerve (according to Beck, Classical Technique)

Landmarks
Greater trochanter, anterior superior iliac spine, pubic tubercle.

Position
The patient lies supine with the leg to be anesthetized extended.

Procedure
The puncture site is found from the intersection of two lines: the perpendicular from the junction of the middle and medial thirds of the line joining the anterior superior iliac spine and the pubic tubercle (inguinal ligament) and a line through the greater trochanter parallel to the line between the iliac spine and the ischial tuberosity (Fig. 10.**5**). A 22G, 12-15 cm needle is advanced from the puncture site in a slightly lateral direction toward the medial side of the femur until it makes contact with bone, and the distance to the femur, usually 4.5-6 cm, is noted. The needle is then withdrawn as far as the subcutis and is then advanced 5 cm further in a vertical direction past the femur. No paresthesia is sought. A motor response of the sciatic nerve distal to the knee or in the foot region (tibial nerve, plantar flexion; fibular nerve, dorsiflexion) shows that the tip of the needle is close to the sciatic nerve. The position of the needle is optimized so that the motor response can be identified at a current of 0.3 mA and a pulse duration of 0.1 ms. Then 20-30 ml of a medium-acting or long-acting local anesthetic (LA) is injected.

Remarks on the Technique
The classical technique of anterior (ventral) sciatic nerve block was described by G. P. Beck in 1963. The technique allows block of the sciatic nerve with the patient in supine position so that the anesthesia can also be performed, e.g., with vertebral fractures, fractures of the pelvis, or the long bones and in the case of obesity, chronic polyarthritis, and other positioning problems. Unsatisfactory anesthesia for a tourniquet at the thigh must be anticipated when this block is combined with a so-called "3-in-1 block" (see Chapter 9), as it is possible that neither the posterior cutaneous nerve of the thigh nor the obturator nerve will be adequately anesthetized. The procedure can be painful because of the deliberate search for the femur and the associated periosteal contact,

and may reduce the patient's acceptance of the procedure.

The problem in the original technique described by Beck is that the needle does not reach the sciatic nerve in over 50% of punctures as the lesser trochanter impedes it (Gligorijevic 2000) (Fig. 10.**6**). Internal rotation of the leg by 45° is said to facilitate finding the sciatic nerve at the level of the lesser trochanter according to Beck's technique, and external rotation should be avoided (Wagner and Mißler 1987). A more distal and medial puncture site is therefore recommended (see Meier modification next).

Anterior (Continuous) Block of the Sciatic Nerve according to Meier (Modification of the Classical Technique)

Landmarks
Anterior superior iliac spine, symphysis, greater trochanter, muscle gap between rectus femoris and sartorius.

Position
The patient lies supine with the leg to be anesthetized in a stretched neutral position.

Procedure
For anatomical orientation, a line is drawn connecting the anterior superior iliac spine and the middle of the symphysis. This line is divided into three equal segments. At the junction of the medial (beside the symphysis) and the middle thirds, a perpendicular line is drawn in the caudal direction. The intersection of this perpendicular with a second line drawn through the greater trochanter parallel to the first line corresponds to the puncture site (Fig. 10.**7**). This is 1-2 cm further medial and 1-2 cm further caudal than in the guidelines given in Beck's classical anterior technique (1963). From here, puncture is performed in a posterior, slightly cranial and lateral direction. The sciatic nerve is readily reached with this technique (Fig. 10.**8**).

In practice, it has proved useful to find the muscle gap between the rectus femoris and the sartorius on the line through the trochanter (Figs. 10.**9**-10.**11**). This point is even further medial and distal than the point according to Meier's method (Fig. 10.**12**). No measurements or drawings are necessary (Fig. 10.**13**). In this muscle gap, vertical pressure is exerted on the femur with two fingers, and the femur is used as an abutment ("two-finger grasp") (Fig. 10.**14**). The blood vessels are pushed medially by this hand grasp and the likelihood of accidental vascu-

lar puncture is reduced. A needle (20G, 10-15 cm insulated needle for single-shot technique, or a 19.5G 15 cm insulated needle for a continuous technique) is then advanced at an angle of 75-85° to the skin in the cranial, posterior and slightly lateral direction (Figs. 10.**14**, 10.**15**). Branches of the femoral nerve are often stimulated after a few centimeters. The position of the needle tip is corrected (usually laterally) until no further response can be detected from the quadriceps muscle and it is then advanced further. Stimulation is initially with a current of 0.8-1.0 mA. After 6-10 cm, the adductor fascia is reached, which is often signaled by an obvious loss of resistance. The needle is advanced further until a motor response is produced in one of the two divisions of the sciatic nerve (fibular nerve, dorsiflexion: tibial nerve, plantar flexion) (Fig. 10.**16**). The correct position of the needle tip is indicated by a motor response in the foot at a current of 0.3 mA and pulse duration of 0.1 ms. If there is a response in the area of the hamstring muscles (contraction of the biceps femoris), the needle must be clearly withdrawn and corrected laterally ("under the femur") (Figs. 10.**17**, 10.**18**). Then 30 ml of a medium-acting or long-acting LA is injected.

- In the continuous technique, following injection of the LA, a 20G catheter is advanced 4 cm proximally through the unipolar needle (Figs. 10.**19**, 10.**20**). Short slight resistance can occur when the catheter tip reaches the end of the needle (Fig. 10.**20**), but this is normally easily overcome, and the catheter can then be advanced smoothly.
- The technique should be performed with peripheral nerve stimulation.
- If sciatic nerve block is combined with a femoral nerve block, anesthetizing the femoral nerve first is rational as this leads to anesthesia of the anterior thigh and helps to improve patient comfort (Fig. 10.**19**).
- The technique can also be performed in obese patients (Figs. 10.**21**, 10.**22**).

Indications and Contraindications (in Combination with Femoral Nerve Block)

Indications
- Operations on the knee, lower leg, or foot (e.g., knee replacement, tibial head osteotomy, arthrodesis, lateral ligament suture, forefoot operation).
- Reposition of fractures in the lower leg and foot area.

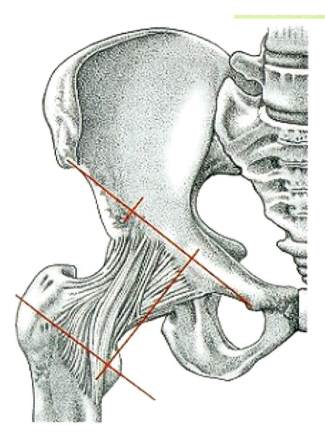

Fig. 10.**5** Anterior sciatic block, landmarks for Beck technique. With the Beck technique the puncture site is found as follows: a line from the anterior superior iliac spine to the pubic tubercle is divided into three; a perpendicular is dropped from the junction of the inner and middle thirds to reach a parallel line through the greater trochanter. The intersection marks the puncture site; the needle direction is perpendicular to the surface on which the patient is lying.

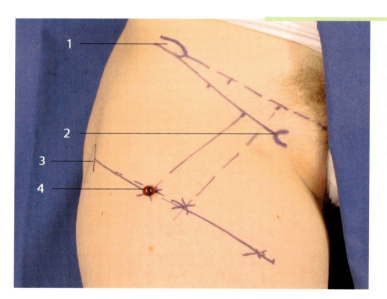

Fig. 10.**6** Needle direction for anterior sciatic nerve block using the Beck technique: note that because of the lesser trochanter the needle very often has to be directed too far medially, which may prevent the sciatic nerve from being found. (With MRI, always imagine seeing the plane from below.) The leg was in neutral position in all investigations.

1   Anterior superior iliac spine
2   Pubic tubercle
3   Greater trochanter
4   Puncture site, Beck technique, marked with nitrocapsule

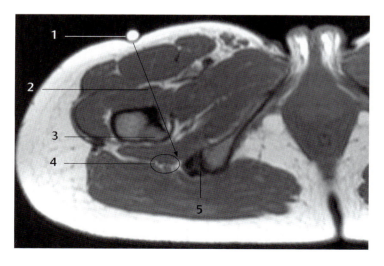

1   Puncture site, Beck technique
2   Needle direction, Beck technique
3   Lesser trochanter
4   Sciatic nerve
5   Ischial tuberosity

Fig. 10.**7** Anterior proximal sciatic nerve block, landmarks for Meier technique: a line is drawn between the anterior superior iliac spine and the middle of the symphysis and a perpendicular through the junction of the inner and middle thirds intersects a parallel line through the greater trochanter at the injection site. In this way, the injection site originally described by Beck is moved medially and caudally, so that it is possible to reach the sciatic nerve.

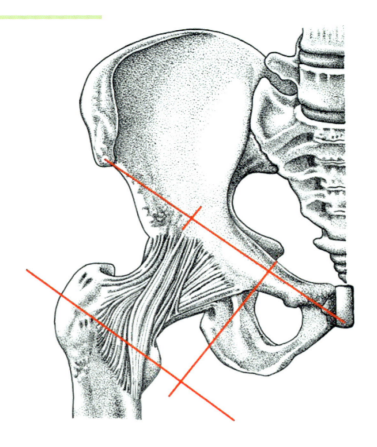

Fig. 10.**8** Anterior proximal sciatic nerve block (landmarks for Meier technique): the line between the anterior superior iliac spine and the middle of the symphysis is divided into three, and a perpendicular is dropped at the junction of the inner and middle thirds toward a parallel line through the greater trochanter. The intersection marks the puncture site. When the needle is relatively perpendicular (sagittal), it encounters the sciatic nerve after 8–12 cm (exactly 8.82 cm here). In practice, the needle is directed cranially as well as sagittally.

  1 Anterior superior iliac spine
  2 Middle of symphysis
  3 Greater trochanter
  4 Puncture site, Meier method, marked
     with nitrocapsule (for MRI)

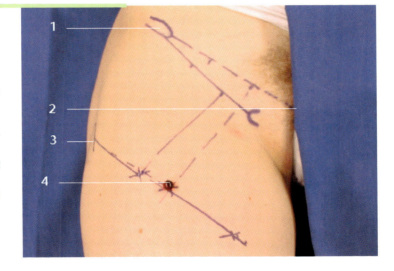

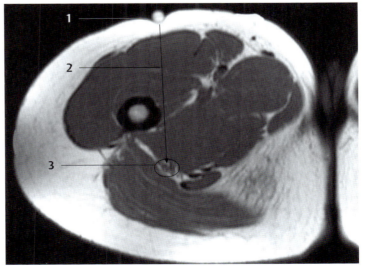

  1 Puncture site, Meier method (marked
     with nitrocapsule)
  2 Needle direction (skin-nerve distance
     8.82 cm with the needle directed ver-
     tically)
  3 Sciatic nerve

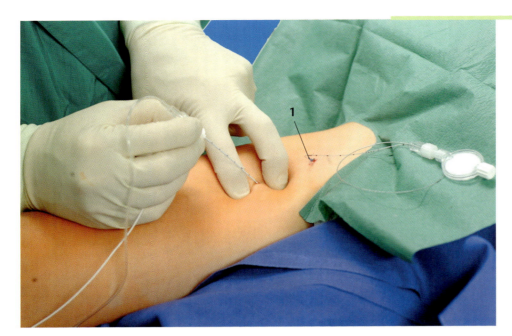

Fig. 10.**9** Anterior sciatic nerve block using the muscle gap between rectus femoris and sartorius muscles for orientation. The puncture site is a good hand's breadth below the puncture site for femoral nerve block. Note: (1) the cranial and slightly lateral needle direction ("below the femur"); (2) the "two-finger grasp" in the muscle gap, which pushes the blood vessels medially.

Right thigh
1 Femoral nerve catheter

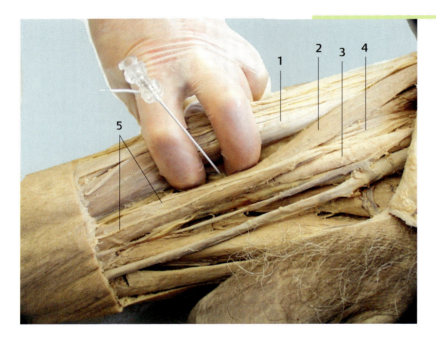

Fig. 10.**10** Anterior sciatic nerve block using the muscle gap between rectus femoris and sartorius for orientation. The puncture site is a good hand's breadth below the femoral nerve block puncture site. Note the "two-finger grasp" in the muscle gap, which pushes the blood vessels medially. When puncture is performed under nerve stimulation, there is occasionally a response in the anterior part of the thigh in the quadriceps muscle after ca. 2–4 cm through stimulation of branches of the femoral nerve.

1 Rectus femoris
2 Sartorius
3 Femoral artery
4 Femoral nerve
5 Nerve fibers from the femoral nerve

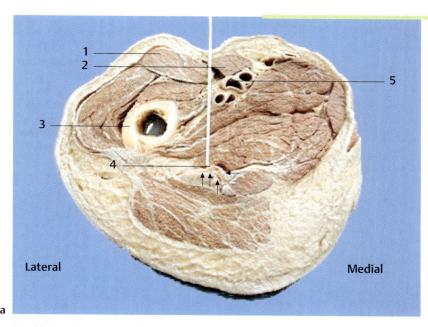

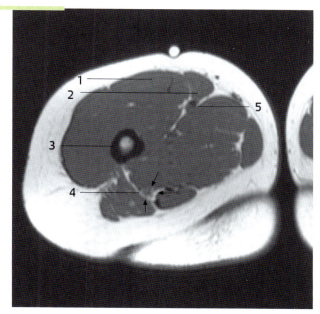

a   b

Fig. 10.**11**   Anterior sciatic nerve block using the muscle gap between rectus femoris and sartorius for orientation: anatomical cross section and MRI at the level of the puncture. **a** Right leg, seen from below, **b** MR image, right thigh.

1 Rectus femoris
2 Sartorius
3 Femur

4 Sciatic nerve
5 Blood vessels

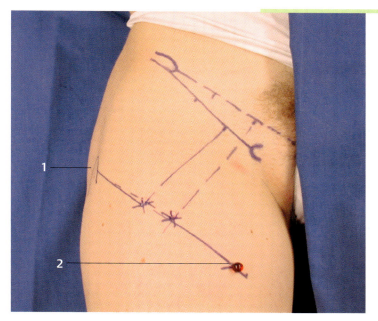

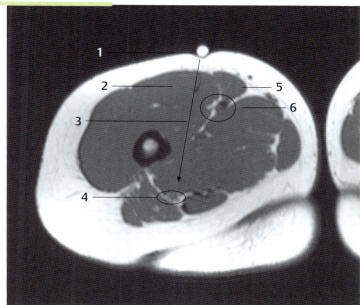

Fig. 10.**12**   Anterior sciatic nerve block using the muscle gap between rectus femoris and sartorius for orientation. Note the slightly lateral needle direction. The nerve is generally reached after 8–12 cm (exactly 9.65 cm here). However, the needle direction should be cranial as well as posterolateral; in this way the skin–nerve distance is increased slightly.

1 Trochanter major
2 Puncture site for anterior sciatic nerve block using the muscle gap between rectus femoris and sartorius for orientation, marked with nitrocapsule.

1 Nitrocapsule marking the injection site
2 Rectus femoris
3 Needle direction
4 Sciatic nerve
5 Sartorius
6 Blood vessels

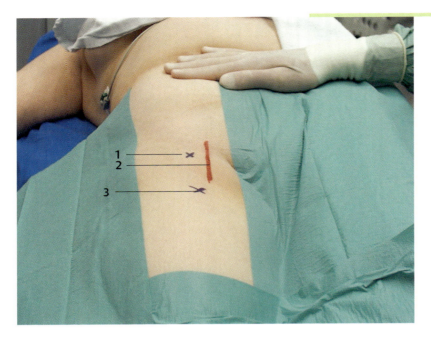

Fig. 10.**13** In practice, it has not proved necessary to exactly define the puncture site for an anterior sciatic nerve block. A sufficient orientation point is a hand's breadth below the puncture site for femoral nerve block. The hand slides medially from the lateral side over the rectus femoris. The first medial muscle gap that can be felt is the gap between rectus femoris and sartorius muscles, and this is where the injection site is located. In many patients, the medial border of the femur can be felt beneath. The puncture site is further medial than the Meier insertion point on the parallel through the greater trochanter, thus usually somewhat medial to the puncture site for the femoral nerve.

1 Puncture site for femoral nerve block
2 Femoral artery
3 Puncture site for anterior sciatic nerve block (variant without measurement)

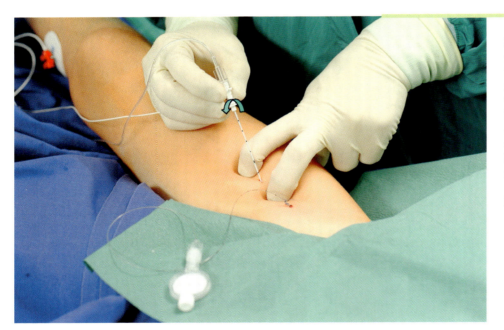

Fig. 10.**14** Two-finger grasp for identification of the muscle gap between rectus femoris and sartorius muscles (right thigh, seen from above). This grasp will also push the blood vessels medially. When the ischiocrural muscles ("hamstring muscles") are stimulated, the needle must be withdrawn and the tip of the needle advanced laterally by also moving the needle hub medially.

Right thigh, seen from above

Fig. 10.**15** Anterior sciatic nerve block (lateral view): when the needle is directed cranially, the sciatic nerve is reached a few centimeters more cranial depending on the needle angle. A more tangential approach to the nerve makes advancement of a catheter easier.

Right thigh, lateral view
   1   Cranial needle direction
   2   Purely sagittal needle direction

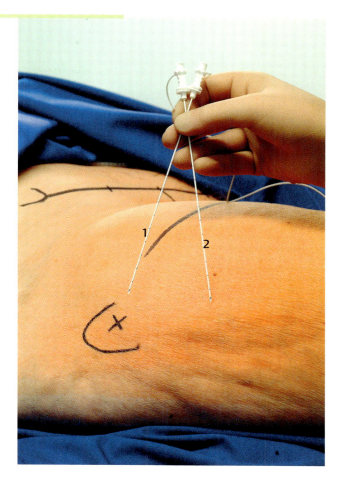

Fig. 10.**16** The correct muscle response for all proximal sciatic nerve blocks should be seen in the foot. Either the (medially located) tibial part (plantar flexors) or the (laterally located) fibular part (dorsiflexors) is stimulated. In the Labat and Mansour techniques, a response by the ischiocrural muscles (thigh flexors or "hamstring muscles") can also be regarded as a correct response.

   1   Response of tibial part of the sciatic nerve: plantar flexion, foot inversion.
   2   Response of fibular part of the sciatic nerve: dorsiflexion, foot eversion.

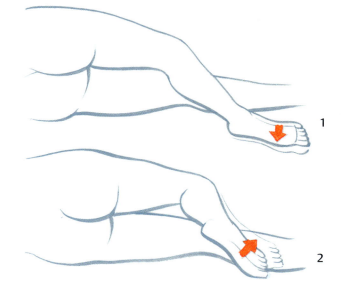

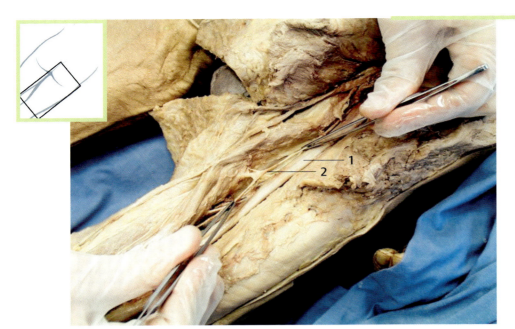

Fig. 10.**17** If the ischiocrural muscles (thigh flexors) are stimulated during anterior sciatic nerve block, the needle tip is too far medial; it must be corrected lateral to the sciatic nerve. To do this, the needle should be withdrawn a few centimeters and then the tip of the needle advanced more laterally ("below the femur") by turning the needle hub medially. The correct response in anterior sciatic nerve blocks should always be sought in the foot.(fibular or tibial division of the sciatic nerve).

Right thigh, posterior view
  1 Sciatic nerve
  2 Motor branches to the ischiocrural muscles

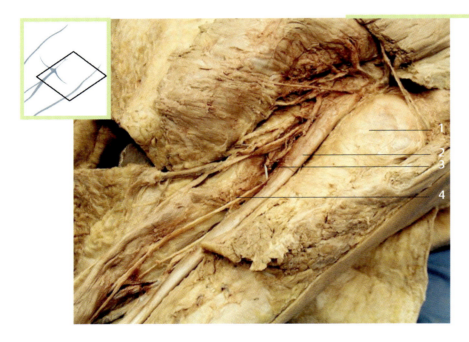

Fig. 10.**18**   (Posterior view.) Demonstration of the motor branches of the sciatic nerve, which supply the ischiocrural muscles and run medial to the sciatic nerve, here with anteriorly advanced needle. See also Fig. 10.**17**.

Right thigh, posterior view
  1 Greater trochanter
  2 Sciatic nerve
  3 Needle tip
  4 Motor branches to the ischiocrural muscles

- Amputations in the thigh (Fig. 10.**23**), lower leg (Fig. 10.**24**) and foot.
- Regional sympathetic block (e.g., perfusion disorders, wound healing disorders, CRPS I).
- Pain therapy (e.g., postoperative, achillodynia, oligoarthritis).
- Postoperative pain therapy after total knee replacement, particularly when there is incomplete extension in the knee joint (Fig. 10.**25**). The benefit of adding a continuous sciatic nerve block to the continuous femoral block to improve analgesia after a total knee replacement is controversial. In most patients, adequate analgesia after total knee arthroplasty cannot be achieved with a continuous femoral nerve block alone. The addition of continuous sciatic nerve block renders a significant improvement in analgesia. (Ben-David 2004; Pham Dang 2005).
- Traumatology (e.g., pain-free positioning for diagnostic investigation).

Contraindications
- General contraindications (see Chapter 15)
- Special contraindications: none.

Fig. 10.**19**   Advancing an indwelling sciatic catheter via the anterior approach. Using a cranial needle direction, the catheter can usually be advanced easily after the slight resistance when the catheter tip has reached the end of the needle.

1   Femoral nerve catheter in situ

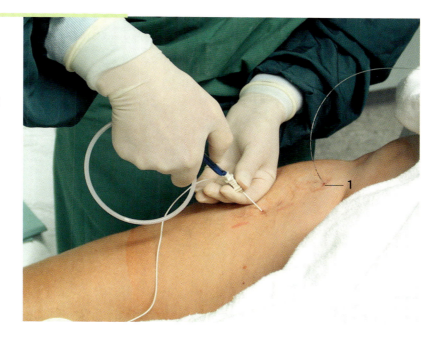

Fig. 10.**20**   An anteriorly introduced needle meeting the sciatic nerve; a catheter was advanced cranially through the needle.

Right thigh, posterolateral view
1   Tip of an anteriorly introduced needle close to the sciatic nerve
2   Part of the catheter advanced through the needle

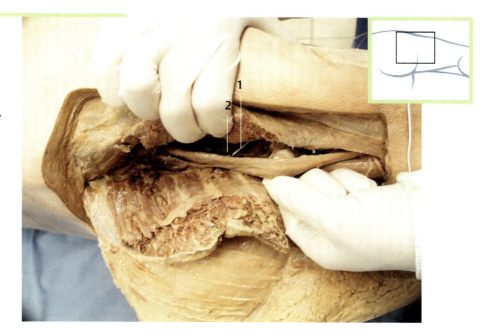

Side Effects and Complications

There are no known special complications of sciatic nerve block. There have been few reports of side effects. Major complications including late sequelae are very rare. Dysesthesia for 1-3 days, which resolved spontaneously, has been described (Fig. 10.**26**).

Practical Notes

• The leg should be in neutral position. According to Vloka et al. (2001), contrary to puncture at the level of the lesser trochanter (Beck technique), external rotation could be of benefit to a puncture performed further distally. This does not concur with our personal experience, however.

• Through digital support ("two-finger grasp") the risk of vascular puncture is markedly reduced and the skin-nerve distance is shortened considerably (Meier 1999 b).

• In contrast to Beck's classical anterior technique, the Meier puncture site is ca. 1-1.5 cm further medial and distal so that contact with the periosteum of the femur is avoided (Meier 1999 a).

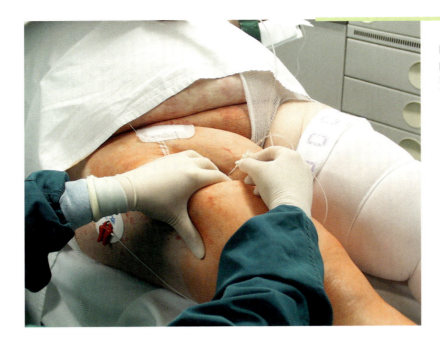

Fig. 10.**21**   Anterior sciatic nerve block is possible even in obese patients, where the sciatic nerve can be expected at a depth of 13–15 cm. Note the hand grasp!

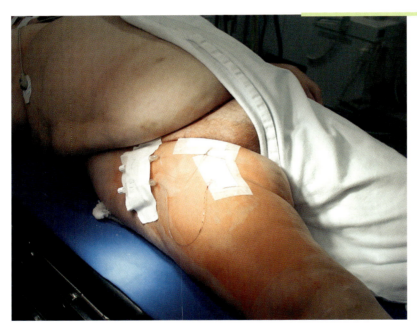

Fig. 10.**22**   Obese patients in particular benefit from the combination of a femoral nerve catheter and a sciatic nerve catheter; this is a patient blocked prior to total knee replacement.

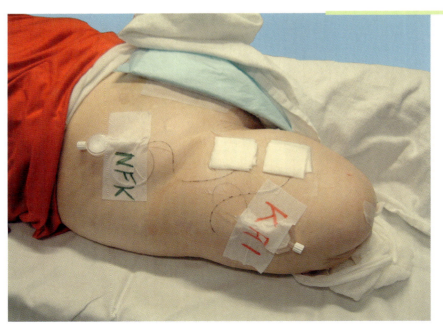

Fig. 10.**23**   Planned thigh amputation, operation on the thigh stump, phantom and/or stump pain are proper indications for continuous proximal sciatic nerve block. If the operative situation does not allow anterior sciatic block, continuous posterior access is possible. When amputation has already taken place, the patient can control the needle passage by giving phantom information about the response to the nerve stimulator ("the foot is now moving downward").

NFK: Femoral nerve catheter
KAI: Continuous anterior sciatic nerve block

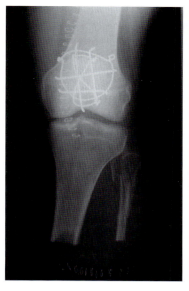 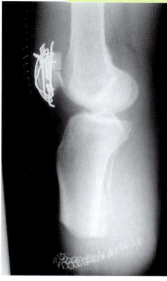 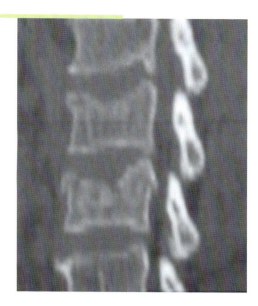

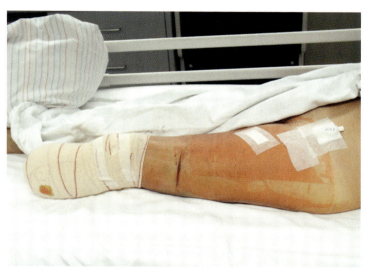 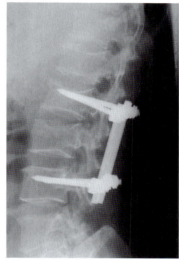 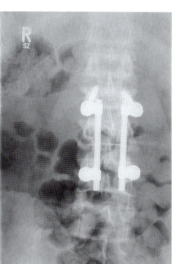

Fig. 10.24 Example of a patient with traumatic lower leg amputation, fracture of the patella and surgically treated L I fracture. Because of uncontrollable phantom pains three days after the trauma, a regional block was urgently indicated. Neuraxial block was ruled out because of the spinal fracture, and it was possible to place an anterior sciatic catheter with the patient's assistance using the nerve stimulator. In conjunction with a femoral nerve block. this rendered the patient pain-free.

Fig. 10.25 Particularly when extension of the knee is prevented, continuous block of the sciatic nerve in conjunction with a femoral nerve block is of great importance to achieve good postoperative mobility after insertion of a total knee replacement.

"3-in-1": femoral nerve block

KAI: Continuous anterior sciatic nerve block

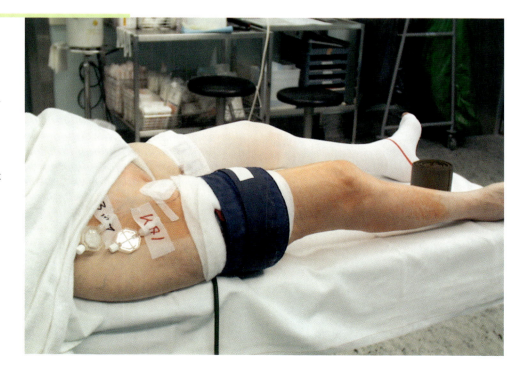

- The course of the deep blood vessels can also be established with a Doppler probe (Büttner and Meier 1999).
- Using the Meier approach, the tip of the needle reaches the nerve 3-4 cm more proximal than with the technique described by Beck. The posterior cutaneous nerve of the thigh can therefore also be anesthetized (Meier 1999b).
- If no stimulation response is produced, the needle should be withdrawn and corrected laterally (Meier 2001).
- The catheter can be advanced more smoothly if the LA has been injected beforehand.
- Advancing the catheter more than 4 cm beyond the tip of the needle has no advantages (Fig. 10.**26**).
- No change in patient position is required when it is combined with a femoral nerve block.
- The onset of the block (as indicated by corrresponding sympathetic block) can be checked through the rise in plantar temperature using a surface thermometer (Büttner and Meier 1999).

Remarks on Technique

In Beck's classical anterior technique (1963) the sciatic nerve is reached relatively distally, and anesthesia of the posterior cutaneous nerve of the thigh is often inadequate. This may cause problems in patients requiring a tourniquet at the thigh. In addition, with Beck's technique the sciatic nerve may be difficult to locate (Fig. 10.**6**). With the modified Meier technique, directing the needle at an angle of 75° to the skin causes needle contact with the sciatic nerve 3-4 cm more proximally, i.e., also with the posterior cutaneous nerve of the thigh (Meier 1999a). The diameter of the sciatic nerve, the largest nerve in the body, is impressive. In anatomical studies only part of the nerve was stained after injection of 10 ml of methylene blue through the catheter (Meier 1999a) (Fig. 10.**27**). To achieve complete anesthesia of the nerve, at least 20 ml of a LA should be injected. When positioning the patient, it should be ensured that the leg to be anesthetized is in neutral position. Bone contact is not necessary and the stimulating needle can be advanced past the femur (lesser trochanter) much more easily when the leg is in neutral position. The distance from the skin of the anterior thigh to the sciatic nerve is ca. 6-10 cm in adults when the needle is directed vertically. With the needle directed cranially, the nerve is reached after 8-12 cm, and sometimes only after 13-15 cm in muscular or obese patients (Bridenbaugh and Wedel 1998; Brown 1996; Chelly et al. 1997; Ericksen et al. 2002). Paresthesia should be avoided. During stimulation, note that contractions of gluteus maximus or tensor fasciae latae do not represent an adequate response. The vicinity of the sciatic nerve is indicated by a response in the area supplied by the nerve (hamstring muscles, triceps surae, tibialis anterior, fibular group), (Kaiser et al. 1990; Wagner 1994; Wagner and Mißler 1987). The motor response should be optimized so that plantar flexion (tibial nerve) or dorsiflexion (common fibular nerve) in the foot is achieved with a current of 0.3 mA and a pulse duration of 0.1 ms. In a study by Neuburger et al. (2001), the stimulated muscle group (whether innervated by the tibial nerve or fibular nerve) had no effect on the block result. With correct stimulation (below 0.5 mA), a success rate over 95% can be achieved (Chelly et al. 1999; Niesel 1994). Performing the block with an immobile needle technique is beneficial as it enables aspiration to exclude vascular puncture and accidental intravascular injection of a LA (Büttner and Meier 1999; Winnie 1975).

For anesthesia, 30 ml of a medium-acting or long-acting LA of adequate concentration should be injected (Bridenbaugh and Wedel 1998; Chelly and Delauny 1999; Wagner and Taeger 1988) (Fig. 10.**28**). In combination with a lumbar plexus block (psoas compartment or "3-in-1 block"), a further 30-40 ml of LA is required. When complete anesthesia of the leg is required, the combination of an anterior sciatic nerve block with femoral nerve block is a good alternative, as both blocks can be performed in the same sterile field without a change in position (Figs. 10.**9**, 10.**14**). The femoral nerve block should be performed before the sciatic nerve block. Placement of a catheter for continuous anesthesia or analgesia is feasible because the sciatic nerve is surrounded by a fascial sheath from its emergence from the infrapiriform foramen until it enters the popliteal fossa (Benninghoff and Goerttler 1975; Clara 1959; Meier 1999a). Advancing the catheter more than 4-5 cm can lead to deviation of the catheter into the true pelvis (pelvis minor) and should be avoided (Fig. 10.**26**). In a study by Meier (1999b) of 85 patients, the catheter was kept in situ for an average of 4 days (up to a maximum of 8 days). Infections at the puncture site were not observed. No side effects, complications, or neurological deficits were found. Sala-Blanch et al. (2004) described two cases using the anterior approach for sciatic nerve block in which, after localizing the nerve with nerve stimulation, CT scanning revealed that the needle (and catheter) had been placed in the epineurial sheath. Despite this, no noticeable nerve damage occurred. Pain therapy through a continuous anterior sciatic nerve block can be provided with 6 ml/h of ropivacaine 0.33% (3.3 mg/ml) or bolus injections of 20 ml of ropivacaine 0.2-0.375% (2-3.75 mg/ml) every 6-8 hours (Meier 2001). The maximum dose of ropivacaine should not exceed 37.5 mg/h. Büttner and Meier (1999) reviewed continuous pain therapy with ropivacaine in clinical practice, which was without complications in over 6000 peripheral catheters.

Summary

The anterior (ventral) technique allows block of the sciatic nerve with the patient in supine position. No change of position is required.. The anesthesia can therefore also be performed, for example, in the presence of vertebral fractures, fractures of the pelvis or long bones, and also in the case of obesity, chronic polyarthritis, and other positioning problems. If a femoral nerve block is performed before the anterior sciatic nerve block and periosteal contact is avoided, the technique can be performed with little pain. The modified technique according to Meier enables anesthesia that includes the posterior cutaneous nerve of the thigh. A catheter can be placed readily without the potential risks seen with transgluteal or parasacral sciatic nerve block (q.v.). As a continuous technique, the procedure can be used for postoperative pain therapy after major surgery on the knee, lower leg, and foot, and for the treatment of pain syndromes distal to the knee and for regional sympathetic block.

Fig. 10.**26** Advancing an anterior sciatic nerve catheter too far can cause it to enter the lesser pelvis through the infrapiriform foramen.

Right gluteal region, posterior view
1 Needle introduced from anterior
2 Sciatic nerve
3 Catheter
4 Infrapiriform foramen with sciatic nerve

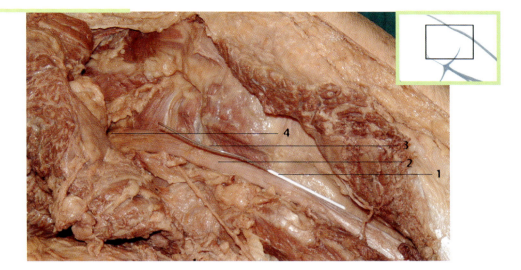

Fig. 10.**27** Posterior view. Our studies with dye (methylene blue) in nonpreserved cadavers have shown that a minimum volume of 20 ml is required to block the entire sciatic nerve.

Right gluteal region, posterior view
1 Sciatic nerve: fibular division, surrounded by dye
2 Sciatic nerve: tibial division, not surrounded by dye

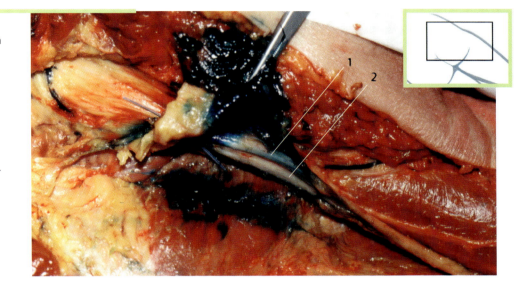

Fig. 10.**28** Distribution of the local anesthetic after anterior sciatic nerve block (contrast was added to the local anesthetic).

→ Catheter

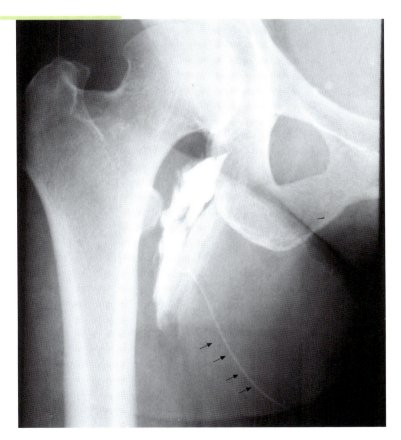

10.3   Dorso-Dorsal (Proximal) Sciatic Nerve Block (According to Raj) (in Supine Position)

The sciatic nerve leaves the pelvis through the greater sciatic foramen and passes to the thigh between the greater trochanter and the ischial tuberosity. When the limb is flexed at the hip, the sciatic nerve is stretched and passes relatively superficially under the gluteus maximus muscle through the groove between the greater trochanter and ischial tuberosity (Figs. 10.**29**, 10.**30**).

Landmarks

The anatomical landmarks of the greater trochanter major and ischial tuberosity are joined by a line. The middle of this line is the puncture site.

Position

The patient lies supine. The limb to be blocked is flexed maximally at the hip (90-120°) and 90° at the knee.

Procedure

A 20G, 10-15 cm needle is connected to a nerve stimulator and advanced proximally vertical to the skin. The vicinity of the sciatic nerve is reached after 5-10 cm. When there is a motor response in the foot (plantar flexion or dorsiflexion) at 0.3 mA/0.1 ms, 30 ml of a medium-acting or long-acting LA is injected (Fig. 10.**31**).
Continuous technique: the catheter is advanced 4-5 cm beyond the needle tip following the injection (Fig. 10.**32**).

Indications and Contraindications

(see under anterior technique)

Side Effects and Complications

There are no known special side effects or complications.

Practical Notes

- Raj et. al. (1975) described the technique as a single-stage procedure, but catheter placement and thus a continuous technique are possible (see below).
- The leg to be blocked can be placed in a stirrup (lithotomy position) (Fig. 10.**31**), (Meier and Büttner 2001).
- The technique is a good alternative to the anterior technique. If the anterior technique proves problematic, it can be performed with the patient in supine position.

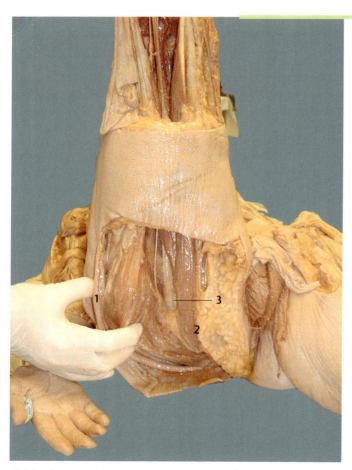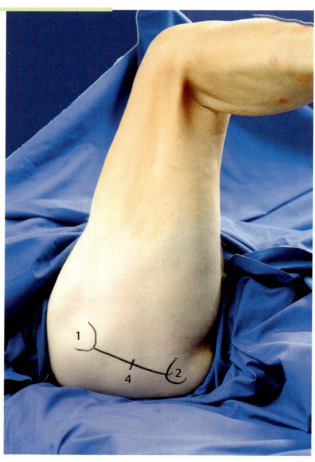

Fig. 10.**29**   (Dorsal) Subgluteal sciatic nerve blockade, Raj technique. The nerve runs in the middle between the greater trochanter and ischial tuberosity. The patient lies supine, the leg is flexed at a right angle at the hip and knee.

1	Greater trochanter	3	Sciatic nerve
2	Ischial tuberosity	4	Puncture site

Remarks on the Technique

The Raj technique, also called the dorso-dorsal technique, was inaugurated in 1975 (Raj et al. 1975). It is easy to perform and is an alternative to the anterior technique (Meier and Heinrich 1995), also with the patient in supine position. Its advantage is the shorter distance to the sciatic nerve. The disadvantage is the necessity of changing the position of the leg to be blocked as the leg has to be held and the change in position can cause pain, e.g., in the case of fractures. Provided the patient is not troubled by pain, the leg to be anesthetized can be elevated in a stirrup. Studies of larger case numbers to provide a scientific evaluation of the technique are lacking. 30 ml of lidocaine 1 % (10 mg/ml) or

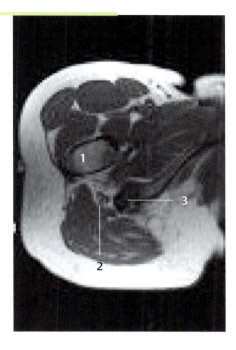 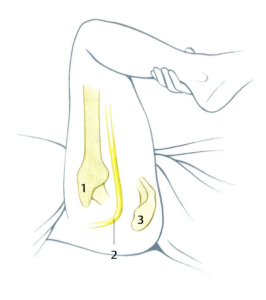

Fig. 10.**30** Subgluteal sciatic nerve blockade, Raj technique. The line connecting the greater trochanter and ischial tuberosity is halved. The midpoint marks the puncture site. The needle is advanced in a cranial direction vertical to the skin surface. After ca. 5 cm (max. 10 cm), the correct needle position is shown by a response in the foot.

1 Greater trochanter
2 Sciatic nerve
3 Ischial tuberosity

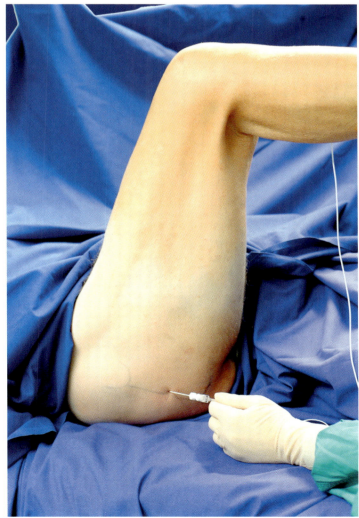

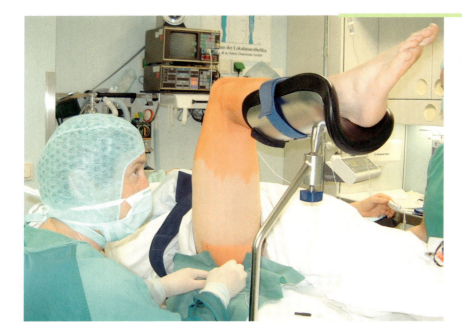

Fig. 10.**31**   Subgluteal sciatic nerve blockade, Raj technique. When the needle is advanced under stimulation, the response target (foot) should be kept in view.

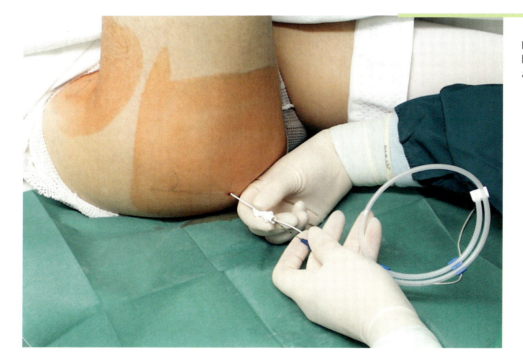

Fig. 10.**32**   Subgluteal sciatic nerve blockade, Raj technique. A catheter can be advanced without difficulty.

mepivacaine 1% (10 mg/ml) or a combination of a medium-acting with a long-acting LA (e.g., 20 ml of mepivacaine 1% [10 mg/ml] with 10 ml ropivacaine 0.75% [7.5 mg/ml]) are suitable for anesthesia. There must be 15–30 minutes allowed for the onset of action, that is, the time from the injection until the operation can commence (Meier and Heinrich 1995). There has so far been no publication regarding the continuous tech-

nique. However, a catheter can be placed readily and without problems because of the direction of the needle (Meier and Büttner 2001). If a continuous technique is planned, the catheter should be advanced 4–5 cm proximally through the insulated needle after injection of the LA. (Comment: the catheter is also very well tolerated subsequently by the patient when sitting [Fig. 10.**33**]).

Summary

Dorso-dorsal sciatic nerve block is an easily performed technique with few complications. Its advantages are the supine patient and the relatively short distance to the sciatic nerve. The method is suitable as an alternative to anterior block, provided the leg to be anesthetized can be adequately positioned without pain.

Fig. 10.**33**   Sciatic nerve catheter in situ, placed according to Raj's subgluteal technique.

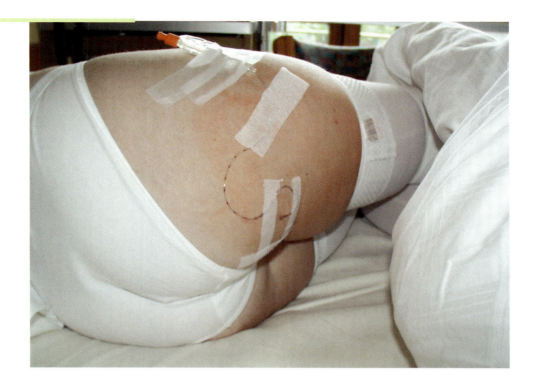

10.4   Proximal Lateral Sciatic Nerve Block (with Patient in Supine Position)

Technique

Landmarks
Greater trochanter, ischial tuberosity.

Position
The patient lies supine with the leg to be anesthetized in neutral position. A small pad is placed under the popliteal fossa so that the greater trochanter is moved slightly forward.

Procedure
The puncture site for the lateral approach to proximal sciatic nerve block is 3-5 cm distal to the most prominent lateral part of the greater trochanter. The skin is entered at the level of the posterior border of the femur and the 20G, 12-15 cm insulated needle is directed dorsally (15-30°) and cranially; the response must be in the foot, as in anterior sciatic nerve block (Figs. 10.**34**-10.**36**). Muscular contractions on the back of the thigh are frequent (Gligorijevic 2000). The sciatic nerve is reached after 8-12 cm (Fig. 10.**37**) and the correct position of the needle tip in the vicinity of the nerve is confirmed by a motor response in the foot region (dorsiflexion or plantar flexion) at 0.3 mA/0.1 ms. After careful aspiration, 20-30 ml of a medium-acting or long-acting LA is injected.

Indications, Contraindications, Complications, Side effects

(see under anterior sciatic nerve block)

Practical Notes

- A hand can be placed beneath the buttocks to palpate the ischial tuberosity in order to improve the anatomical orientation.
- If no motor response is produced, the needle should be withdrawn and corrected in the anterior direction when it is advanced again.
- The fibular nerve is stimulated first with the described needle direction. The motor response with this technique is therefore usually dorsiflexion of the foot initially.

Remarks on the Technique

The first description of a lateral, proximal approach by Ichiyanagi (1959) did not become widely used; the technique was taken up again in 1985 by Guardini et al. in a modified form. Guardini reported a success rate of 95%. The method can be performed without changing the patient's position. The procedure is unsuitable for patients with fractures of the neck of the femur, hematoma in this region, or previous total hip replacement on the side to be anesthetized (anatomical orientation may be impaired). At the level at which the sciatic nerve is reached, the nerve runs together with the inferior gluteal artery behind the quadratus femoris. The artery is medial to the sciatic nerve. The posterior cutaneous nerve of the thigh, which usually separates from the sciatic nerve further cranially, is sometimes not blocked sufficiently and pain can then occur on the back of the thigh during operation with a thigh tourniquet.

Summary
Lateral proximal sciatic nerve block in combination with lumbar plexus anesthesia is suitable for operations on the knee and lower leg. Anatomical orientation can present problems when the thigh is of large circumference.

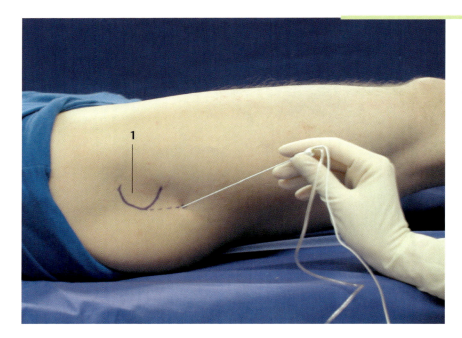

Fig. 10.**34**   The puncture site for the proximal lateral approach to proximal sciatic nerve block is 3–5 cm distal to the most prominent lateral part of the greater trochanter. The needle enters at the level of the posterior border of the femur and is directed dorsally (15–30°) and cranially; as in anterior sciatic nerve block, the stimulation response must be in the foot.

1   Greater trochanter

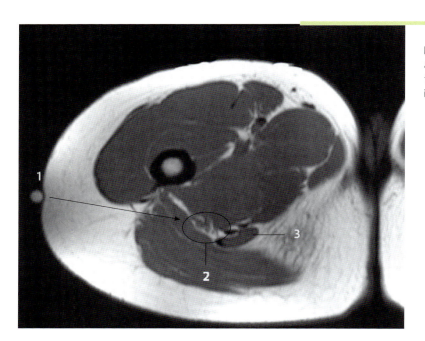

Fig. 10.**35**   Transverse MR image for lateral approach to the proximal sciatic nerve: note the somewhat dorsal needle direction, which is necessary for contacting the sciatic nerve.

1   Nitrocapsule marking the puncture site
2   Sciatic nerve
3   Ischial tuberosity

1   Greater trochanter
2   Puncture site

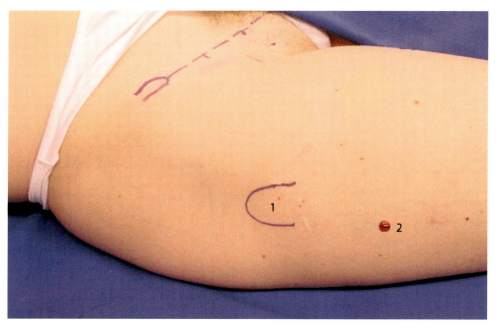

Fig. 10.**36**   Sciatic nerve, lateral view.

1   Sciatic nerve
2   Ischial tuberosity
3   Greater trochanter

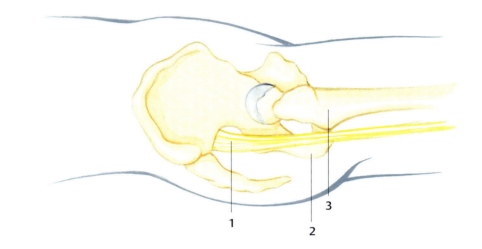

Fig. 10.**37**   Lateral approach to the proximal
sciatic nerve (dissection in left lateral position, posterior view). The slightly dorsal
needle direction makes it possible to
approach the sciatic nerve tangentially, so
that the tibial division may be stimulated
instead of the lateral fibular division.

1   Greater trochanter
2   Sciatic nerve
3   Ischial tuberosity

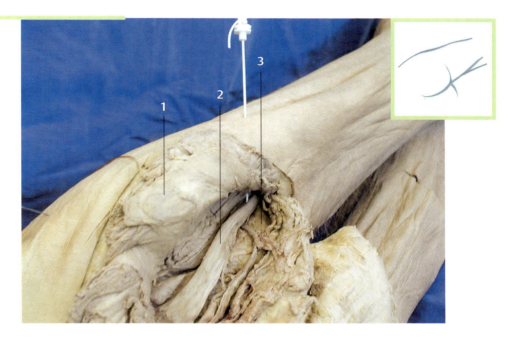

10.5   Proximal Sciatic Nerve Block (with Patient Lying on Side)

The gluteal region is limited by a triangle,
the apex of which is formed by the posterior
superior iliac spine, the medial corner by the
ischial tuberosity, and the lateral corner by
the greater trochanter (Fig. 10.**38**). The two
sides and the base of the triangle form *three
orientation lines*: the spine-tuberosity line,
the spine-trochanter line, and tuberosity-trochanter line. These lines are the basis of anatomical orientation in all proximal dorsal
techniques of sciatic nerve block.

Techniques of Dorsal Transgluteal Sciatic Nerve Block

**Dorsal Transgluteal Sciatic Nerve Block
(according to Labat, Classical Technique)**

The posterior Labat technique is called the
standard technique and is performed with
the patient lying on his or her side. The procedure can be combined particularly well
with a psoas compartment block as the
patient's position does not have to be
changed further.

Landmarks
Posterior superior iliac spine, greater trochanter.

Position
The patient lies on his or her side with the
side to be blocked uppermost. The leg
underneath can be extended, and the leg to
be blocked is flexed ca. 30-40° at the hip and
ca. 70° at the knee. The posterior superior
iliac spine and greater trochanter are sought
as anatomical landmarks, marked and joined
by a line.

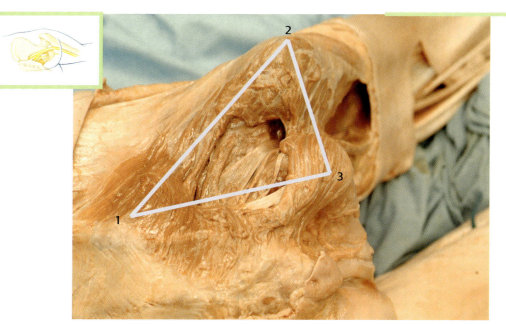

Fig. 10.**38**   Right leg, posterior view: the triangle between the superior posterior iliac spine, greater trochanter and ischial tuberosity is used for orientation in all proximal blocks of the sciatic nerve that are performed from behind. The sciatic nerve leaves the pelvis minor through the infrapiriform foramen; it crosses the spine–tuberosity line ca. 6 cm caudal to the spine (puncture site according to Mansour technique), and it leaves the triangle in the middle of the tuberosity–trochanter line (puncture site according to Raj's dorsal subgluteal technique). Labat's classical technique uses the spine–trochanter line for orientation. For a continuous dorsal technique with the patient in lateral position, the puncture site is selected according to either Mansour or Labat, and the needle is directed toward the middle of the tuberosity–trochanter line.

Right pelvis, posterior view
   1   Posterior superior iliac spine
   2   Greater trochanter
   3   Ischial tuberosity

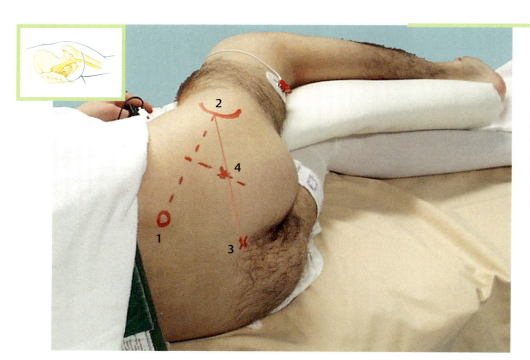

Fig. 10.**39**   Posterior sciatic nerve block, Labat technique. The leg to be blocked is positioned so that the shaft of the femur lies in the continuation of the tuberosity–trochanter line. The injection site is 4–5 cm caudal on the perpendicular through the midpoint of the line between the posterior superior iliac spine and the greater trochanter. A line connecting the sacral hiatus and the greater trochanter intersects this perpendicular at the injection site.

   1   Posterior superior iliac spine
   2   Greater trochanter
   3   Sacral hiatus
   4   Injection site

The hip flexion of the leg to be blocked is adjusted so that the shaft of the femur forms a straight line with the connecting line that has been drawn.

Procedure
The midpoint of the line connecting the spine and the trochanter is marked; a line is then drawn caudally from the midpoint at a right angle and the puncture site is marked after 4 (max. 5) cm (Fig. 10.**39**). As an additional aid to orientation, a line can be drawn joining the greater trochanter and the sacral

hiatus (Winnie 1975). This line will intersect the previously drawn perpendicular line at the established puncture site (Fig. 10.**39**). A 20G, 10-15 cm insulated needle is advanced vertically to the skin surface (Figs. 10.**40**, 10.**41**). An immobile needle technique enables aspiration (Winnie 1969) (Fig. 10.**42**). On bone contact, the skin-bone distance is recorded and the needle is then withdrawn sufficiently to allow correction of its position when it is advanced again. The needle should not be advanced further than the measured skin-bone distance so as to

exclude puncture of the pelvis minor. The needle direction is corrected in a fan pattern along the Labat line until a distal motor response is visible in the sciatic nerve area (tibial nerve, fibular nerve). The nerve is reached after 7.5-15 cm (Chelly and Delauny 1999). Then 30-40 ml of a medium-acting or long-acting LA of adequate concentration is injected.
A continuous technique can also be performed from the same puncture site with a modification of the needle direction. In this case, the direction of the needle is not per-

Fig. 10.**40** Posterior sciatic nerve block, Labat technique. The puncture is made perpendicular to the skin surface. The nerve is reached after 7.5–12 cm. The stimulation response should be in the foot, but with this approach a response in the ischiocrural muscles (thigh flexors or "hamstring muscles") can also be regarded as adequate. A response in the gluteal muscles, which is often produced when the needle is advanced, is not adequate; the needle must be advanced further.

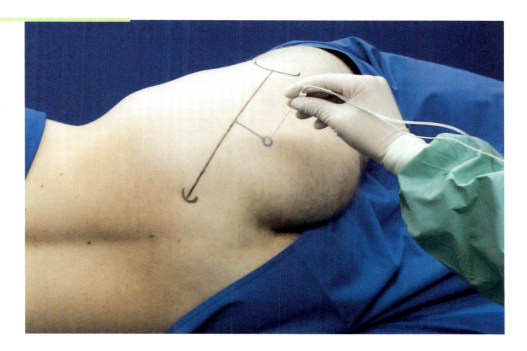

Fig. 10.**41** Posterior sciatic nerve block, Labat technique. The puncture is made perpendicular to the skin surface. The nerve is reached after 7.5–12 cm.

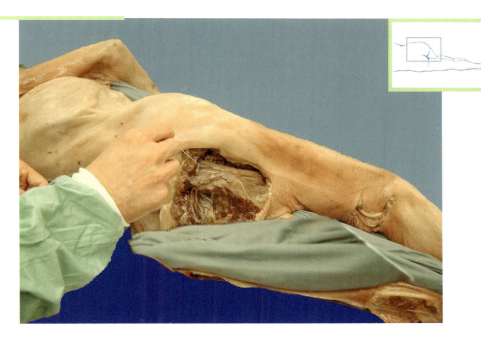

Fig. 10.**42** Posterior sciatic nerve block, Labat technique. The puncture is made perpendicular to the skin surface. The nerve is reached after 7.5–12 cm. Aspiration must be performed at intervals during injection of the local anesthetic to exclude intravascular injection.

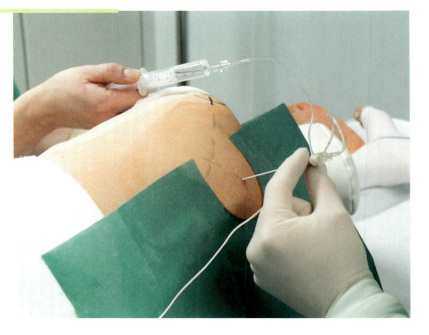

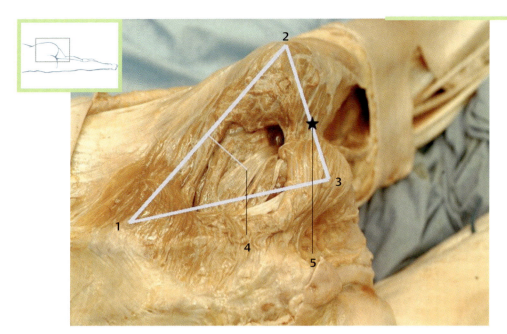

Fig. 10.**43**   For continuous posterior sciatic nerve block using the Labat technique, the tip of the needle should be directed to follow the course of the sciatic nerve, i.e., toward the middle of the line between the ischial tuberosity and greater trochanter. In this way, a tangential approach to the nerve is achieved, which enables the catheter to be advanced without problems.

Right pelvis, posterior view
1 Posterior superior iliac spine
2 Greater trochanter
3 Ischial tuberosity
4 Classical puncture site, Labat method
5 Target for continuous posterior sciatic nerve block

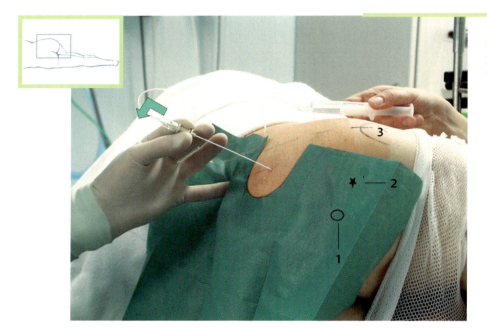

Fig. 10.**44**   Needle direction for continuous posterior sciatic nerve block via catheter, see also Fig. 10.**43**.

1 Ischial tuberosity
2 Needle target
3 Greater trochanter

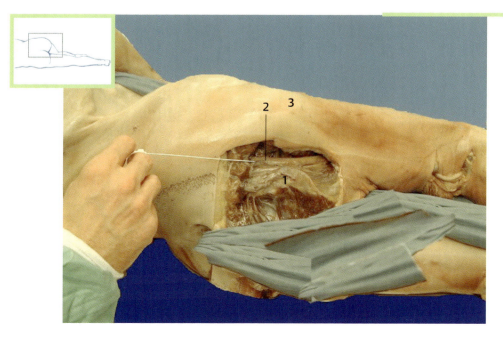

Fig. 10.**45**   As Fig. 10.**44**, here in an anatomical dissection.

1 Ischial tuberosity
2 Sciatic nerve
3 Greater trochanter

Fig. 10.**46** Continuous posterior sciatic nerve block. The tip of the needle should be directed according to the course of the sciatic nerve toward the middle third between the ischial tuberosity and the greater trochanter.

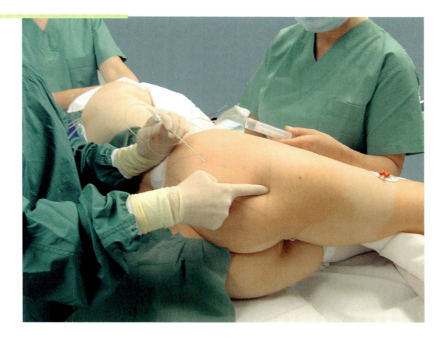

Fig. 10.**47** Easy advancement of a catheter in continuous posterior sciatic nerve block.

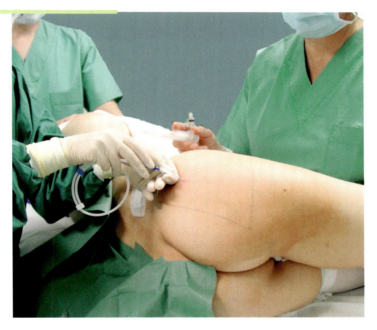

pendicular to the skin but is directed toward the middle third between the ischial tuberosity and the greater trochanter where the sciatic nerve passes from the gluteal region to the back of the thigh (Figs. 10.**43**-10.**47**). The nerve is reached after ca. 8-12 cm at an angle of ca. 45° to the skin.

Dorsal (Transgluteal) Continuous Sciatic Nerve Block (according to Meier)

Landmarks
Posterior superior iliac spine, greater trochanter, ischial tuberosity.
The landmarks are established by the spine-tuberosity line and the tuberosity-trochanter line (Polino et al. 2000; Rongstad et al.

1996). The spine-tuberosity line is the line from the posterior superior iliac spine to the ischial tuberosity. The infrapiriform foramen is in the middle of this line. The midpoint of the spine-tuberosity line marks the puncture site. The tuberosity-trochanter line is the line from the ischial tuberosity to the greater trochanter and this is divided in three. The sciatic nerve runs between the inner and middle thirds (Figs. 10.**48**-10.**50**).

Position
The patient lies on his or her side with the side to be blocked uppermost. The leg underneath is extended, and the leg to be blocked is flexed ca. 30-40° at the hip and ca. 70° at the knee.

Procedure
A 20G, 10-15 cm insulated needle is advanced at an angle of about 45° to the skin in the direction of the junction of the inner and middle thirds of the tuberosity-trochanter line. It reaches the sciatic nerve after 10-12 cm. If the direction of the needle has to be corrected, this should be done medially. A response in the foot at 0.3 mA/0.1 ms indicates that the tip of the needle is in the correct position; 20-30 ml of a medium-acting or long-acting LA is injected. The tangential approach of the needle to the sciatic nerve enables placement of a catheter (Fig. 10.**51**). The catheter is advanced 3-5 cm caudally beyond the needle tip.

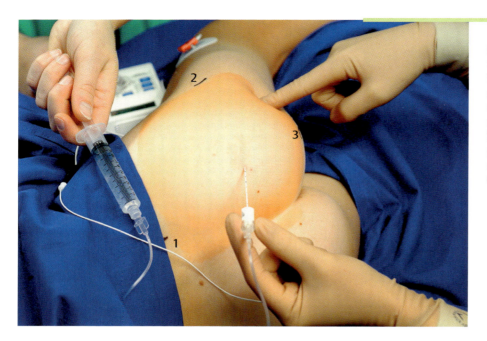

Fig. 10.**48**   Posterior continuous technique to block the sciatic nerve (as modified by Meier). The puncture site is the middle of the spine–tuberosity line; the needle should be directed to follow the course of the sciatic nerve, i.e., toward the middle of the line between the ischial tuberosity and the greater trochanter. In this way, a tangential approach to the nerve is achieved, which enables the catheter to be advanced easily.

1   Posterior superior iliac spine
2   Greater trochanter
3   Ischial tuberosity

Indications and Contraindications for Proximal Dorsal Sciatic Nerve Blocks

Indications
(in combination with psoas compartment block)

- Operations on the knee, lower leg or foot (including tourniquet at the thigh during, e.g., total knee replacement, tibial head osteotomy, arthrodesis, lateral ligament suture, forefoot operations)
- Repositioning of fractures of the lower leg and foot
- Amputation in the thigh, lower leg, and foot
- Regional sympathetic block (perfusion disorders, wound healing disorders, CRPS 1)
- Pain therapy (e.g., postoperative, achillodynia, oligoarthritis)
- Traumatology (e.g., pain-free positioning for diagnostic investigations)

Contraindications
- General contraindications (see Chapter 15)
- Coagulation disorders

Complications and Side Effects

Very little has been reported regarding complications or side effects. Major complications and late sequelae are regarded as very rare.

Practical Notes

- Combination with a psoas compartment block enables sufficient anesthesia of the entire leg.
- As the posterior cutaneous nerve of the thigh is usually also anesthetized, the technique ensures that a thigh tourniquet will be well tolerated.
- The method should be performed with a nerve stimulator. In contrast to sciatic nerve blocks performed with the patient supine, a response in the ischiocrural muscles is here also regarded as adequate.
- The gluteus maximus muscle is often stimulated directly initially, but the adequate motor response is in the lower leg and foot region.
- Puncture of large vessels is possible and can be avoided by the use of a Doppler probe.
- To establish the onset of the block, the rise in plantar temperature can be measured with a surface thermometer.

Remarks on the Technique

The dorsal transgluteal technique of sciatic nerve block was first described in 1924 by Labat. The most important addition to the method was a further guide line added by Winnie (1975). This line from the greater trochanter major to the sacral hiatus facili-

tates establishment of the puncture site. The transgluteal technique of sciatic nerve block ensures good to very good quality of anesthesia. Practically the whole sacral plexus can be blocked. However, complete sacral plexus anesthesia also means that the inferior gluteal nerve and pudendal nerve are anesthetized (Mansour and Benetts 1996; Wagner 1994). This leads to hypoesthesia in the perineal region and possibly also to urinary retention. Impairment of bladder function should therefore be watched for. With the Labat technique, misplacement of the needle into the pelvis minor is a possibility. Blood vessels can also be accidentally punctured, particularly the inferior gluteal artery (Meier 2001; Wagner 1994) (Fig. 10.**52**). The inferior gluteal artery, the largest artery from the internal iliac artery, runs 1-2 cm medial to the line from the puncture site using the proximal technique in the lateral position (Fig. 10.**53**). The length of the perpendicular line showing the puncture site should therefore not exceed 4 cm. If it is necessary to perform a transgluteal sciatic nerve block in a patient with a coagulation disorder, a Doppler probe can be used to avoid accidental vascular puncture (Fig. 10.**54**). The block should always be performed with peripheral nerve stimulation. The motor response must be in the lower leg and foot. Whether the stimulated muscle group (tibial nerve or common fibular nerve) has an influence on the result of the block is controversial. In contrast to sciatic nerve

Fig. 10.**49**   As Fig. 10.**48**, posteroinferior view.

1   Greater trochanter
2   Ischial tuberosity

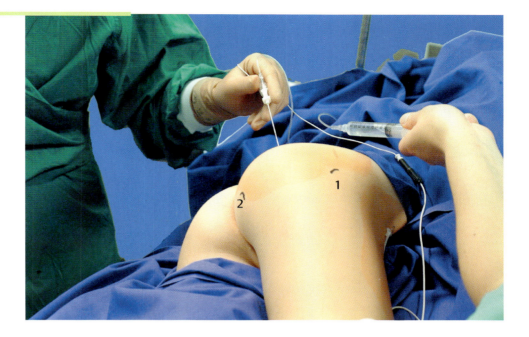

Fig. 10.**50**   As Fig. 10.**49**, here in an anatomical dissection.

Right thigh, posteroinferior view
1   Greater trochanter
2   Ischial tuberosity
3   Sciatic nerve

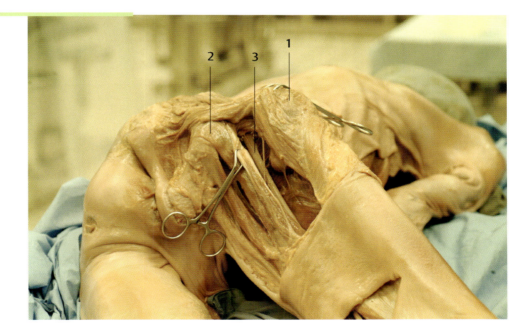

Fig. 10.**51**   Catheter in situ in posterior sciatic nerve block.

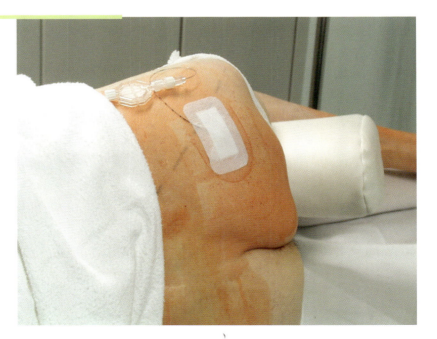

blocks performed in supine position, a response of the ischiocrural muscles is here regarded as adequate.

Sciatic nerve block as a selective anesthesia for surgery is indicated in just a few situations (e.g., foot surgery). When using a thigh tourniquet, it must be combined with a lumbar plexus block. In this case, a combination of the psoas compartment block and the dorsal technique is most rational, as the patient's position does not have to be changed. If an operation is performed with a calf tourniquet, a saphenous nerve block provides adequate supplementary anesthesia.

When two block techniques are combined (lumbar plexus and sacral plexus) 60 ml of a local anesthetic of adequate concentration is usually necessary (Fig. 10.**55**).

A disadvantage of the Labat technique is the direction of the stimulation needle vertical to the course of the nerve, which means that a catheter often cannot be advanced or can be advanced only with difficulty. For smoother catheter placement, the needle direction has to be changed. Meier et al. routinely perform continuous dorsal sciatic blocks using simple anatomical landmarks for orientation: the lines through the spine-tuberosity line and the tuberosity-trochanter line. This is a technique that is easy to follow in clinical practice and has been performed in large numbers (Meier 1999b). Similar results can also be obtained if the needle is

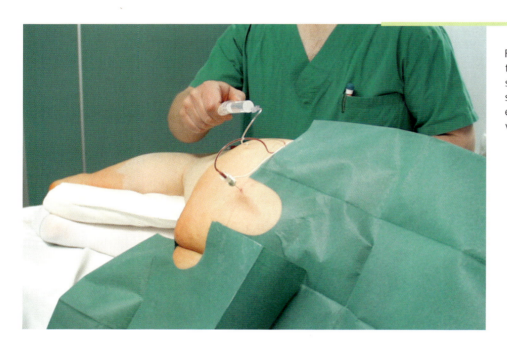

Fig. 10.**52** With the Labat technique, puncture too far medially may end intravascularly, so a maximum distance of 5 cm from the spine-trochanter line should not be exceeded. Here: bloody aspiration after vascular puncture.

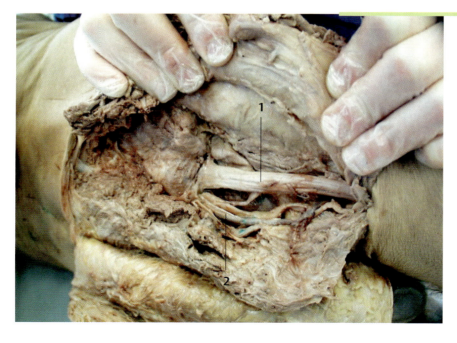

Fig. 10.**53** Using the Labat technique, needle puncture too far medially should be avoided as blood vessels pass here.

Right gluteal region, posterior view
  1 Sciatic nerve
  2 Inferior gluteal artery

directed from the classical puncture site in the Labat technique to the middle third between the ischial tuberosity and the trochanter major. Catheter placement is useful only when pain lasting longer than 24 hours can be anticipated (pain therapy, sympathetic block). This applies, for example, to total knee replacement. Particularly if there has been a flexion contracture previously, this operation can be associated with very severe pain postoperatively in the posterior

region of the knee. As the sciatic nerve has a large proportion of sympathetic fibers, it is rational to use the continuous sciatic nerve block for therapeutic and diagnostic sympathetic block (Smith and Siggins 1988). The onset of the block can be checked by measuring the increase in plantar temperature with surface thermometer. The rise in temperature occurs after a few minutes and in the absence of previous vascular disease can nearly reach core body temperature when the sympathetic block is complete.

Summary

Transgluteal sciatic nerve block is a highly effective standard anesthesia. In combination, e.g., with psoas compartment block (see Chapter 8) the method provides complete anesthesia of the leg. A disadvantage is the need for a change in patient position. Complications are very rare.

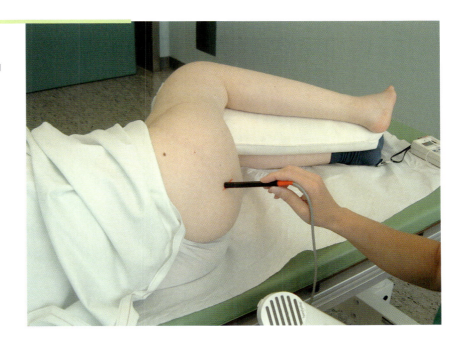

Fig. 10.**54** The blood vessels (inferior gluteal artery and vein) can be located using Doppler; they run about 1–2 cm medial to the puncture site in the Labat technique.

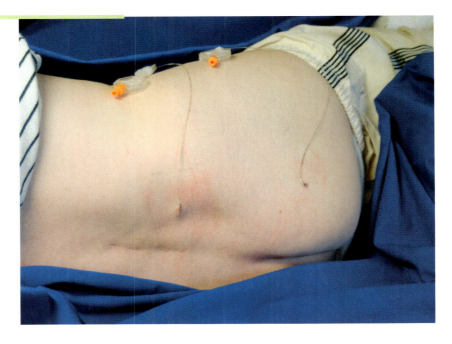

Fig. 10.**55** Posterior sciatic nerve catheter in situ in conjunction with a psoas compartment catheter.

10.6   Parasacral Sciatic Nerve Block (Mansour Technique)

Technique

Landmarks
Posterior superior iliac spine, ischial tuberosity.

Position
The patient lies on his or her side with the leg to be anesthetized uppermost. The leg underneath can be extended, and the leg to be blocked is flexed ca. 30-40° at the hip and ca. 70° at the knee (Fig. 10.**56**).

Procedure
The posterior superior iliac spine and the ischial tuberosity are identified and joined by a line. Six centimeters caudal to posterior superior iliac spine on this line is the puncture site (Figs. 10.**57**-10.**59**).
A 21G, 10 cm insulated needle is advanced in a sagittal direction (perpendicular to the skin) until the motor response in the foot at a minimal current of 0.3 mA and a pulse duration of 0.1 ms at a depth of 6-8 cm (max. 10 cm) is seen (Fig. 10.**56**). Then 30 ml of a medium-acting or long-acting LA is injected. A continuous technique can also be performed from the puncture site in the Mansour technique by changing the needle direction toward the middle third of the line between the greater trochanter and the ischial tuberosity. The catheter is advanced 4-5 cm caudally through the needle (Fig. 10.**58**) (e.g., 22G, 110 mm insulated needles [Contiplex D; B. Braun]; 19.5G, 120 mm insulated needle with pencil-point tip [Plexolong catheter set. Pajunk, Geisingen, Germany]).

Indications and Contraindications

(see transgluteal technique)

Side Effects and Complications

(see transgluteal technique)

Practical Notes

- As the greater trochanter is not required for anatomical orientation, the technique is suitable for patients with a total hip replacement on the side to be anesthetized.
- If there is no response at a needle depth of up to 10 cm, the needle direction should be corrected 5-10° caudally (Meier 2001).
- If there is bony contact during the procedure, the needle should be withdrawn and advanced again 1-2 cm further caudally on the spine-tuberosity line (Morris and Lang 1999; Morris et al. 1997). In this case, care has to be taken not to advance past a depth of 2.5 cm beyond the bony surface.
- The onset of all sciatic nerve block techniques can be tested by checking the rise in plantar temperature using a surface thermometer (Büttner and Meier 1999).

Remarks on the Technique

The parasacral technique of sciatic nerve block was described by Mansour in 1993. In parasacral anesthesia of the sciatic nerve, the nerve is reached so far proximally that block of the entire sacral plexus occurs. Morris and Lang assume that the obturator nerve is also anesthetized due to its anatomical vicinity. In their view the parasacral block of the sciatic nerve together with a so-called "3-in-1 block" will cause complete anesthesia of the leg (Morris and Lang 1997). However, as the technique is performed in the lateral position, combination of parasacral sciatic nerve block with psoas compartment block is more rational, as a change of patient position is not necessary.

Summary

Parasacral anesthesia of the sciatic nerve is easy to learn and has a high success rate (Ripart et al. 2005). The technique is performed with the patient in lateral position. Catheter placement is easily performed (Gaertner et al. 2004) (Fig. 10.**59**) and the analgesia is also effective in preventing a chronic pain syndrome. Because of the anatomical vicinity of the pelvis minor with its blood vessels and organs, radiographic imaging using contrast should be considered to check the position of a catheter. 20-30 ml of a medium-acting or long-acting LA is needed to achieve adequate anesthesia. Ropivacaine 0.33% [3.3 mg/ml] 6 ml/h or 20 ml of ropivacaine 0.2-0.375% [2-3.75 mg/ml] every 6-8 hours is suitable for a continuous block.

Fig. 10.**56** Posterior sciatic nerve block, Mansour technique. Puncture is performed in a sagittal direction and the nerve is reached after ca. 10 cm. The leg does not have to be flexed at the hip for this technique.

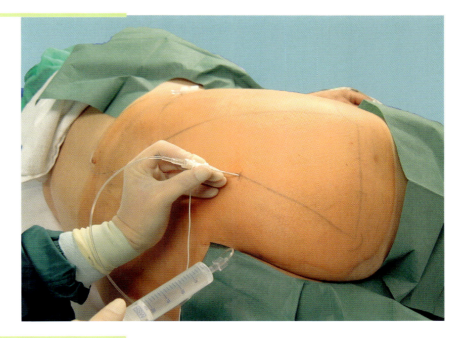

Fig. 10.**57** Posterior sciatic nerve block according to the Mansour technique is oriented by the spine–tuberosity line. The puncture site is located 6 cm distal to the posterior superior iliac spine. The nerve is reached so far proximally that block of the entire sacral plexus may result.

1 Piriformis
2 Sciatic nerve

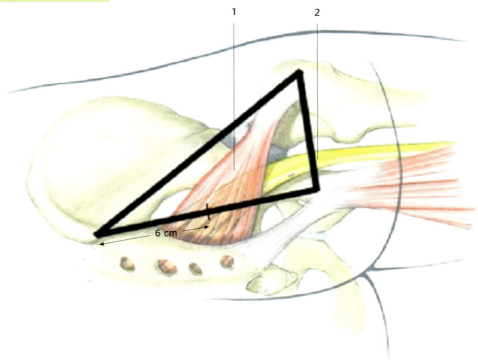

Fig. 10.**58** A continuous technique can also be performed from the Mansour puncture site by lowering the needle hub and altering the needle direction toward the middle between the greater trochanter and ischial tuberosity.

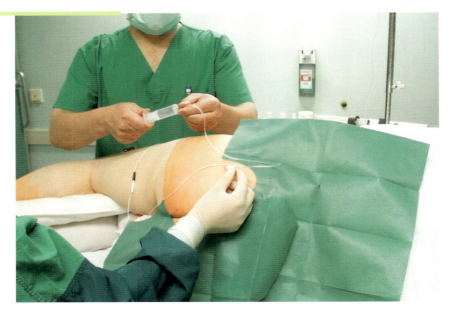

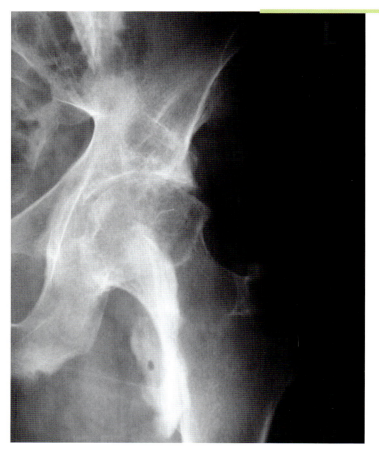

Fig. 10.**59** Injection of contrast through a posterior sciatic nerve catheter (modified Mansour technique): note the spread along the course of the nerve in the middle third between the ischial tuberosity and greater trochanter. The course behind the lesser trochanter is also worth noting (see also anterior sciatic nerve block, Beck technique).

References

Beck GP. Anterior approach to sciatic nerve block. Anesthesiology. 1963;24:222-4.

Ben-David B, Schmalenberger K, Chelly JE. Analgesia after total knee arthroplasty. Is continuous sciatic blockade needed in addition to continuous femoral blockade? Anesth Analg. 2004;98:747-9

Benninghoff A, Goerttler K. Lehrbuch der Anatomie des Menschen. 11 th ed. Munich: Urban & Schwarzenberg; 1975.

Bridenbaugh PhO, Wedel DJ. The lower extremity. In: Cousins MJ, Bridenbaugh PhO, eds.. Neural blockade in clinical anesthesia and management of pain. 3rd ed. Philadelphia: Lippincott-Raven; 1998:373-409.

Brown DL. Regional anesthesia and analgesia. Philadelphia: Saunders; 1996:279-88.

Büttner J, Meier G. Kontinuierliche periphere Techniken zur Regionalanästhesie und Schmerztherapie - Obere und untere Extremität. Bremen: Uni-Med-Verlag; 1999.

Chelly JE, Delaunay L. A new anterior approach to the sciatic nerve block. Anesthesiology. 1999;6:1655-60.

Chelly JE, Greger J, Howart G. Simple anterior approach for sciatic blockade. Reg Anesth. 1997;(A)22:114.

Chelly JE, Delaunay L, Matuszczak M, Hagberg C. Sciatic nerve blocks. Techniques in Regional Anesthesia and Pain Management 1999;3:39-46.

Clara M. Das Nervensystem des Menschen. 3 rd ed. Leipzig: Barth; 1959.

Ericksen NL, Swenson JD, Pace NL. The anatomic relationship of the sciatic nerve to the lesser trochanter: Implications for anterior nerve block. Anesth Analg. 2002;95:1071-4.

Gaertner E, Laseurain P, Venet C, et al. Continuous parasacral sciatic block: A radiographic study. Anesth Analg. 2004;98:831-4

Gligorijevic S. Lower extremity blocks for day surgery. Techniques in Regional Anesthesia and Pain Management 2000;4:30-7.

Guardini R, Waldron BA. Sciatic nerve block: A new lateral approach. Acta Anaesthesiol Scand. 1985;29:515-9.

Ichiyanagi K. Sciatic nerve block: Lateral approach with the patient supine. Anesthesiology. 1959;20:601.

Kaiser H, Niesel HCh, Klimpel L. Grundlagen und Anforderungen der peripheren elektrischen Nervenstimulation. Ein Beitrag zur Erhöhung des Sicherheitsstandards in der Regionalanästhesie. Reg Anaesth. 1990;13:143-4.

Labat G. Regional anesthesia: Its technique and clinical application. Philadelphia: Saunders; 1924:45.

Mansour NY, Benetts FE. An observational study of combined continuous lumbar plexus and single-shot sciatic nerve blocks for post-knee surgery analgesia. Reg Anesth. 1996;21:287-91.

Meier G. Der kontinuierliche anteriore Ischiadicuskatheter (KAI). In: Mehrkens HH, Büttner J, eds. Kontinuierliche periphere Leitungsblockaden. Munich: Arcis; 1999 a;47-8.

Meier G. Technik der kontinuierlichen anterioren Ischiadicusblockade (KAI). In: Büttner J, Meier G, eds. Kontinuierliche periphere Techniken zur Regionalanästhesie und Schmerztherapie - Obere und untere Extremität. Bremen: Uni-Med-Verlag; 1999 b;132-7.

Meier G. Periphere Blockaden der unteren Extremität. Anaesthesist. 2001;50:536-59.

Meier G, Büttner J. Regionalanästhesie - Kompendium der peripheren Blockaden. Munich: Arcis; 2001.

Meier G, Heinrich Ch. Sciatic nerve block: A comparison of three different techniques. 24 th Central European Congress on Anesthesiology. Bologna: Monduzzi; 1995:509-12.

Morris GF, Lang SA. Continuous parasacral sciatic nerve block: Two case reports. Reg Anesth. 1997;22:469-72.

Morris GF, Lang SA. Innovations in lower extremity blockade. Techniques in Regional Anesthesia and Pain Management 1999;3:9-18.

Morris GF, Lang SA, Dust WN, Van der Wal M. The parasacral sciatic nerve block. Reg Anesth. 1997;22:100-4.

Neuburger M, Rotzinger M, Kaiser H. Elektrische Nervenstimulation in Abhängigkeit von der benutzten Impulsbreite - Eine quantitative Untersuchung zur Annäherung der Nadelspitze an den Nerven. Anesthesist. 2001;50:181-6.

Niesel H Ch., eds. Regionalanästhesie, Lokalanästhesie, regionale Schmerztherapie. Stuttgart: Thieme; 1994.

Pham Dang C, Gautheron E, Guilly J, et al. The value of adding sciatic block to continuous femoral block for analgesia after total knee replacement. Reg Anesth Pain Med. 2005;30:128-33.

Polino F, Castro A, Bello R, Sanchez Pena J, Ojeda R, Fornes C. Postoperative analgesia by continuous 3-in-1-blockade in total hip arthroplasty. Int Monitor Reg Anesth. 2000;(A)12:245.

Raj PP, Parks RI, Watson TD, Jenkins MT. A new single position supine approach to sciatic nerve block. Anesth Analg. 1975;54:489-93.

Ripart J, Cuvillon P, Nouvellon E, Gaertner E, Eledjam JJ. Parasacral approach to block the sciatic nerve: A 400-case survey. Reg Anesth Pain Med 2005;30:193-7

Rongstad K, Mann RA, Prieskorn D. Popliteal sciatic nerve block for postoperative analgesia. Foot Ankle Int. 1996;17:378-82.

Sala-Blanch X, Pomés J, Matute P, et al. Intraneural injection during anterior approach for sciatic nerve block. Anesthesiology. 2004;101:1027-30

Smith BE, Siggins D. Low volume, high concentration block of the sciatic nerve. Anaesthesia. 1988;43:8-11.

Vloka Jd, Hadzic A, April E, Thys DM. Anterior approach to the sciatic nerve block: The effects of leg rotation. Anesth Analg. 2001;92:460-2.

Wagner F. Beinnervenblockaden In: Niesel HC, eds. Regionalanästhesie, Lokalanästhesie, regionale Schmerztherapie. Stuttgart: Thieme; 1994:417-521.

Wagner F, Mißler B. Kombinierter Ischiadicus/3-in-1-Block. Anaesthesist. 1987;46:195-200.

Wagner F, Taeger L. Kombinierter Ischiadicus/3 in 1-Block III: Prilocain 1% vs. Mepivacain 1%. Reg Anaesth. 1988;11:61.

Winnie AP. An immobile needle for nerve blocks. Anesthesiology. 1969;31:577.

Winnie AP. Regional Anesthesia. Surg Clin North Am. 1975;54:861.

11   Blocks at the Knee

11.1   Anatomical Overview

The *sciatic nerve* (L4-S3) consists of two components, the common *fibular nerve* (synonym: common peroneal nerve) and the *tibial nerve*, which are surrounded in the pelvis minor and thigh by a common connective-tissue sheath and therefore give the impression of a single nerve trunk. The division into the two branches can take place at a variable level. The common connective-tissue sheath ends at the latest on entry to the popliteal fossa and the nerve divides into the tibial nerve and the common fibular nerve (Fig. 11.1).

The *common fibular nerve* (L4-S2) divides below the popliteal fossa into the *deep fibular nerve* and the *superficial fibular nerve*. The deep fibular nerve innervates the extensor muscles of the lower leg and foot. The superficial fibular nerve supplies the muscles of the fibular group. The *tibial nerve* (L4-S3) is responsible for the motor supply of the toe and foot flexors.

The tibial nerve innervates the skin of the lateral lower leg and the sole of the foot and, after joining the communicating branch of the fibular nerve to form the sural nerve, it supplies the lateral border of the heel and foot. The dorsum of the foot is innervated by the superficial fibular nerve, apart from the area between the great toe and second toe (deep fibular nerve) (see Fig. 7.7).

Fig. 11.**1**   The sciatic nerve, which often divides very proximal into the tibial nerve and fibular nerve, leaves the common that which surrounds the two divisions at the latest on entering the popliteal fossa (ca. 8–10 cm above the popliteal crease), and the tibial nerve and fibular nerves separate here. In order to block both divisions of the sciatic nerve in the region of the popliteal fossa with one injection, this must be performed at least 8–10 cm above the popliteal crease. A continuous technique can also be performed here without difficulty. A complete block distal to the knee requires an additional block of the saphenous nerve, a main branch of the femoral nerve which provides sensory innervation of the medial lower leg.

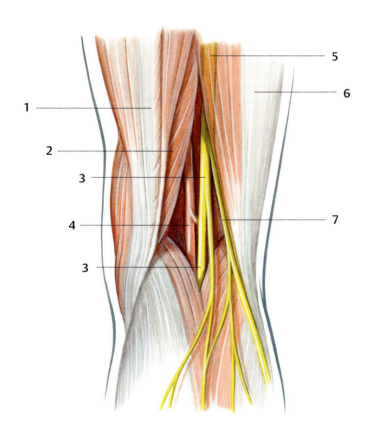
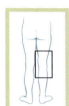

1   Semitendinosus
2   Semimembranosus
3   Tibial nerve
4   Popliteal artery
5   Sciatic nerve (covered by muscle)
6   Biceps femoris
7   Common fibular nerve

11.2   Classical Popliteal Block, Dorsal Approach

For historical reasons the classical popliteal approach is mentioned here. For several reasons (see below) it is not recommended as the first choice for a distal sciatic approach.

Landmarks
Popliteal fossa, knee crease.

Position
The patient lies prone. With the knee extended, puncture is performed at the level of the popliteal crease or slightly cranial to it (Fig. 11.**2**). The tibial nerve is found ca. 1 cm lateral to the artery. It is situated at a depth of 1-3 cm. To block the common fibular nerve from the same puncture site, the needle is withdrawn under the skin and advanced again further laterally toward the head of the fibula. After ca. 3-4 cm a response will be obtained from the nerve.

Remarks on the Technique

Anesthesia of the sciatic nerve or of its two divisions (fibular nerve and tibial nerve) in the region of the popliteal fossa is often called popliteal block or "knee block." It is a

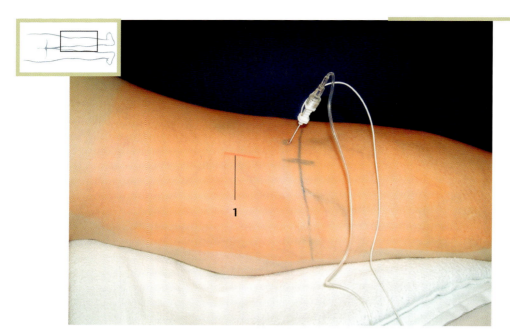

Fig. 11.**2**   Right popliteal fossa, posterome-dial view. The classical "popliteal block" is performed in the popliteal crease where the tibial nerve and fibular nerve are already sep-arated, so that the two nerves have to be found and blocked individually to obtain a complete block of the lower leg. Here block of the tibial nerve.

1   Popliteal artery

highly effective technique and is easily per-formed without problems. The disadvantage of the classical popliteal block is the neces-sity of finding two nerves separately in order to be able to anesthetize the entire foot. The fibular and tibial nerves can be separately blocked in the popliteal fossa from one puncture site because of the close vicinity of the two nerves. This requires a change in the direction of the needle for selective stimula-tion of the two nerves.
This "double injection technique" should be a quick procedure, as the risk of intraneural

injection increases with the time required (Gligorijevic 2000). Administration of the local anesthetic after finding the first nerve can result in partial anesthesia of the second nerve even before it has been localized, because of its proximity. This reduces ade-quate response by the nerve stimulator and perception of inadvertent paresthesia, and thus increases the risk of accidental intraneural injection of the local anesthetic. However, the popliteal block is regarded as a safe technique (Jan et al. 2000). The "double injection technique" leads to an onset period

and an effective block (Bailey et al. 1994). Singelyn et al. (1991) performed 625 blocks with nerve stimulation in a prospective study; 30 ml of mepivacaine 1 % [10 mg/ml] or bupivacaine 0.5 % [5 mg/ml] was injected. An adequate block was achieved in 92 % of the patients and in a further 5 % the block could be supplemented successfully. The popliteal artery was punctured in two patients (0.3 %). Patient satisfaction was 95 %.

11.3   Distal Block of the Sciatic Nerve

Technique

Posterior Approach, Continuous Technique According to Meier

The sciatic nerve divides on entry into the popliteal fossa at the latest into its two main branches, the tibial nerve and the common fibular nerve. The common fascial sheath can no longer be found in the popliteal fossa. For reasons of efficacy, this suggests finding and anesthetizing the sciatic nerve as far cranially as possible in the popliteal fossa, i.e., before it divides—that is, performing a distal sciatic nerve block (Fig. 11.**3**).

Landmarks
Cranial to the popliteal crease, the popliteal fossa is bounded above the popliteal crease laterally by the tendon of biceps femoris, and medially by semimembranosus and the tendon of semitendinosus. The puncture is made at the lateral boundary of the popliteal fossa (corresponding to the inside of the biceps femoris tendon) ca. 8-12 cm above the popliteal crease (Figs. 11.**4**-11.**6**).

Position
The patient lies on his or her side with the leg to be blocked uppermost. The leg beneath is flexed at the knee, and the over-

lying one is extended but relaxed (Fig. 11.**5**). (Positioning variant: The patient lies supine and the limb to be blocked is elevated and flexed at the hip and knee, "lithotomy posi-tion," Fig. 11.**7**)

Procedure (in Lateral Position)
The patient is asked to bend the knee. The tendon of the biceps femoris can then readily be palpated on the lateral side. The leg is then extended. A line is drawn about 8-12 cm proximal and parallel to the popliteal crease. The intersection with the tendon of the biceps femoris marks the puncture site (Fig. 11.**6**). The puncture site is

Fig. 11.**3** Right popliteal fossa, posterior view. The sciatic nerve, which often
splits very proximal into the tibial and
fibular nerves, leaves the common
sheath that surrounds the two divisions
at the latest on entering the popliteal
fossa (ca. 8–10 cm above the popliteal
crease) where the two main branches
separate. In order to block both divisions
of the sciatic nerve in the region of the
popliteal fossa with one injection, this
must be performed at least 8–10 cm
above the popliteal crease. A continuous
catheter technique can also be used
here without difficulty.

  1 Semimembranosus
  2 Tibial nerve
  3 Popliteal crease
  4 Sciatic nerve
  5 Biceps femoris, reflected laterally
  6 Fibular nerve

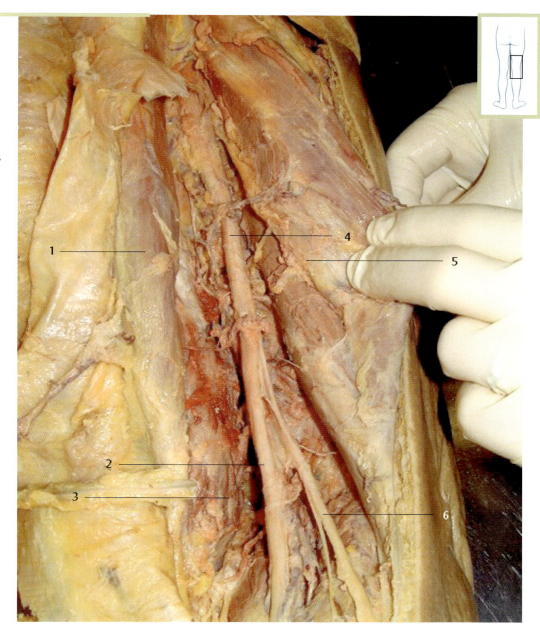

Fig. 11.**4** Cross section through the
right thigh at the level of puncture
(here 9 cm above the popliteal crease)
for distal sciatic nerve block, and MRI
at the same level in prone position.
The plane through the right thigh is
seen from below.

  1   Biceps femoris
  2   Semimembranosus/
       semitendinosus
  3   Sciatic nerve
  3 a Fibular nerve
  3 b Tibial nerve
  4   Popliteal artery

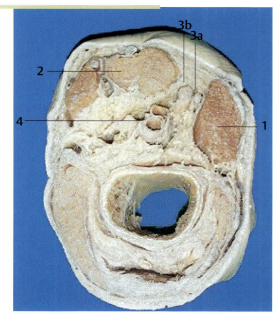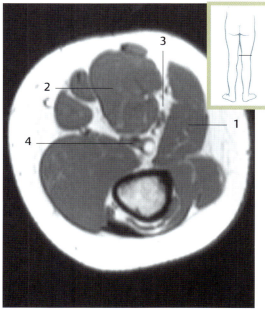

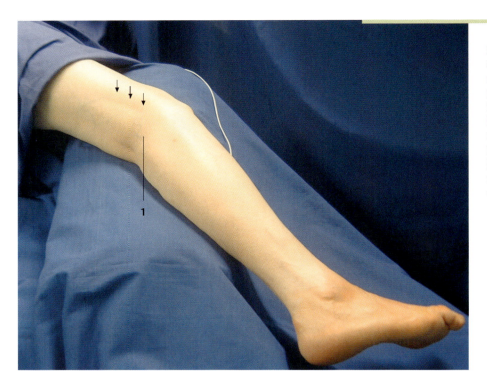

Fig. 11.**5**   Distal sciatic nerve block, distal approach in lateral position: there is a posterior and a lateral approach to distal sciatic nerve block. The dorsal approach can be performed in the lateral or supine position (see below). The tendon of the biceps femoris is used for orientation. A skin groove can often be identified medial to the tendon and for better orientation the patient can be asked to flex the lower leg against resistance, which makes the tendon more prominent.

1   Popliteal crease
→   Skin groove medial to the tendon of
→   biceps femoris

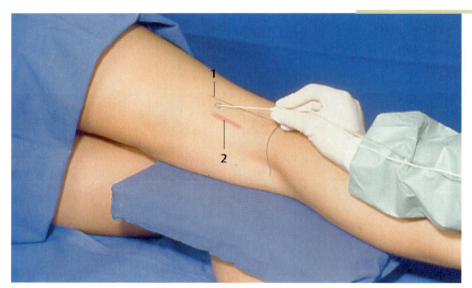

Fig. 11.**6**   The injection site for posterior distal sciatic nerve block is located immediately medial to the tendon of biceps femoris ca. 10 cm cranial to the popliteal crease. The needle is directed slightly medially and cranially. Note that the artery runs lateral to the midline and that the sciatic artery is still lateral to the artery.

1   Tendon of biceps femoris
2   Popliteal artery (does not absolutely have to be found for this technique)

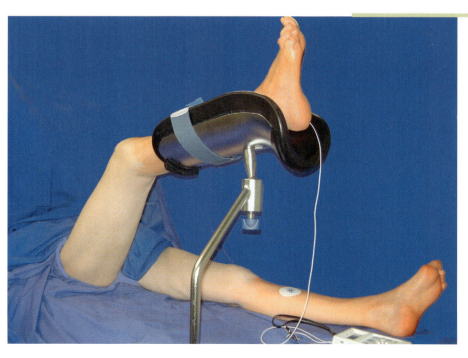

Fig. 11.**7**   If the leg is positioned appropriately, dorsal distal sciatic nerve block can also be performed on a patient in supine position.

Fig. 11.**8** Right popliteal fossa, posterior view. Dorsal distal sciatic nerve block: the puncture site is medial to the tendon of biceps femoris and lateral to the popliteal vessels.

1 Biceps femoris
2 Tibial division of the sciatic nerve
3 Fibular division of the sciatic nerve
4 Semitendinosus
5 Popliteal artery
6 Semimembranosus

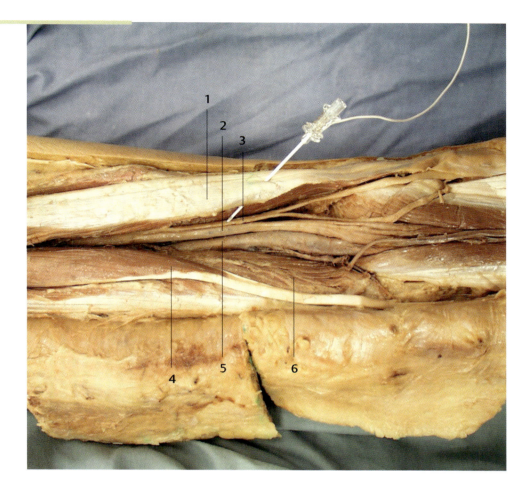

Fig. 11.**9** Orientation and performance of a distal posterior sciatic nerve block is also possible in obese patients, here in the left leg. A 6 cm needle may be too short in obese patients.

1 Popliteal artery
2 Puncture site

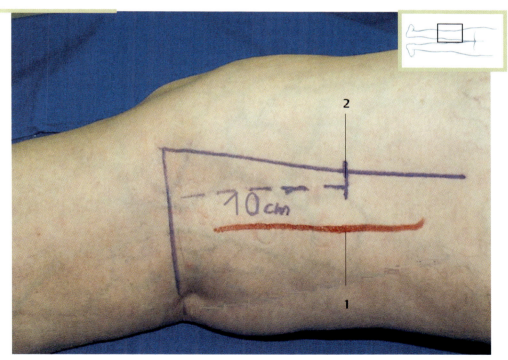

medial to the tendon of the biceps femoris and lateral to the popliteal vessels (Meier 1996) (Fig. 11.**8**).
Following disinfection, infiltration, and pre-puncture of the skin at the puncture site, a 6-10 cm long 19.5G insulated needle is advanced cranially and slightly medially at an angle of 30-45° to the skin. When the fascia is reached, obvious resistance (a "click") can often be felt. The sciatic nerve or its divisions are reached after 4-6 cm. In obese patients a distance of >6 cm may be possible (Fig. 11.**9**). Because of the laterally situated puncture site, the fibular nerve is usually reached first and then the tibial nerve when the needle is advanced further medially. The position of the needle tip is optimal when pronation of the foot with

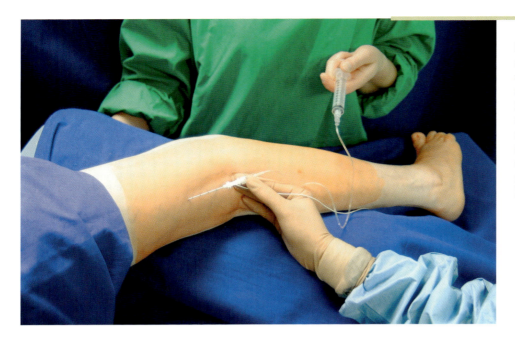

Fig. 11.**10** Using the distal posterior approach, the sciatic nerve is reached after 4–6 cm depending on the angle. The response is due to stimulation of either the lateral fibular division (dorsiflexors) or the medial tibial division (plantar flexors). It is often possible to stimulate both divisions by slight wobbling movements. The optimal response is from the foot. After the nerve is successfully found, the nerve 30–40 ml of local anesthetic is injected intermittently.

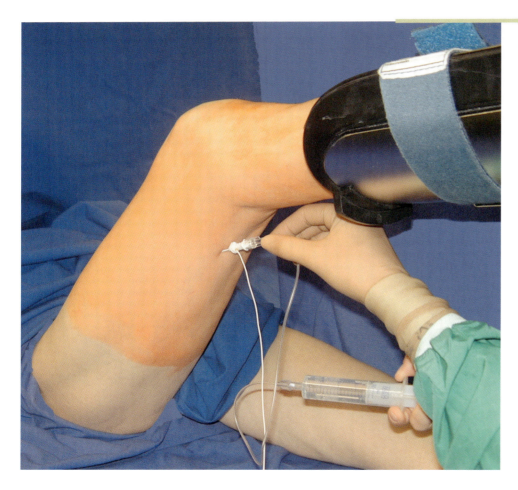

Fig. 11.**11** Performing dorsal distal sciatic nerve block in supine position.

dorsiflexion (fibular division) or a motor response of the tibial nerve (supination of the foot with plantar flexion) can be produced at 0.3 mA and pulse duration of 0.1 ms. Both responses can often be achieved by a minimal shift of the needle tip. Then 30-40 ml of local

anesthetic (LA) is injected (e.g., mepivacaine or lidocaine 1 % [10 mg/ml] or ropivacaine 0.75 % [7.5 mg/ml]) (Fig. 11.**10**). If the leg is in the appropriate position, dorsal distal sciatic nerve block can also be performed with the patient supine (Fig. 11.**11**).

For a continuous block, the catheter is advanced cranially 4-5 cm beyond the tip of the needle after LA is injected (Figs. 11.**12**, 11.**13**).

Fig. 11.**12**   A catheter can be advanced usually without difficulty with this technique.

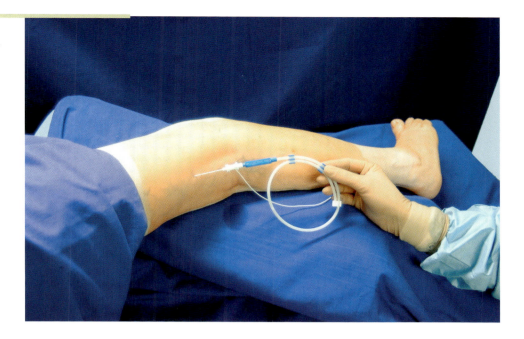

Fig. 11.**13**   Indwelling catheter for continuous dorsal distal sciatic nerve block.

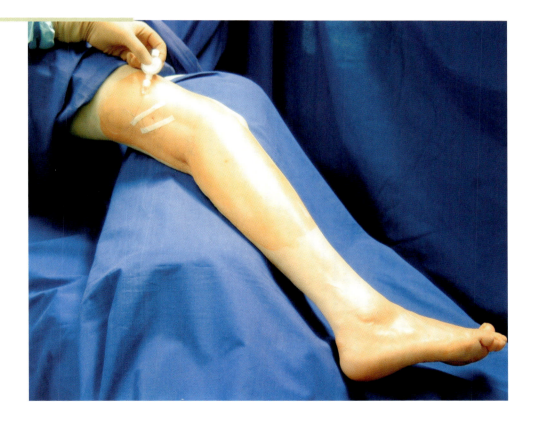

Practical Notes

- If the tibial nerve is stimulated first, the position of the needle tip should be directed more laterally in order to reach the fibular nerve.

- Vascular puncture is not anticipated with this technique (Fig. 11.**14**).

Lateral Approach

Landmarks and Position
Lateral femoral epicondyle, vastus lateralis, biceps femoris.

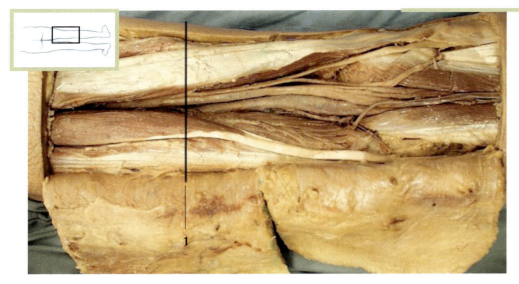

Fig. 11.**14** MRI of right thigh in lateral position, 9 cm above the popliteal crease (seen
from below). As the nerve is reached first
with the described needle direction, vascular
puncture is normally excluded.

1 Plane for MRI
(12 cm above the popliteal crease)

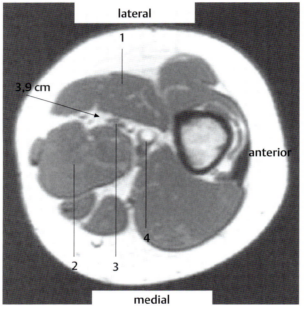

1 Biceps femoris
2 Semimembranosus/semitendinosus
3 Sciatic nerve
4 Popliteal artery

The skin–nerve distance is 3.9 cm, when the
needle passed directly. A more cranial direction should be preferred.

Supine, the leg should be supported at the
foot so that the muscles of the thigh can sag
freely (Fig. 11.**15**).

Procedure
The puncture site is 8-12 cm cranial to the
lateral femoral epicondyle in the groove
between the biceps femoris and vastus lateralis (Fig. 11.**16**). The angle of puncture in the
transverse plane varies with the distance
from the lateral femoral epicondyle: the
further cranial the puncture site, the lower
the angle posteriorly (Figs. 11.**17**-11.**21**); the
minimum distance from the femoral condyle

is 8 cm. Distal to this, the sciatic nerve has
already separated into the common fibular
nerve and tibial nerve and runs without the
common connective-tissue sheath (Fig.
11.**22**). As well as the variable posterior
needle angle, the needle should be directed
in the cranial direction (Fig. 11.**23**), as this
will facilitate advancement of a catheter . At a
distance of 8-12 cm proximal to the lateral
femoral condyle, the nerve is reached from in
front, so there can be a response from the
tibial nerve first, although the common fibular nerve lies more lateral (and somewhat
posterior) to the tibial nerve. The skin-nerve

distance can be up to 8 cm, sometimes even
more, so a 10-12 cm needle should be used
(Fig. 11.**24**).

Indications and Contraindications

Indications for Single-Stage and Continuous Sciatic Nerve Blocks
(sometimes in combination with a
saphenous nerve block)
• Anesthesia for operation on the foot or
ankle (e.g., lateral ligament suture, resection arthroplasty, arthrodesis, amputation

Fig. 11.**15** Besides the posterior approach, there is also a lateral approach to the distal sciatic nerve. For this approach, the lower leg should be supported with a pad so that the dorsal muscles sag as freely as possible.

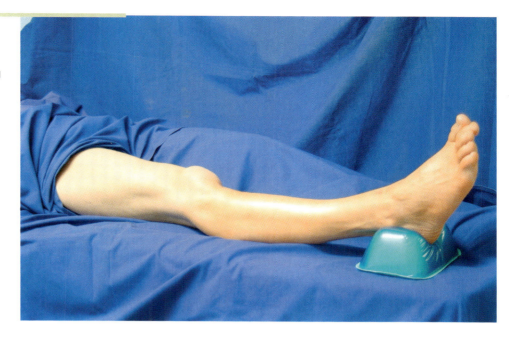

Fig. 11.**16** Distal sciatic nerve block, lateral approach with the patient in supine position: for orientation, the muscle gap between the vastus lateralis and the biceps femoris is localized ca. 12 cm above the popliteal crease.

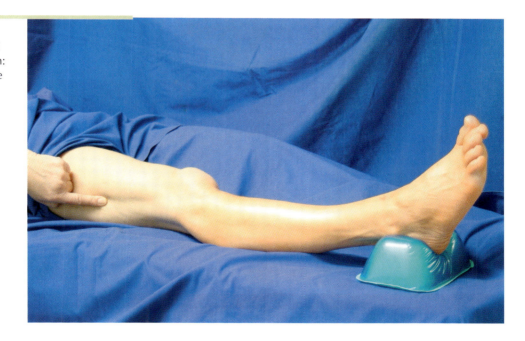

[Fig. 11.**25**], free tissue transfer/transplantation with microvascular-vascular attachment to the lower leg/foot region [e.g., latissimus dorsi flaps] [Fig. 11.**26**]).
- Anesthesia/pain therapy for fractures distal to the knee.
- Postoperative pain therapy (e.g., ankle and foot region).
- Pain therapy (e.g., diabetic gangrene, CRPS I).
- Regional sympathetic block (perfusion and wound healing disorders, CRPS I; Figs. 11.**27**, 11.**28**).

Contraindications
- General contraindications (see Chapter 15).
- Previous peripheral vascular surgery in the legs (relative).

Side Effects and Complications

There are no reported special complications and side effects.

Practical Notes

- Vascular puncture is not to be expected with the lateral technique and a distal sciatic nerve block.
- In polyneuropathy, peripheral nerve stimulation should be performed with a pulse duration of 1.0 ms.
- If the operation is performed with lower leg tourniquet, it is rational to perform supplementary block of the saphenous nerve (the sensory terminal branch of the femoral nerve, q.v.).

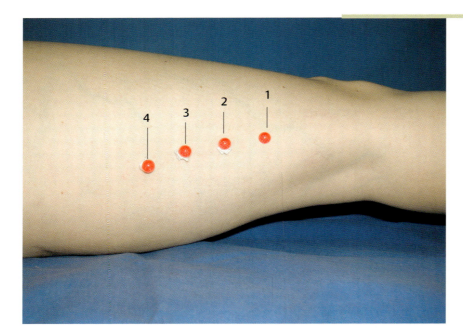

Fig. 11.**17** In general the lateral approach to the sciatic nerve can be used at any level, but the level of puncture has a considerable influence on the puncture angle in the dorsal direction. MRI investigations at three different levels proximal to the popliteal crease (12, 16, 20 cm) were used to determine the angle between the marked puncture site (between the vastus lateralis and the biceps femoris) and the sciatic nerve. As the gap between the vastus lateralis and the biceps femoris moves dorsally from distal to proximal, the angle of needle direction decreases as the distance from the popliteal crease increases.

Distance from popliteal crease to puncture site:

    1   9 cm
    2   12 cm
    3   16 cm
    4   20 cm

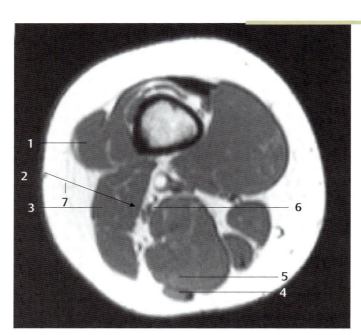

Fig. 11.**18** Lateral puncture of the sciatic nerve 9 cm above the popliteal crease. The angle dorsally is ca. 22°; the skin–nerve distance is 5.2 cm when the needle passes directly. However, a more cranial needle direction should be selected.

    1   Vastus lateralis
    2   Marker 9 cm proximal to the popliteal crease
    3   Biceps femoris
    4   Semitendinosus
    5   Semimembranosus
    6   Sciatic nerve
    7   Needle direction

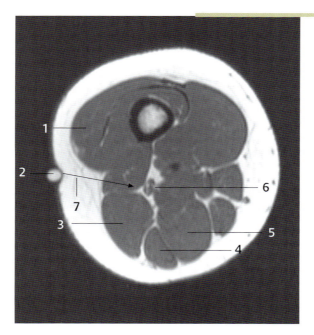

Fig. 11.**19** Lateral approach to the sciatic nerve 12 cm above the popliteal crease. The angle dorsally is 9°; the skin–nerve distance is 4.8 cm when the needle passes directly. However, a more cranial needle direction should always be selected.

    1   Vastus lateralis
    2   Marker 12 cm proximal to the popliteal crease
    3   Biceps femoris
    4   Semitendinosus
    5   Semimembranosus
    6   Sciatic nerve
    7   Needle direction

Fig. 11.**20**   Lateral approach to the sciatic nerve 16 cm above the popliteal crease: the dorsal angle is 6°, the skin–nerve distance is 5.9 cm when the needle passes directly. However, a more cranial needle direction should be preferred.

1   Vastus lateralis
2   Marker 16 cm proximal to the popliteal crease
3   Biceps femoris
4   Semitendinosus
5   Semimembranosus
6   Sciatic nerve
7   Needle direction

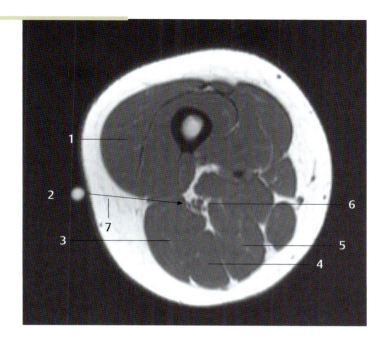

Fig. 11.**21**   Lateral approach for puncture of the sciatic nerve 20 cm above the popliteal crease. The dorsal angle is 0°; the skin–nerve distance is 5.6 cm when the needle passes directly. However, a more cranial needle direction should be selected.

1   Vastus lateralis
2   Marker 20 cm proximal to the popliteal crease
3   Biceps femoris
4   Semitendinosus
5   Semimembranosus
6   Sciatic nerve
7   Needle direction

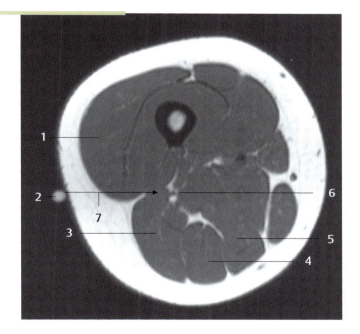

- If there is an indication for sympathetic block, a response from the tibial nerve should be sought.
- If it is not possible to position the needle in closer proximity to the nerve despite a motor response at higher current, the needle must be changed in a medial (fibular motor response) or a lateral (tibial motor response) direction respectively.

Remarks on the Technique

Labat described block of the sciatic nerve in the popliteal fossa for the first time in 1924. Different variants of popliteal block are employed in clinical practice.
Operations on the foot can be very painful postoperatively. Opioids are often inadequate for pain therapy and have disturbing side effects (Bonica 1980, 1984). The use of con-

tinuous regional techniques for postoperative pain therapy is therefore particularly indicated in painful operations on the ankle and foot.
The existence of a fascial sheath around the nerve(s) is an important requirement for the success of a continuous technique (catheter technique). The fascia has been demonstrated in several anatomical studies on dissected specimens (Meier et al. 1999 a; Rorie

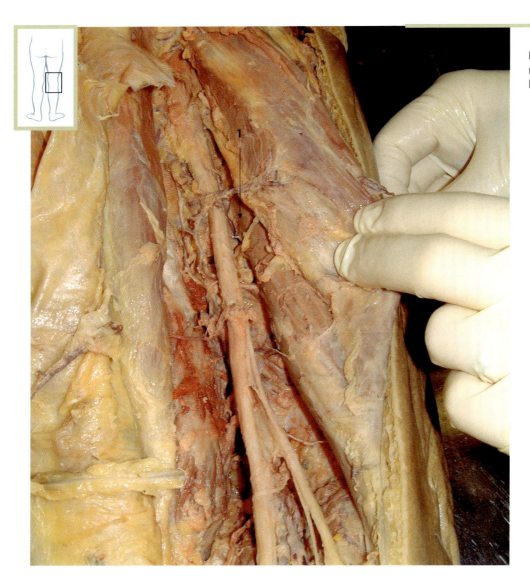

Fig. 11.**22** Distal lateral approach for sciatic nerve block, posterior view, right thigh, the biceps femoris muscle reflected laterally.

1 Needle tip

et al. 1980; Vloka et al. 1996 a, 1996 b). Radiological examination with contrast reproducibly shows the uniform distribution in a space limited by the fascial sheath (Bauereis and Meier 1997) (Fig. 11.**29**). Injection and placement of the catheter within this fascial sheath therefore optimizes anesthesia/ analgesia.

As the selected injection site is quite proximal, and where the two divisions of the sciatic nerve lie very close together, a "double injection technique" is not necessary . The best response for a successful block is the subject of much discussion. Mach (2000)

found no differences in success rates between stimulation of the tibial nerve and fibular nerve in a study of 112 patients with a posterior popliteal block. As the diameter of the tibial nerve is about twice that of the fibular nerve, it can be expected that the time required to complete a block of the tibial nerve will be longer. As with all techniques, where the local anesthetic is injected into a space bounded by connective tissue or fascia, an adequate volume and adequate concentration of the LA should be selected. For distal sciatic nerve blocks 30-40 ml of, e.g., lidocaine 1 % or mepivacaine 1 % (10 mg/

ml) or of ropivacaine 0.5 % (5 mg/ml) or 0.75 % (7.5 mg/ml) is recommended (Meier 1999 b, Meier et al. 1999 b).

In 1997 Singelyn et al. investigated the course and effectiveness of a continuous dorsal sciatic nerve block in 30 patients operated on the foot. In 93 % of cases, the technique was performed without problems. A motor response was produced at a needle depth of 4-5.5 cm. The patients were given 40 ml of mepivacaine 1 % (10 mg/ml) with epinephrine and a continuous infusion of bupivacaine 0.25 % (2.5 mg/ml). The anesthesia was sufficient in 28 patients (93 %). Fewer

Fig. 11.**23** Distal lateral sciatic nerve block: ca. 12 cm proximal to the popliteal crease in the groove between vastus lateralis and biceps femoris muscle.

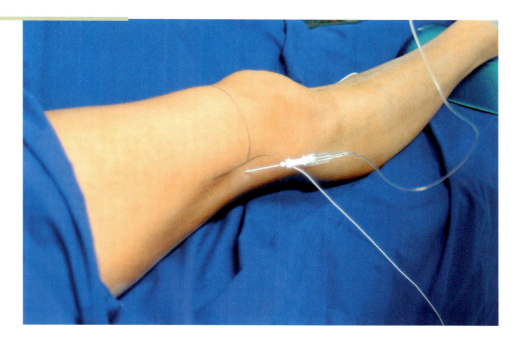

Fig. 11.**24** Distal lateral sciatic nerve block. The needle is directed ca. 10° dorsally and 30° cranially and the nerve is reached after 5–8 cm.

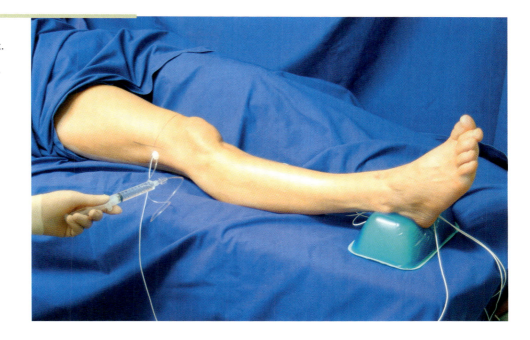

than 10% of the patients required an opioid in the postoperative period. Singelyn recommends 0.125% (1.25 mg/ml) bupivacaine 7 ml/h for continuous administration and additional patient controlled boluses of 2.5 ml/30 min for 48-72 hours if needed (Singelyn 1998).

With the continuous technique for distal sciatic nerve block as described by Meier in 1996, the puncture site is rather proximal. The puncture site lateral to the artery was selected in order to avoid artificial vascular puncture. The sciatic nerve is reached at a depth of 5-6 cm when the needle is directed cranially at

an angle of 30-40° to the skin (Meier et al. 1999 a). In large thighs, the distance to the sciatic nerve can be greater, particularly with a more tangential needle direction; 10-12 cm needles are needed for these patients. Advancing the needle at an acute angle to the nerve rather than perpendicular facilitates the insertion of a catheter (Bauereis and Meier 1997; Meier 1999 a, 2001).

In a study by Meier et al. (1999 b) of 303 patients, a distal sciatic nerve catheter was placed for operation on the foot or ankle and subsequent pain therapy. The patients were given 10 ml of mepivacaine 2% (20 mg/ml)

and 20 ml of mepivacaine 1% (10 mg/ml) for anesthesia. The postoperative pain therapy consisted of ropivacaine 0.375% (3.75 mg/ml) or bupivacaine 0.25% (2.5 mg/ml). The catheter was in used situ for an average of 4.5 days (max. 21 days). Side effects or complications were not observed. Patient acceptability of this procedure was extraordinarily high: 94% of the patients were satisfied or very satisfied.

The main advantage of the lateral approach to distal sciatic nerve block is the fact that the patient can remain in supine position. Orientation is simple. It is important that the

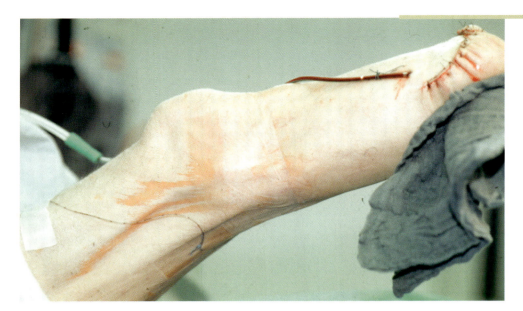

Fig. 11.**25** Distal sciatic nerve block is an ideal alternative to a lumbar epidural catheter for pain therapy and prophylaxis before and after lower leg amputations.

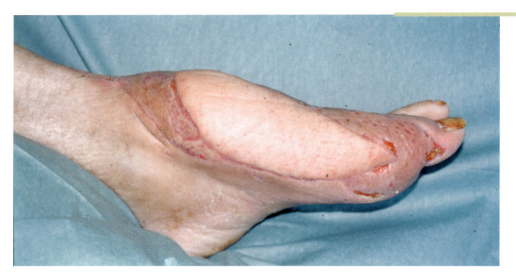

Fig. 11.**26** For free tissue transfer (e.g., latissimus dorsi flap) to the lower leg and foot region, anesthesia, postoperative analgesia, and sympathetic block via a distal sciatic nerve catheter are the ideal alternative to a lumbar epidural catheter.

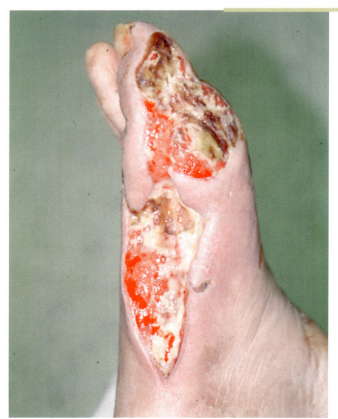

Fig. 11.**27** Wound healing disorders due to a poor blood perfusion can be an indication for a blockade via a distal sciatic nerve catheter.

Fig. 11.**28** The sciatic nerve is rich in sympathetic fibers. After successful injection of the local anesthetic there is a marked sympathetic block with a rise in temperature and vasodilatation which can also be used therapeutically. Continuous sciatic nerve block is an ideal alternative to a continuous lumbar epidural block for various indications.

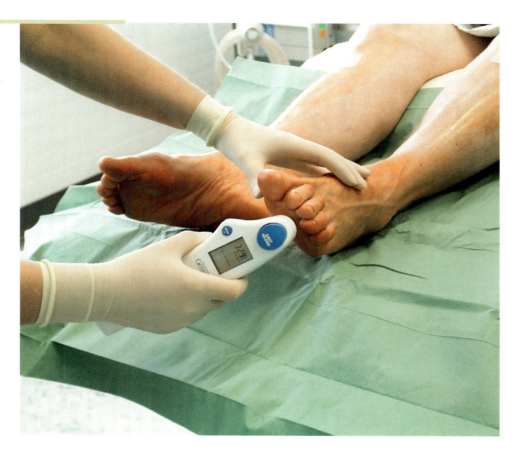

Fig. 11.**29** Spread of contrast along the sciatic nerve after injection via an indwelling catheter.

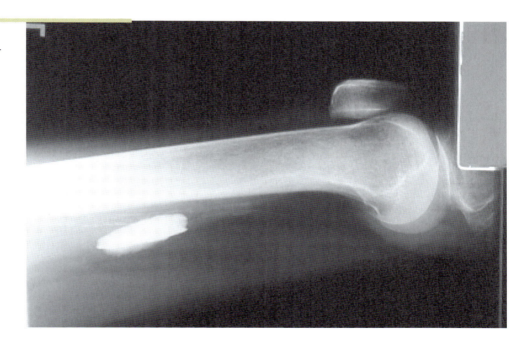

leg sags freely; the distance to the nerve can be 8 cm or more, so that a 10–12 cm-long needle should be selected.

The extent to which distal sciatic nerve block can be employed in conjunction with a saphenous nerve block for anesthesia for operations in the ankle region (ankle fracture, Achilles tendon rupture) depends essentially on whether space will allow lower leg tourniquet. Lower leg exsanguina-

tion should not be less than 6 cm from the head of the fibula.. However, in ankle fractures or Achilles tendon rupture, disinfection and draping are so far proximal that there is no room for a tourniquet on the lower leg. Otherwise, all operations on the foot can be performed with lower leg tourniquet using distal sciatic nerve block in conjunction with saphenous nerve block. For pain therapy and sympathetic block, however, the distal sciatic

block is ideal for the lower leg. The block may be performed on both legs at the same time without problems (Fig. 11.**30**).

Summary

Distal techniques of sciatic nerve block are excellent for operations on the lower leg and in the foot region. In combination with a

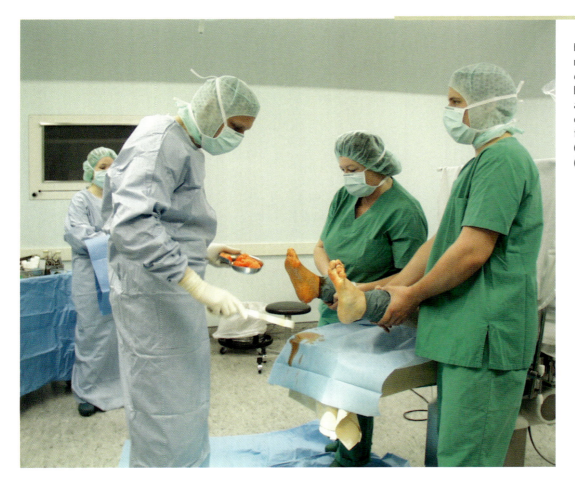

Fig. 11.**30** Bilateral distal sciatic nerve block can be performed in conjunction with saphenous nerve blocks for operation on both feet at the same time. A tourniquet can be applied to the leg about four fingers above the malleoli or 6 cm below the head of the fibula (avoid fibular nerve injury!).

saphenous nerve block (q.v.), surgery can be performed on a blood-free lower leg. The continuous techniques are suitable for pain therapy and regional sympathetic block. The procedures have few complications and are safe and effective when performed with nerve stimulation.

References

Bailey SL, Parkinson S, Little WL. Sciatic nerve block. A comparison of single versus double injection technique. Reg Anesth. 1994;19:9-13.

Bauereis Ch, Meier G. The continuous distal sciatic nerve block for anaesthesia and post-operative pain management. Int Monitor Reg Anesth. 1997;(A)9:96.

Bonica JJ. The management of pain. Philadelphia: Lea and Febiger; 1980:1205-9.

Bonica JJ. Local anaesthesia and regional blocks. In: Wall PD, Melzack R, eds. Textbook of pain. Edinburgh: Churchill Livingstone; 1984:541-57.

Gligorijevic S. Lower extremity blocks for day surgery. Techniques in Regional Anesthesia and Pain Management 2000;4:30-7.

Jan RA, Kerner M, Provenzano DA, Adams SB, Viscusi ER. Popliteal nerve block and its safety in foot and ankle surgery. Anesth Analg. 2000;59:371-6.

Labat G. Regional anesthesia: Its technique and clinical application. Philadelphia: Saunders; 1924:45.

Mach D. Is the type of motor response an important factor in determining the quality of the sciatic nerve block with a relatively small volume of local anaesthetics? Int Monitor Reg Anesth. 2000;(A)12:203.

Meier G. Der kontinuierliche Ischiadikusblock zur Anaesthesia und postoperativen Schmerztherapie. Anaesthesist. 1996;(S2)45:100.

Meier G. Der distale Ischiadikusblock (DIB) mit Katheter (DIK). In: Büttner J, Meier G, eds. Kontinuierliche periphere Techniken zur Regionalanästhesie und Schmerztherapie - Obere und untere Extremität. Bremen: Uni-Med-Verlag; 1999a:140-4.

Meier G. Der distale Sciatickatheter (DIK). In: Mehrkens HH, Büttner J, eds. Kontinuierliche periphere Leitungsblockaden. München: Arcis-Verlag; 1999b:43-6.

Meier G. Periphere Blockaden der unteren Extremität. Anaesthesist. 2001;50:536-59.

Meier G, Bauereis Ch, Meier Th, Maurer H, Huber Ch. Schmerztherapie mit distalen Ischiadikuskathetern - Anatomische Voraussetzungen. Schmerz. 1999a;(S1):75.

Meier G, Bauereis Ch, Meier Th: Kontinuierliche distale Sciatic nerve blockaden zur Schmerztherapie. Schmerz. 1999b;(S1):74-5.

Rorie DK, Byer DE, Nelson DO. Assessment of block of the sciatic nerve in the popliteal fossa. Anesth Analg. 1980;59:371-6.

Singelyn FJ. Continuous femoral and popliteal sciatic nerve blockades. Techniques in Regional Anesthesia and Pain Management 1998;2:90-5.

Singelyn FJ, Gouverneur JM, Gribomont BF. Popliteal sciatic nerve block aided by a nerve stimulator: a reliable technique for foot and ankle surgery. Reg Anesth. 1991;16:278-81.

Singelyn FJ, Aye F, Gouverneur JM. Continuous popliteal sciatic nerve block: An original technique to provide postoperative analgesia after foot surgery. Anesth Analg. 1997;84:383-6.

Vloka J, Hadzic A, Kitain E, et al. Anatomic considerations for sciatic nerve block in the popliteal fossa through the lateral approach. Reg Anesth. 1996a;21:414-8.

Vloka J, Hadzic A, Lesser J, et al. Presence and anatomical characteristics of a common perineural sheath in the popliteal fossa. Reg Anesth. 1996b;21(2):13.

12 Peripheral Block (Conduction Block) of Individual Nerves of the Lower Limb

12.1 Lateral Cutaneous Nerve of the Thigh

Anatomical Overview

The lateral cutaneous nerve of the thigh (L2-L3) is a purely sensory nerve; after leaving the lumbar plexus it crosses the iliacus muscle lateral to the psoas. The nerve lies below the iliac fascia here and emerges through the fascia immediately below and medial to the anterior superior iliac spine, where it divides into anterior and posterior fibers that run a few centimeters subcutaneously distal to the anterior superior iliac spine. The anterior fibers supply the skin of the lateral thigh and end in the prepatellar plexus. The posterior fibers innervate the skin of the lateral hip region below the greater trochanter as far as the middle of the thigh (Figs. 12.**1**-12.**4**).

Technique

Block of the Lateral Cutaneous Nerve of the Thigh (Classical Technique)

Landmarks and Position
Anterior superior iliac spine: the puncture site is 2 cm distal and 2 cm medial to the anterior superior iliac spine.
The patient lies supine (Fig. 12.**5**).

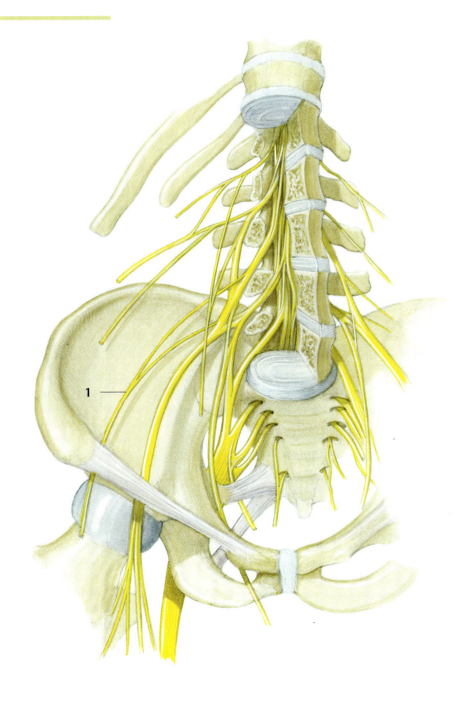

Fig. 12.**1** The lateral cutaneous nerve of the thigh arises from the lumbar plexus.

1 Lateral cutaneous nerve of the thigh

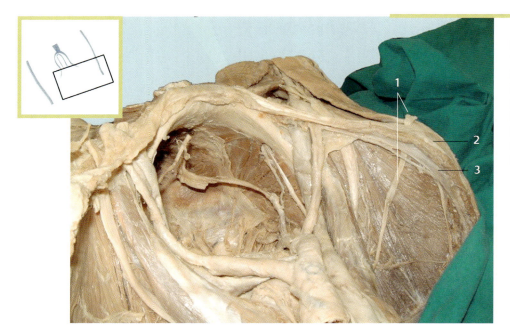

Fig. 12.**2** Cranial view into the lesser pelvis. The lateral cutaneous nerve of the thigh (L2–L3) is a purely sensory nerve and crosses the iliacus muscle lateral to the psoas muscle after leaving the lumbar plexus. The nerve lies under the iliac fascia and passes through the fascia immediately below and medial to the anterior superior iliac spine and divides into anterior and posterior branches.

1 Lateral cutaneous nerve of the thigh
2 Anterior superior iliac spine
3 Iliac fascia

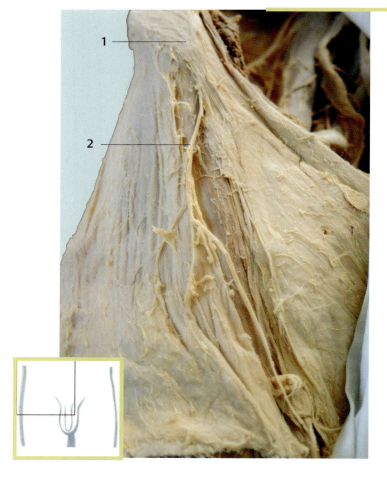

Fig. 12.**3** Right iliac crest (anterior view). The lateral cutaneous nerve of the thigh passes through the fascia immediately below and medial to the anterior superior iliac spine and divides into anterior and posterior branches, which run subcutaneously for a few centimeters distal to the anterior superior iliac spine. The anterior branches supply the skin of the lateral thigh and terminate the prepatellar plexus. The posterior branches innervate the skin of the lateral hip region below the greater trochanter as far as the middle of the thigh.

1 Anterior superior iliac spine
2 Lateral cutaneous nerve of the thigh

Procedure

The anterior superior iliac spine on the side to be anesthetized is palpated and the puncture site is established 2 cm caudally and 2 cm medially. Following disinfection, local infiltration anesthesia is given. At the marked site, a 4-6 cm long 24G needle is advanced vertical to the skin (Fig. 12.**5**). A loss of resistance can be felt when the needle passes through the fascia. Following negative aspiration, a total of 15 ml of a medium-acting or long-acting local anesthetic (LA) is injected, subfascially at first and then in a fan pattern above the fascia after withdrawing the needle. The procedure corresponds to a field block (Cousins et al. 1998; Hallén et al. 1991; Rosenquist and Lederhaas 1999).

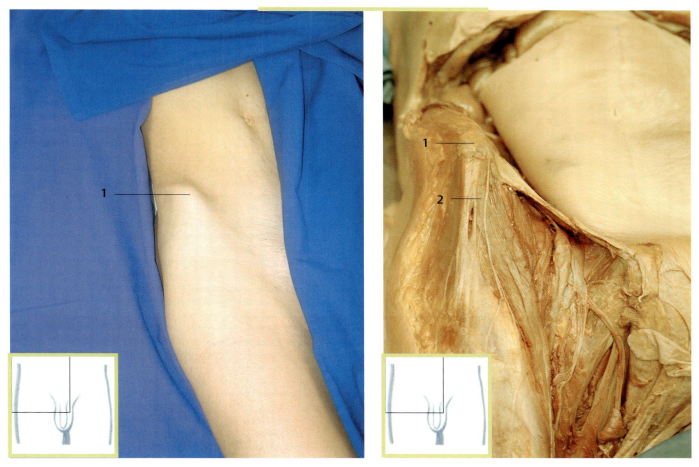

Fig. 12.**4**   Right iliac crest. The lateral cutaneous nerve of the thigh passes through the fascia immediately below and medial to the anterior superior iliac spine and divides here into anterior and posterior branches, which run subcutaneously for a few centimeters distal to the anterior superior iliac spine.

   1   Anterior superior iliac spine
   2   Lateral cutaneous nerve of the thigh

Fig. 12.**5**   Right iliac crest. The anterior superior iliac spine on the side to be anesthetized is palpated and the puncture site is located 2 cm caudally and 2 cm medially At the marked site, a 4–6 cm long 24G needle is advanced vertical to the skin. A loss of resistance can be felt when the tip of the needle passes through the fascia. Following negative aspiration, a total of 15 ml of a medium-acting or long-acting LA is injected, subfascially at first and then in a fan pattern above the fascia after withdrawing the needle. The procedure corresponds to a field block.

   1   Anterior superior iliac spine

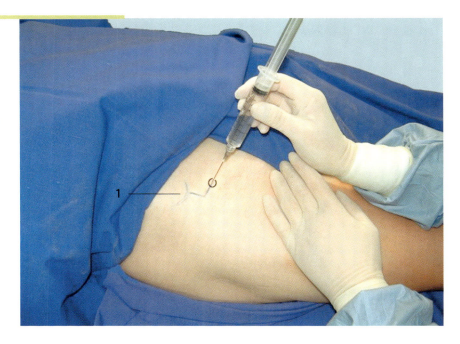

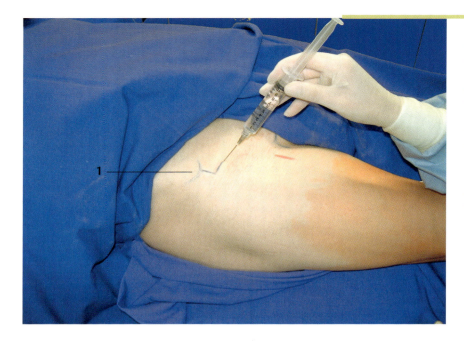

Fig. 12.**6** Right iliac crest. Block of the lateral cutaneous nerve of the thigh (alternative technique): 2 cm caudal and 2 cm medial to the anterior superior iliac spine a 6 cm needle is advanced cranially until after it pierces the fascia lata and bony resistance indicates that the iliac crest has been reached. Then 5 ml of LA is injected between the fascia lata and the iliac crest. This is repeated twice with 5 ml of LA each time and the needle is directed further medially each time. This produces a depot of 15 ml of LA below the inguinal ligament.

1 Anterior superior iliac spine

Block of the Lateral Cutaneous Nerve of the Thigh (Alternative Technique)

Procedure

The point 2 cm caudal and 2 cm medial to the anterior superior iliac spine is again selected as the puncture site. The 6 cm needle is directed cranially, pierces the fascia lata, and is advanced until bony resistance indicates that the iliac crest has been reached (Fig. 12.**6**). Local anesthetic (5 ml) is injected between the fascia lata and the iliac crest. This is repeated twice with 5 ml of LA each time and the needle is directed further medially each time. This produces a depot of 15 ml of LA below the inguinal ligament.

Indications, Contraindications, Side Effects

Indications

- Supplemental analgesia of the lateral side of the thigh in the case of incomplete lumbar plexus block.
- Skin graft harvesting on the lateral thigh, muscle biopsy.
- Meralgia paresthetica (diagnostic and therapeutic e.g., after total hip replacement).

Contraindications and Side Effects

No specific contraindications, no known clinically important side effects.

Practical Notes

- As the anterior parts of the nerve end in the prepatellar area, block of the lateral cutaneous nerve is usually necessary for extensive (open) operations on the knee (Ellis and Feldman 1996).
- The majority of the local anesthetic must be injected under the fascia.
- The procedure is also possible with peripheral nerve stimulation (PNS) (Shannon and Lang 1995). The pulse duration must be set to 1.0 ms (Fig. 12.**7**). If the insulated needle is in the correct location, the patient feels tingling paresthesia in the lateral part of the thigh (see below).

Remarks on the Technique

The course of the nerve is very variable. This refers both to its individual division and to its area of innervation. In 4-6% of cases it is believed not to be present at all and can possibly be regarded as a branch of the femoral nerve (Bonniot 1922/23; Hovelacque 1927). Failure of anesthesia after a selective block can thus be explained anatomically. The close relationship between the femoral nerve and the lateral cutaneous nerve of the thigh is emphasized by reports on block effects in the region of the femoral nerve after conduction anesthesia of the lateral cutaneous nerve of the thigh (Konder et al.

1990; Lonsdale 1988; Sharrock 1980). To ensure a higher success rate, Shannon et al. (1995) described an alternative PNS technique, which is initially performed transdermally. The electrodes are placed medial to the anterior superior iliac spine and directly below the inguinal ligament (Fig. 12.**8**). Starting from a current of 20 mA and a pulse frequency of 2 Hz, paresthesia is sought in the lateral thigh. At the site where the most marked paresthesia can be produced, a 22G insulated needle is introduced and the position of the needle tip is further optimized with PNS until the patient still reports ("tingling") paresthesia even at 0.6 mA/1 Hz. Morris and Lang (1999) point out that the paresthesia is reported synchronously with the nerve stimulator pulse and that injection of only 6 ml of LA leads to successful anesthesia. The possible advantages are a lower volume of LA and a higher success rate. Shannon reports an increase in the success rate from 85% to 100%. However, Rosenquist regards the procedure as relatively complex. For this reason, PNS is not recommended for routine use (Rosenquist and Lederhaas 1999). An isolated block of the lateral cutaneous nerve of the thigh finds its place in pain therapy for the treatment meralgia paresthetica and for anesthesia, e.g., for muscle biopsy and superficial operations on the lateral thigh (Bonica 1984; Jenkner 1983; Rybock 1989).

Fig. 12.**7** Finding the lateral cutaneous nerve of the thigh by means of peripheral nerve stimulation.

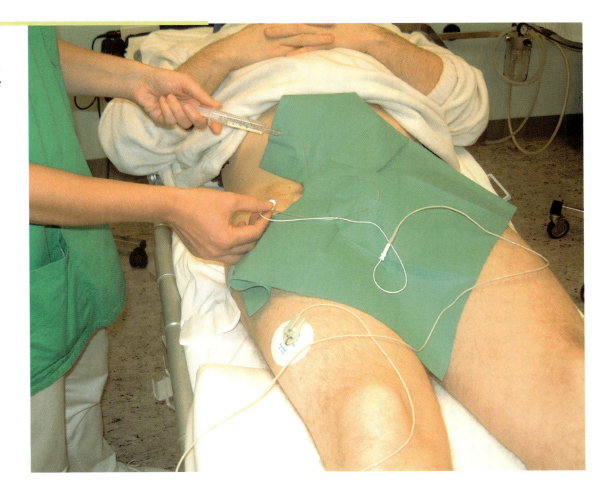

Fig. 12.**8** Finding the lateral cutaneous nerve of the thigh by means of transdermal nerve stimulation.

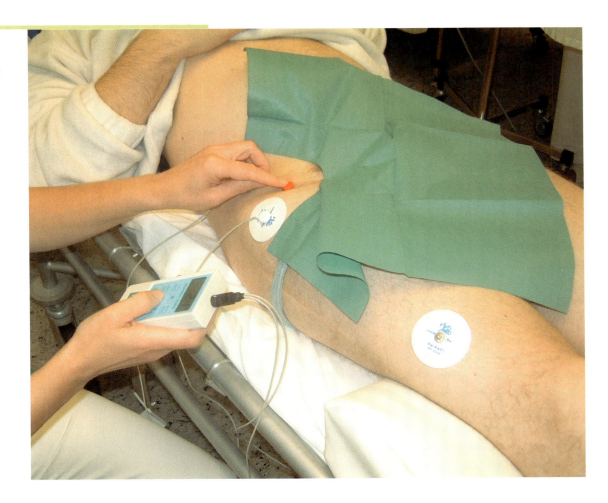

12.2 Infiltration of the Iliac Crest

Indication
Anesthesia and pain therapy for iliac crest bone graft harvesting.

Procedure
The area intended for removal of bone chips from the iliac crest is first infiltrated subcutaneously with a medium-acting or long-acting LA (Fig. 12.**9**). This is followed by injection as far as the periosteum of the iliac crest (Fig. 12.**10**). This injection is given as a field block in order to infiltrate the entire harvesting area.

When bone graft harvesting is complete, the surgeon can place an epidural catheter between the subcutaneous fat and the reconstructed musculofascial and periosteal tissue, bringing the catheter out through the skin (Fig. 12.**11**). Pain therapy can commence postoperatively with an intermittent injection of 20 ml of a long-acting LA. Alternatively continuous local infiltration of the periosteum through an elastomer pump has proved useful. With this type of system, subcutaneous tunneling of the catheter outside the operation area (Fig. 12.**12**) is possible.

Local Anesthetics, Dosage:
Anesthesia (single shot): 20 ml of ropivacaine 0.75 % (7.5 mg/ml).

Analgesia: 20 ml of ropivacaine 0.375 % (3.75 mg/ml) bolus or 5 ml of ropivacaine 0.2 % (2 mg/ml) continuously.

Practical Notes
- Bone chip harvesting from the iliac crest is an operation that causes severe pain postoperatively. Anesthesia should therefore be provided with a long-acting LA.
- Continuous administration is very effective. The elastomer pump system enables insertion outside the operation field and is therefore preferred by some surgeons.

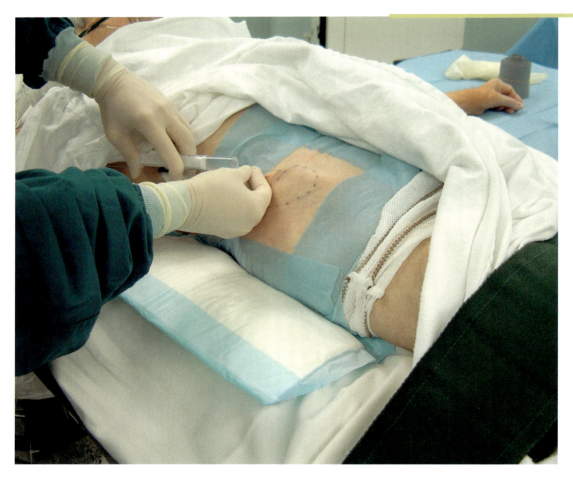

Fig. 12.**9** Infiltration of the iliac crest.

Fig. 12.**10** Infiltration of the iliac crest; the injection must encompass the periosteum.

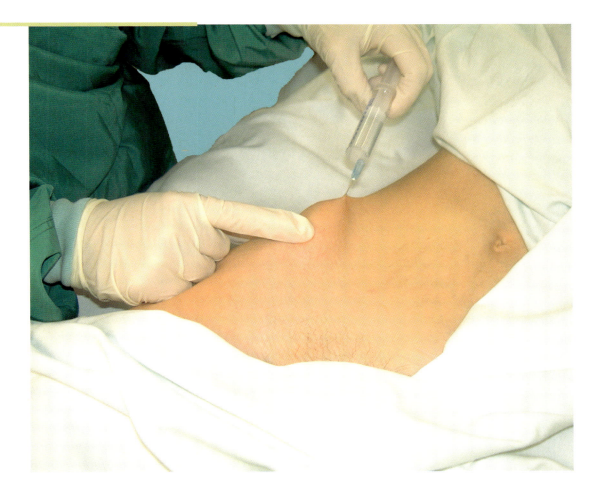

Fig. 12.**11** Inserting a catheter for local pain therapy after harvesting bone chips from the iliac crest.

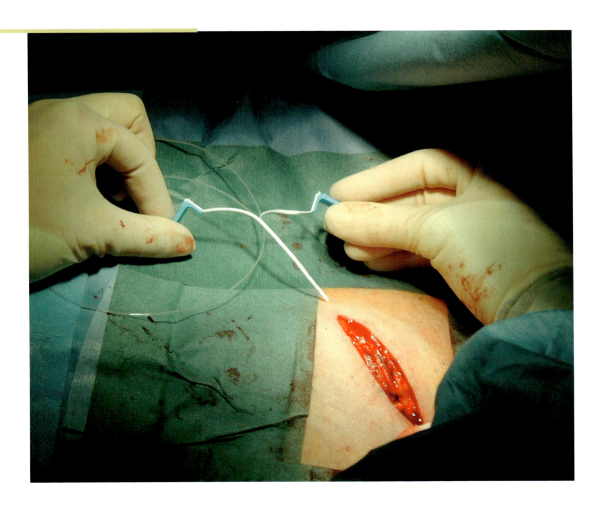

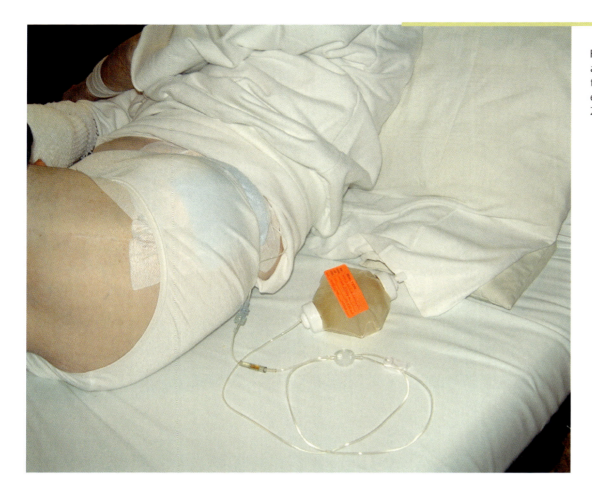

Fig. 12.**12**   Continuous administration of local anesthetic by means of an elastomer pump (ropivacaine 2 mg/ml; 5 ml/h).

12.3   Obturator Nerve Block

Anatomical Overview

The obturator nerve (L2–L4) arises from the lumbar plexus and is a nerve with both sensory and motor fibers. It runs on the medial border of the psoas muscle down through the pelvis, accompanied by the obturator artery and vein. It passes together with these through the obturator foramen and obturator canal to the thigh (Fig. 12.**13**).

Here the nerve divides into the anterior (superficial) branch, which innervates the anterior adductors and the hip joint and ends in a cutaneous main branch that provides a variable sensory supply to the medial side of the thigh; and the posterior (deep) branch (Fig. 12.**14**), which is

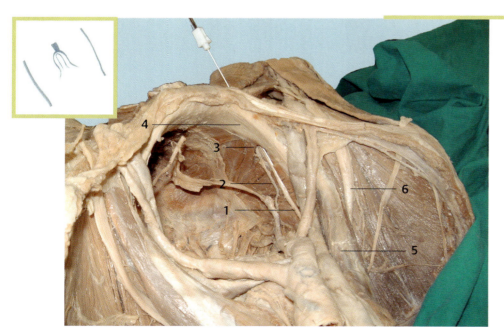

Fig. 12.**13**   View from above into the pelvis minor: the obturator nerve leaves the pelvis minor through the obturator canal together with blood vessels. The further course of the nerve is indicated by a needle introduced into the obturator canal from the external end.

1   Obturator nerve
2   Blood vessels
3   Obturator canal
4   Pubic bone
5   Psoas major
6   Femoral nerve

Fig. 12.**14** The obturator nerve comes from the lumbar plexus, passes separately from the other nerves of the lumbar plexus on the inside of the psoas major muscle, and leaves the pelvis minor through the obturator canal, from where it provides the motor supply to the adductor muscles. The sensory innervation of the obturator nerve is variable: occasionally it is responsible for the sensory supply of medial parts of the knee joint. Whether it can be assigned a sensory area of skin is doubtful; if so, it is on the medial side of the knee. However, there is obvious overlapping with the areas of innervation of other nerves.

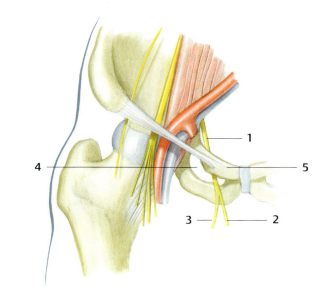

1 Obturator nerve
2 Anterior branch (superficial)
3 Posterior branch (deep)
4 Obturator foramen
5 Pubic bone

Fig. 12.**15** The pubic tubercle is used for orientation in the classical technique of obturator nerve block. The puncture site is located 1.5 cm lateral and 1.5 cm caudal to the pubic tubercle. Note the femoral nerve and sciatic nerve catheters already in situ.

1 Pubic tubercle

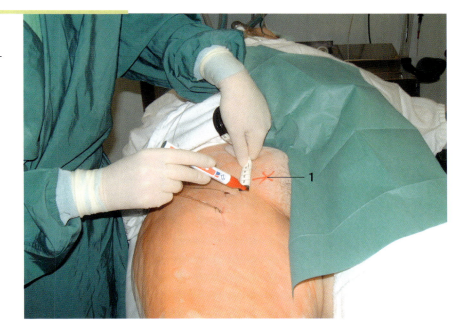

responsible for the posterior adductors and sends a branch to the posterior knee joint.

Technique

Obturator Nerve Block (Classical Technique)

Landmarks and Position
The pubic tubercle is the bony landmark for obturator nerve block. The pubic tubercle on the side to be blocked is palpated and the puncture site is marked 1.5 cm lateral and caudal to the pubic tubercle (Fig. 12.**15**).

The patient lies supine. The leg is slightly abducted.

Procedure
A 22G, 8 cm insulated needle is inserted perpendicular to the underlying surface at the puncture site and advanced (Fig. 12.**16**). After 2-5 cm it reaches the superior ramus of the pubic bone. The distance to the pubic ramus is recorded and the needle is withdrawn somewhat; then the needle is slowly advanced in a more latero-caudal direction (more laterally and only slightly caudally) to 2-3 cm beyond the previously recorded depth. Here it passes the lower border of the pubic ramus and is close to the obturator canal (Figs. 12.**17**, 12.**18**). Following contractions of the adductors at 0.3 mA/0.1 ms and after negative aspiration, 15 ml of a medium-acting or long-acting LA is injected. Because of the proximity of the obturator artery, there is a risk of accidental intravascular injection (Figs. 12.**19**, 12.**20**) and a hematoma may develop. If the needle is advanced too far, it can pass through the obturator canal into the pelvis minor, with the risk of injuring internal organs (Fig. 12.**19**).

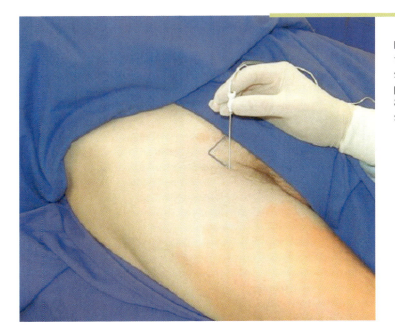

Fig. 12.**16** Obturator nerve block is performed in supine position with the leg slightly abducted. Puncture is performed perpendicular to the underlying surface with an 8 cm insulated needle connected to a nerve stimulator.

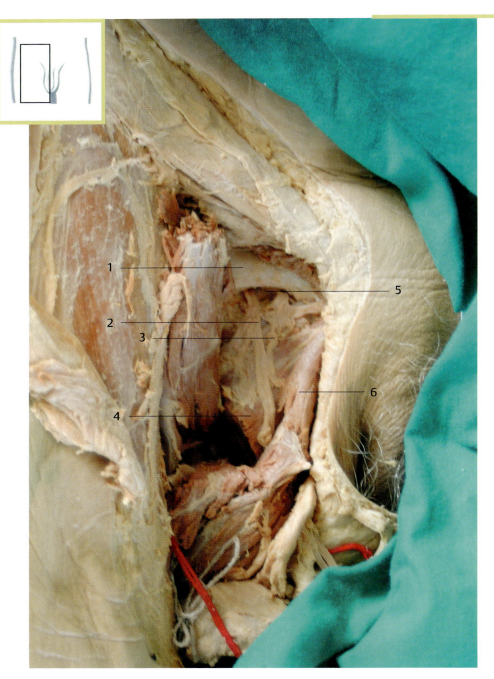

Fig. 12.**17** Right groin region. The obturator nerve leaves the pelvis minor through the obturator canal and immediately divides into its two branches.

1 Superior pubic ramus
2 Obturator nerve
3 Obturator artery
4 Adductor brevis
5 Obturator canal
6 Adductor longus

Fig. 12.**18** Right leg, cranial view. Classical technique of obturator nerve block. After ca. 2–5 cm, the horizontal superior pubic ramus is reached. Following bone contact, the needle is withdrawn somewhat, the distance to the pubic ramus is recorded, and the needle is again advanced in the latero-caudal direction (more laterally and only slightly caudally) 2–3 cm beyond the previously recorded distance. It passes the lower border of the pubic ramus and lies close to the obturator canal. Following contractions of the adductors at a stimulus of 0.3 mA/0.1 ms and after negative aspiration, 15 ml of medium-acting or long-acting LA is injected.

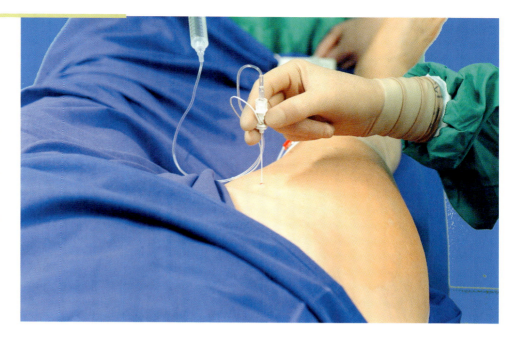

Fig. 12.**19** View from above into the pelvis minor. If the needle is advanced too far, the needle can pass through the obturator canal into the pelvis minor with the risk of injury of internal organs.

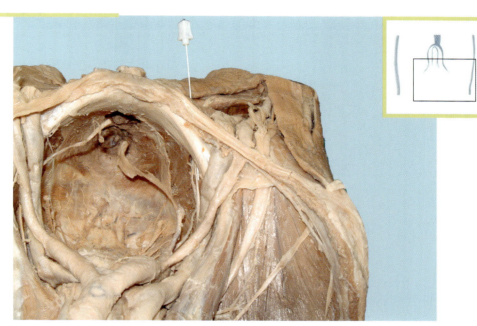

Fig. 12.**20** As the obturator nerve is accompanied by blood vessels when it passes through the obturator canal, vascular puncture with hematoma or intravascular injection of the LA is possible.

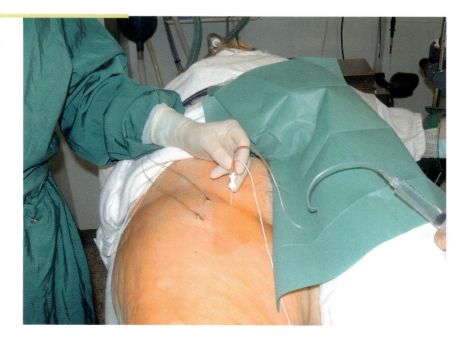

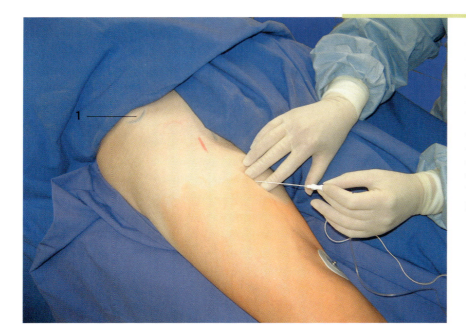

Fig. 12.**21** Alternative technique of obturator nerve block. The proximal attachment (origin) of adductor longus is palpated. Puncture is performed immediately laterally to the tendon origin with an 8–12 cm needle. The needle is directed toward the ipsilateral anterior superior iliac spine; the puncture angle to the long axis of the leg is thus about 45°; the needle direction is slightly dorsal. At a depth of 3–8 cm, contractions of the adductors at 0.3 mA/0.1 ms indicate the proximity of the obturator nerve.

1 Anterior superior iliac spine

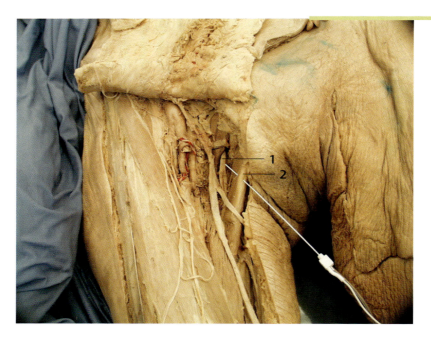

Fig. 12.**22** As Fig. 12.**21**, here in an anatomical dissection.

1 Obturator nerve
2 Tendon of adductor longus

Obturator Nerve Block (Alternative Technique)

Landmarks and Position
Proximal attachment of the tendon of adductor longus, femoral artery, anterior superior iliac spine.
The patient lies supine. The leg on the side to be anesthetized is abducted and externally rotated (Fig. 12.**21**).

Procedure
The proximal attachment (origin) of the tendon of adductor longus is palpated. After disinfection and local anesthesia , puncture is performed with a 22G, 8-12 cm insulated needle immediately lateral to or above the tendon's medial end (Fig. 12.**22**). The needle is directed toward the ipsilateral anterior superior iliac spine. The puncture angle to the long axis of the leg is thus ca. 45°. The needle is then advanced slightly dorsally at an angle of ca. 15-20° (Figs. 12.**21**-12.**24**). At a depth of 3-8 cm, contractions of the adductors at 0.3 mA/0.1 ms indicate contact with the anterior branch of the obturator nerve (Bridenbaugh and Wedel 1998; Meier 1999) (Fig. 12.**25**). After negative aspiration, 15 ml of a medium-acting or long-acting LA is injected. This produces a complete block of both divisions of the obturator nerve. Figure 12.**26** shows the spread toward the obturator canal using a contrast agent. When a continuous technique is performed, the catheter is advanced 3-5 cm cranially through the needle following the main dose injection (Fig. 12.**27**).

Fig. 12.**23** Needle direction for obturator nerve block (alternative technique).

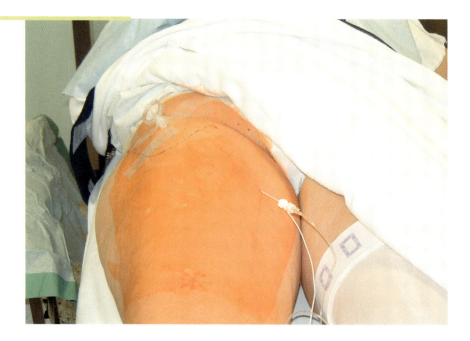

Fig. 12.**24** Obturator nerve block (alternative technique). Right-handed person at the patient's left leg; note indwelling needle for femoral nerve and catheter in situ for sciatic nerve.

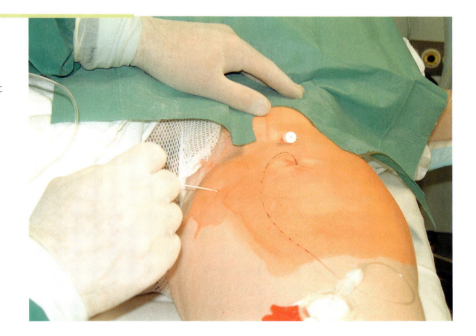

Indications and Contraindications

Indications
- Supplementation for incomplete lumbar plexus blockade.
- Diagnosis and treatment of pain syndromes in the hip and groin (subinguinal) region (Hong et al. 1996).
- Adductor spasm (Vloka and Hadzic 1999).
- Transurethral resection of bladder wall tumors (to eliminate the obturator reflex in spinal anesthesia) (Augspurger and Donohue 1980).

Contraindications
- General contraindications (q.v.).
- Coagulation disorders.

Complications and Side Effects

Intravascular injection, hematoma (mainly with the classical technique), nerve injury (Sunderland 1968).

Practical Notes

- In the classical technique, the contact between the needle tip and the superior pubic ramus ensures that the needle has reached the obturator canal and has not perforated adjacent soft tissues (bladder, vagina) (Bridenbaugh and Wedel 1998) (Fig. 12.**20**).

- Successful block can be identified by the reduced adduction force (Platzer 1999).
- During preparation, it should be ensured that the skin and mucous membranes of the genital region do not come into contact with the disinfectant.
- The *modified technique* has the advantage that the needle direction does not have to be altered and the usually painful contact with periosteum is avoided.
- The *modified technique* enables catheter placement (Meier 1999) (e.g., 19.5G, 120 mm Plexolong catheter set, Pajunk, Germany).
- When the thigh is abducted (*modified technique*) the origin of the adductor longus projects obviously under the skin and

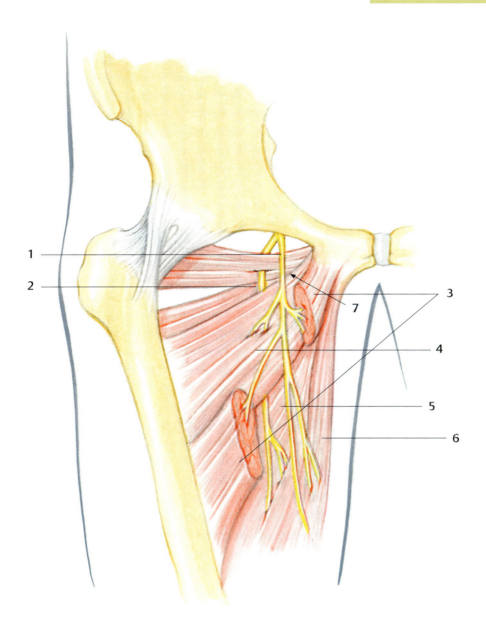

Fig. 12.**25** An alternative technique for blocking the obturator nerve by localizing the nerve behind the tendon of adductor longus. The anterior branch is reached and stimulated; after injection of 10–15 ml of LA there should be a complete block of the two divisions of the nerve. The tendon of adductor longus can always be palpated readily when the leg is slightly abducted.

1 Obturator nerve, anterior branch (superficial)
2 Obturator nerve, posterior branch (deep)
3 Adductor longus
4 Adductor brevis
5 Adductor magnus
6 Gracilis
7 Site of puncture for the alternative technique

the muscle gap between adductor longus and sartorius can be readily palpated (Platzer 1999).

Remarks on the Technique

An accessory obturator nerve arises from the roots of L3 and L4 in 30% of patients (Falsenthal 1974; Sunderland 1968). This was described for the first time by Schmitt in 1744 (Bier 1908). The accessory nerve gives branches to the hip and does not pass through the obturator foramen but runs together with the femoral nerve and can thus also be blocked by a femoral nerve block (Cousins and Bridenbaugh 1998). If adductor spasm persists although the obturator nerve has been anesthetized, this can be attributable to the accessory branch of

the nerve (Vloka and Hadzic 1999). To achieve adequate block of the obturator nerve, a volume of 10-15 ml of LA is required (Auberger and Niesel 1982; Bonica 1980; Hoffmann and Meyer 1980; Jenkner 1983; Löfström 1980; Paul et al. 1996). Yazaki et al. (1985) injected 1% (10 mg/ml) lidocaine at the point of maximum adductor contraction with electrical stimulation until the muscle response disappeared completely. With this procedure 96% of 78 blocks were successful. This agrees with the results of Parks and Kennedy (1967), who have reported a success rate of over 95%.

It is often assumed that neuraxial anesthesia leads to elimination of the obturator reflex. This is not the case as the interruption of nerve is blocked proximal to the transurethral electrical stimulus. Particularly in urological operations (e.g., transurethral

resection of bladder wall tumors) under spinal anesthesia, a supplementary obturator nerve block can therefore be rational in order to suppress an obturator reflex (Augspurger and Donohue 1980; Gasparich et al. 1984).

An important practical indication is selective block of the obturator nerve in incomplete lumbar plexus anesthesia. This applies particularly to the so-called "3-in-1 block". The sensory supply of the medial side of the thigh is very variable and is therefore unsuitable for monitoring the success of an obturator block (Bergmann 1994; Geiger et al. 2000; Morris and Lang 1999). The spread of the zone of analgesia can extend from the medial side of the thigh to the upper tibial third of the lower leg, but in some cases the sensory area of skin can be so small that cutaneous anesthesia is absent, even though

Fig. 12.**26** Spread of contrast after obturator nerve block (alternative technique).

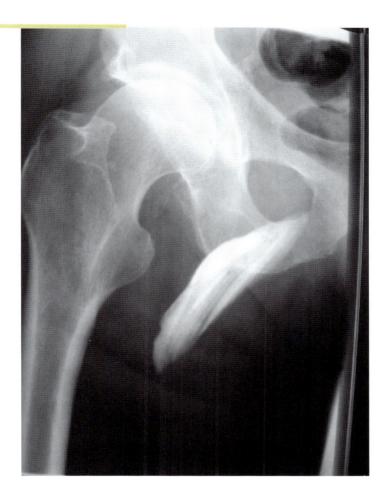

Fig. 12.**27** With the alternative technique of obturator nerve block, an indwelling catheter can also be introduced.

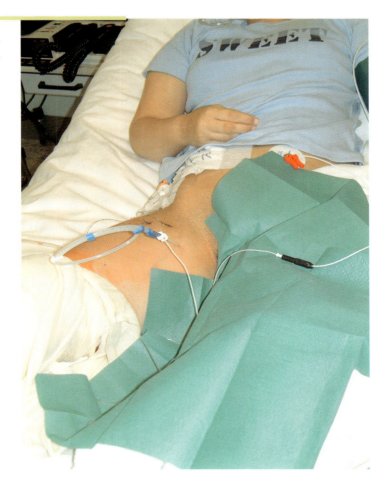

motor block of the adductors indicates an adequate block. However, an insufficient block can lead to pain problems when using a thigh tourniquet, depending on the extent of skin innervation (Vloka and Hadzic 1999). The extent to which the knee joint periosteum is supplied by the obturator nerve is not completely clear. If a patient complains of pain particularly on the medial side of the knee after an inguinal paravascular 3-in-1 block for a knee operation, an insufficient

block of the obturator nerve should be suspected (see also Chapter 9? on inguinal paravascular block). If selective anesthesia of the nerve is successfully performed in this case, the block serves as both diagnosis and pain therapy . This also applies for the diagnosis of pain in the hip region (Trainer et al. 1986). Anesthesia of the obturator nerve in patients with hemiparesis and adductor spasm can be very effective. The variant of the technique (see above) is a development

of a technique described by Wassef (1992), who described it as an "interadductor approach"; this has been performed successfully in quadriplegia and multiple sclerosis for the treatment of adductor spasm. The development leads to simplification of the technical procedure, enables placement of a catheter, and expands the range of indications for the method (Büttner and Meier 1999; Meier and Büttner 2001).

12.4   Saphenous Nerve Block

Anatomical Overview

The saphenous nerve (L2/L4) is the sensory terminal branch of the femoral nerve. The saphenous nerve passes as far as the adductor hiatus together with the femoral artery and femoral vein. In this region, the blood vessels pass further through the adductor canal into the popliteal fossa.

However, the nerve continues behind the sartorius muscle in the subsartorial fat, separated from the blood vessels (Fig. 12.**28**) and penetrates the fascia lata (knee fascia) medial to the sartorius tendon at the level of the patella (Fig. 12.**29**). As a superficial cutaneous nerve, it divides below the knee (Figs. 12.**30**, 12.**31**) and the main branch accompanies the long saphenous vein as far

as the medial malleolus or even beyond it (Fig. 12.**32**).
The saphenous nerve innervates the skin of the inside of the lower leg from the knee to just below the medial malleolus on the dorsum of the foot and even reaches as far as the great toe in up to 20% of cases (Morris and Lang 1999).

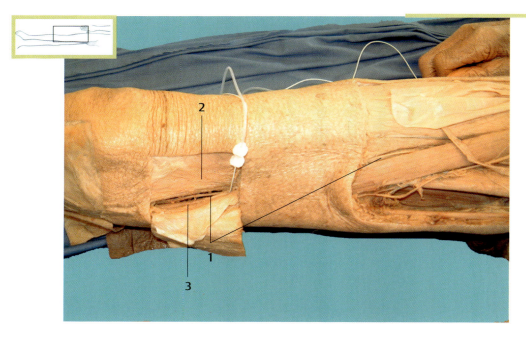

Fig. 12.**28**   Right thigh, medial view. The saphenous nerve (L2/L4) is the sensory terminal branch of the femoral nerve. It runs together with the femoral artery and femoral vein as far as the adductor hiatus. In this region, the blood vessels run further through the adductor canal into the popliteal fossa. However, the saphenous nerve continues separately from the vessels behind the sartorius in the subsartorial fat through the gap between vastus medialis and sartorius. It provides the sensory supply to the inside of the lower leg, and occasionally the area of innervation can extend as far as the great toe.

1   Saphenous nerve
2   Vastus medialis
3   Sartorius

Fig. 12.**29** Right knee, medial view. The
saphenous nerve runs under the sartorius
muscle, crosses under it, and passes through
the fascia lata (knee fascia) behind its tendon
at the level of the patella.

1 Saphenous nerve
2 Sartorius

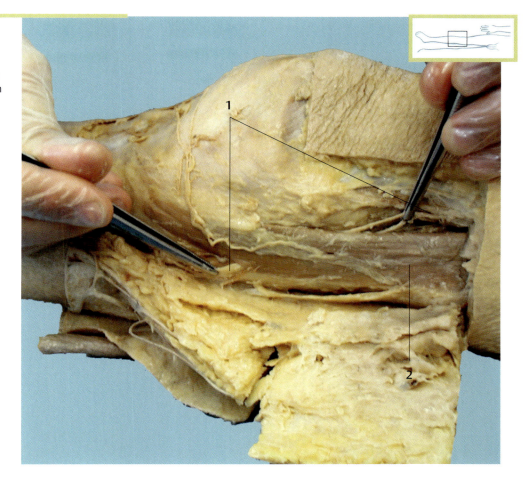

Fig. 12.**30** The saphenous nerve runs under
the sartorius muscle, crosses under it, and
passes through the fascia lata (knee fascia)
behind its tendon at the level of the patella.
As a superficial cutaneous nerve, it branches
below the knee and accompanies the long
saphenous vein as far as the medial malleolus or beyond it.

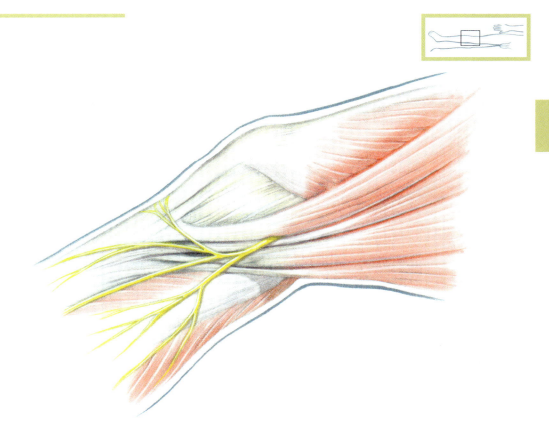

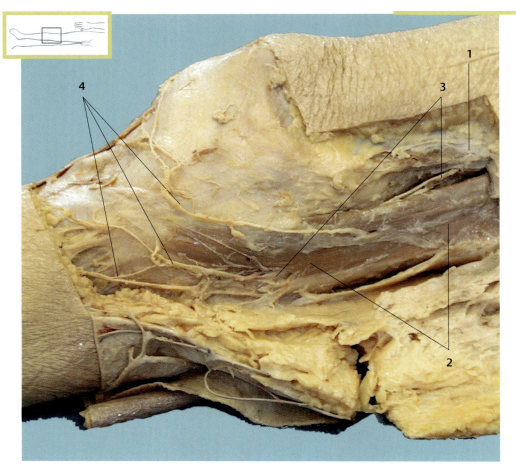

Fig. 12.**31** Anatomical dissection, same view as Fig. 12.**30**.

1 Vastus medialis
2 Sartorius
3 Saphenous nerve
4 Prepatellar branches of the saphenous nerve

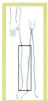

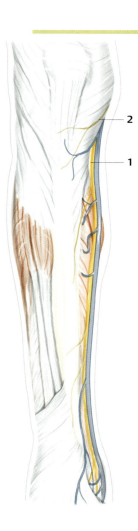

Fig. 12.**32** The main branch of the saphenous nerve runs superficially together with the long saphenous vein on the belly of gastrocnemius. (From Platzer: *Taschenatlas der Anatomie* [*Pocket Atlas of Anatomy*], Vol. 7. Stuttgart: Thieme; 1999.)

1 Long saphenous vein with saphenous nerve
2 Prepatellar branches of the saphenous nerve

Fig. 12.**33**   Technique of (classical) saphenous nerve block. The tibial tuberosity is palpated. Following disinfection, subcutaneous infiltration with 5–10 ml of LA is performed with a 6 cm long 24G needle from the tuberosity toward the medial head of gastrocnemius.

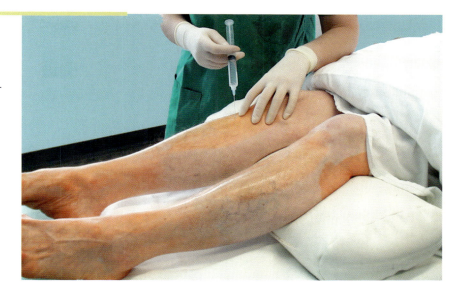

Fig. 12.**34**   The injection must extend to the border of gastrocnemius (see also Fig. 12.**35**). Depending on the length of the needle, moving the needle (new puncture) may be necessary (possibly several times).

1   Tibial tuberosity
2   Belly of the gastrocnemius

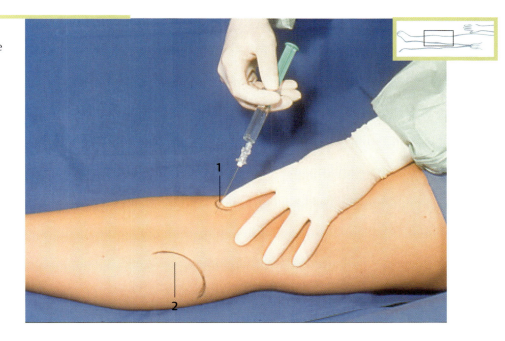

Fig. 12.**35**   The main branch of the saphenous nerve runs superficially together with the long saphenous vein on the belly of gastrocnemius and this is where the main depot of LA must be placed.

1   Long saphenous vein with saphenous nerve
2   Prepatellar branches of the saphenous nerve
3   Location of main depot of local anesthetic

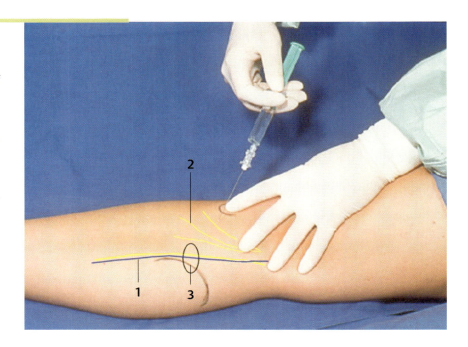

Technique

Saphenous Nerve Block (Classical Technique "Below-the-Knee Field Block")

Landmarks and Position

Tibial tuberosity, medial head of gastrocnemius.
The patient lies supine with the leg extended. A small pad (or pillow) can be placed under the knee (Fig. 12.**33**).

Procedure

The tibial tuberosity is palpated. After disinfecting the skin, a subcutaneous infiltration is performed between the tuberosity toward the medial head of gastrocnemius with a 6 cm long 24G needle and 5-10 ml of LA (Fig. 12.**34**).

- The technique is simple infiltration anesthesia.
- The main depot should be injected around the long saphenous vein, which runs in the angle between the belly of gastrocnemius and the tibia; this is where the main branch of the saphenous nerve runs (Fig. 12.**35**).

- Intermittent aspiration tests should be performed to exclude accidental injection into the saphenous vein.
- The injection can be painful due to periosteal contact by the needle tip, as there is very thin subcutaneous tissue over the tibia.

Transsartorial Technique of Saphenous Nerve Block

The transsartorial technique is a compartment block of the saphenous nerve between the sartorius muscle and vastus medialis (intermuscular vastoadductor septum) (Platzer 1999) (Fig. 12.**36**).

Landmarks and Position

Medial side of the thigh, patella, vastus medialis and sartorius muscles.
The patient lies supine and the leg to be anesthetized is stretched and relaxed.

Procedure

For anatomical orientation, the patient is asked to extend the leg actively. This causes the sartorius and vastus medialis muscles to contract. The outlines of the two muscles are readily palpable on the medial side of the thigh (Fig. 12.**37**). The puncture site is 3-4 cm superior and 6-8 cm posterior to the superomedial border cranial to the upper border of the patella in the muscle gap between the sartorius and vastus medialis (Benzon 2005).

Following disinfection, infiltration anesthesia, and skin prepuncture, a 22G or 19.5G needle is advanced on the medial side of the thigh in the gap between the sartorius muscle and vastus medialis until a loss of resistance after ca. 2-4 cm indicates that the needle tip is in the correct position in the subsartorial fat (Figs. 12.**38**-12.**40**). Following successful aspiration, 10 ml of a medium-acting to long-acting LA is injected. For the continuous technique, a 20G catheter is advanced 3-5 cm through the 19.5G needle following the LA injection (Fig. 12.**41**). Alternatively, the space can be found through the sartorius muscle; in this case the needle passes through the sartorius until an appropriate loss of resistance is felt after 2-4 cm. This is the explanation of the term "transsartorial technique."

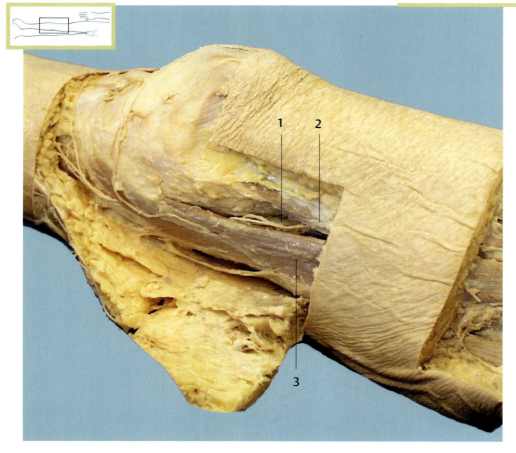

Fig. 12.**36** Right knee, medial view. Transsartorial technique of saphenous nerve block. The transsartorial technique is a compartment block of the saphenous nerve between the sartorius muscle and the intermuscular vastoadductor septum. About two fingers above the upper border of the patella the space between vastus medialis and sartorius is found. The saphenous nerve runs in this space behind the sartorius muscle.

1 Saphenous nerve
2 Vastus medialis
3 Sartorius

Fig. 12.**37** Transsartorial technique of saphenous nerve block. The transsartorial technique is a compartment block of the saphenous nerve between the sartorius and the intermuscular vastoadductor septum. About two fingers above the upper border of the patella the space between vastus medialis and sartorius is found. The saphenous nerve runs in this space behind the sartorius muscle.

1 Patella
2 Vastus medialis
3 Sartorius

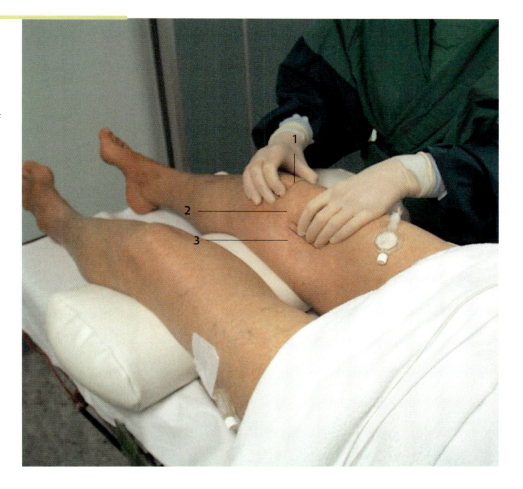

Fig. 12.**38** In the gap between vastus medialis and sartorius the needle is advanced about 3–4 cm superior and 6–8 cm posterior to the superomedial border of the patella behind the sartorius until a loss of resistance after ca. 2–4 cm, which indicates that the tip of the needle is in the correct position in the subsartorial fat. Following negative aspiration, 10 ml of a medium-acting to long-acting LA is injected.

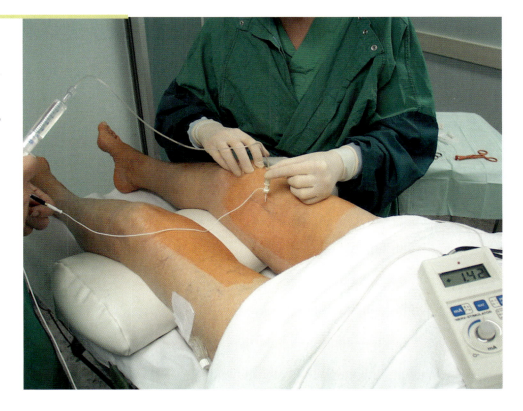

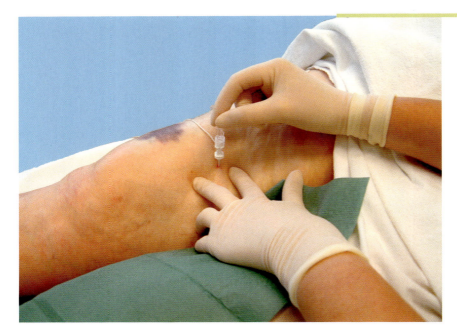

Fig. 12.**39** In the gap between vastus medialis and sartorius the needle is advanced about three fingers proximal to the medial knee joint line behind the sartorius until a loss of resistance after ca. 2–4 cm indicates that the tip of the needle is in the correct position in the subsartorial fat. Following negative aspiration, 10 ml of a medium-acting to long-acting LA is injected. Right-handed persons can stand on the patient's left side to perform a block of the right leg.

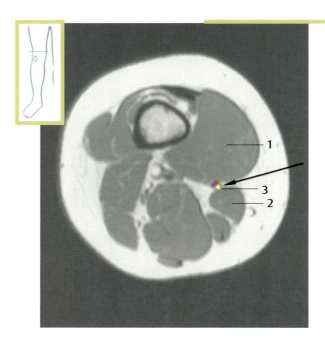

Fig. 12.**40** MRI section through the right thigh at the level of transsartorial saphenous nerve block, caudal view.

1　Vastus medialis
2　Sartorius
3　Saphenous nerve

- The advantage of this technique is that it is almost pain-free (no periosteal contact) and has a greater success rate than the classical approach (Benzon 2005; Morris et al. 1997).
- As this is a "loss-of-resistance technique," use of a needle with a short bevel is recommended.
- The technique can also be performed with PNS (Comfort et al. 1996), (Fig. 12.**42**).
- The technique enables a perineural catheter to be placed (Meier and Büttner 2001) (Fig. 12.**41**).

Indications and Contraindications

Indications
- Supplement for incomplete lumbar plexus block (in the distal innervation region of the femoral nerve).
- Combination with distal sciatic block (q.v.) or popliteal block (lower leg tourniquet, operations in the region of the medial lower leg, varicose vein surgery).
- Operations and pain therapy in the region of the medial lower leg (e.g., muscle biopsy, skin graft harvesting) (Fig. 12.**43**).

Contraindications
No special contraindications. Relative: marked varicosity.

Complications and Side Effects

There are no reported special side effects or complications.

Remarks on the Technique

The transsartorial technique was described in 1993 by Van der Wahl as a "loss-of-resistance" (LOR) method. In 1997 Morris et al. reported a 100% success rate with transsartorial saphenous nerve block in 80 patients. The block was performed with 10 ml lidocaine 1.5% (15 mg/ml) with epinephrine 1 : 200000, and the onset of effect was within 5 minutes.

Fig. 12.**41** The transsartorial technique can also be performed as a continuous technique with a catheter.

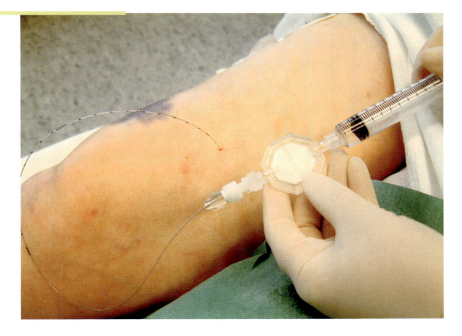

Fig. 12.**42** The transsartorial technique can usefully be assisted by a nerve stimulator. The sensory saphenous nerve runs together with a motor branch from the femoral nerve, which innervates the vastus medialis muscle, so the nerve branch to vastus medialis can be stimulated. Contractions of vastus medialis indicate that the tip of the needle is in the correct position and injection of the LA will block both nerves.

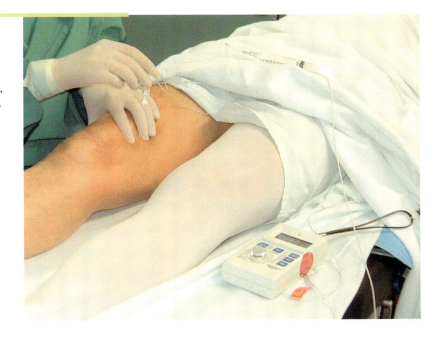

Fig. 12.**43** Case example of a patient with an extremely painful soft-tissue disease in the lower leg. A distal sciatic catheter alone did not bring adequate relief; complete freedom from pain was not achieved until after a saphenous nerve block via a transsartorial catheter.

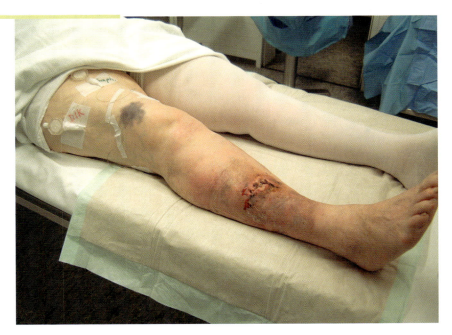

For the patient, the transsartorial technique offers the advantage of an almost pain-free procedure as the periosteum of the tibia is not touched by the needle. Saphenous nerve block below the knee (classical technique) has the relatively common disadvantage of resulting in an inadequate block. According to Morris, the classical technique of saphenous nerve block has a success rate of only 39% (Morris and Lang 1999). Mansour reported on subsartorial block of the saphenous nerve in 1993. In comparison with the transsartorial technique, the subsartorial technique described by Mansour is difficult to perform with regard to the given landmarks and position of the patient (Bouaziz et al. 1999). However, an interesting observation of Mansour's was the combination with peripheral nerve stimulation. Here he made use of the fact that the sensory saphenous nerve runs together with a motor branch from the femoral nerve which innervates the vastus medialis muscle. The motor nerve to the vastus medialis can be found by nerve stimulation. Contractions of vastus medialis indicate the correct position of the needle tip, and injection 5–10 ml of LA will block the two nerves. In a pilot study, the success rate was 80% (Bouaziz et al. 1999). Another possibility for verifying that the needle is in the correct position is stimulation of the sensory saphenous nerve; a pulse duration of 1.0 ms should be selected. If the tip of the needle is in the correct position, the patient reports tingling paresthesia in the innervation area of the saphenous nerve. For clinical practice, a combination of the LOR method (van der Wahl) with peripheral nerve stimulation (contractions of the vastus muscle) as described by Mansour is optimal for saphenous nerve block. In this way, the advantages of both methods are exploited (Meier and Büttner 2001).

Peripheral nerve stimulation can be used for diagnostic block of the saphenous nerve, e.g., in saphenous neuralgia. If the sensory saphenous nerve is sought exclusively, a pulse duration of 1.0 ms and cooperation of the patient under instruction are required (Defalque and McDanal 1994).

The transsartorial technique was originally described as a single-shot technique. So far, no study has been published of a continuous technique of transsartorial saphenous nerve block. However, catheter placement is easy to perform with the transsartorial approach (e.g., 19.5G, 60 mm Plexolong catheter set, Pajunk, Germany) (Büttner and Meier 1999). The catheter is advanced 3 cm into the subsartorial space. This possibility expands the indications for saphenous nerve block beyond supplementary block in the case of incomplete lumbar plexus anesthesia or combined anesthesia in foot block. A catheter technique can usefully be employed, e.g., in neuralgic disorders or inadequate wound healing or for plastic surgery (skin grafting, ulcers, burns, etc.).

12.5 Fibular Nerve Block

(Synonym: peroneal nerve block. Note on anatomical nomenclature: the terms fibular nerve and peroneal nerve are synonymous.)

Anatomical Overview

The common fibular nerve (L4–L5 and S1–S2) has both sensory and motor nerve fibers and is the smaller of the two terminal branches of the sciatic nerve. It runs initially between the tendon of the biceps femoris and the lateral head of gastrocnemius, then passes around the head of the fibula and subsequently lies on the bone immediately under the fascia (Figs. 12.**44**, 12.**45**).

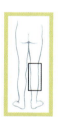

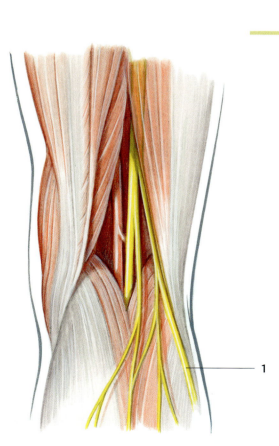

Fig. 12.**44**   Right popliteal fossa. The common fibular nerve (L4–L5 and S1–S2) has both sensory and motor nerve fibers and is the smaller of the two terminal branches of the sciatic nerve. It runs initially between the tendon of the biceps femoris muscle and the lateral head of the gastrocnemius muscle, then passes around the head of the fibula and subsequently lies on the bone immediately under the fascia. The common fibular nerve provides the sensory supply to the knee, the skin of the lateral lower leg, the ankle, and the heel. It provides motor innervation to the muscles of the anterolateral lower leg and is responsible for dorsiflexion and pronation of the foot.

1   Common fibular nerve

The common fibular nerve is the sensory supply to parts of the knee, the skin of the lateral lower leg, the ankle, and the heel (see Fig. 7.**7**). It provides motor innervation to the muscles of the anterolateral lower leg and is responsible for dorsiflexion and pronation of the foot (Fig. 12.**46**).

Technique

Fibular Nerve Block (Dorsal Technique)

Landmarks and Position
The leg to be anesthetized is bent slightly and the head of the fibula is marked. The patient lies supine.

Procedure
The head of the fibula is palpated. Following disinfection and local infiltration anesthesia, the puncture is made 2 cm caudal and dorsal to the head of the fibula vertically to the skin (Figs. 12.**47**, 12.**48**). The short 24G or 22G insulated needle is advanced cautiously until it is felt to penetrate the fascia or the

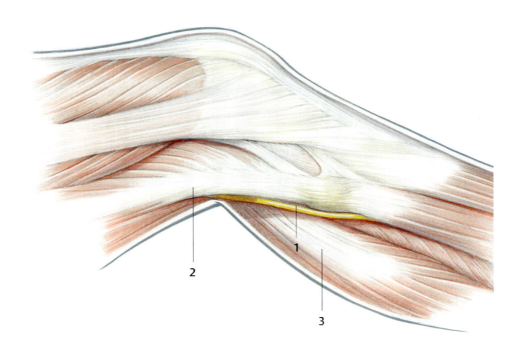

Fig. 12.**45**   Right knee, lateral view. The common fibular nerve runs initially between the tendon of the biceps femoris muscle and the lateral head of the gastrocnemius muscle, then passes around the head of the fibula and subsequently lies on the bone immediately under the fascia.

   1   Common fibular nerve
   2   Tendon of biceps femoris
   3   Lateral head of gastrocnemius muscle

Fig. 12.**46**   The response to stimulation of the common fibular nerve consists of dorsiflexion and pronation of the foot.

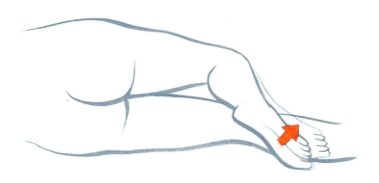

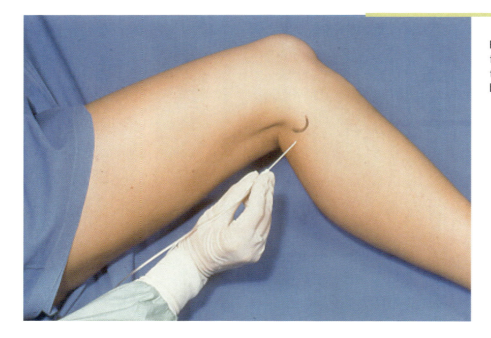

Fig. 12.**47** The common fibular nerve is found immediately distal and posterior to the head of the fibula. To do this, the leg is bent slightly.

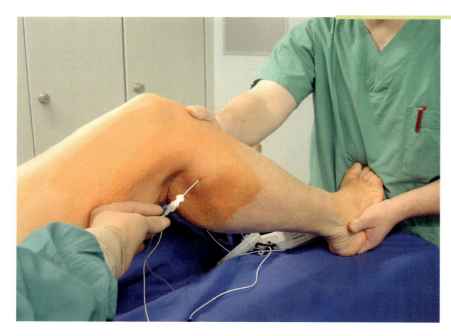

Fig. 12.**48** An assistant to hold the leg can be helpful.

motor response of the common fibular nerve (dorsiflexion of the foot) becomes visible (Fig. 12.**49**). This is followed by injection of 2–5 ml of LA (Fig. 12.**50**). Paresthesia should not occur.

Fibular Nerve Block (Lateral Technique)

Landmarks and Position
The patient lies supine with the legs extended (or bent slightly).

Procedure
Following skin disinfection, a fine needle is inserted ca. 2 cm distal and dorsal to the head of the fibula (Fig. 12.**51**). The needle is advanced ca. 1 cm in a mediocaudal direction until a response is produced and a LA depot is placed in the space behind the head of the fibula (Hoerster 1988).

Indications and Contraindications

Indications
- Incomplete anesthesia after proximal block of the sciatic nerve
- Diagnostic block.
- Pain therapy

Contraindication
Relative: nerve lesion (previous documentation required).

Complications and Side Effects

Neuropathy (intraneural injection and pressure injury due to excessive volume of local anesthetic must be avoided).

Practical Notes

- As the nerve reacts very sensitively to paresthesia—in the literature there are reports of persistent dysesthesia—PNS is recommended.
- Successful block leads to paresis of the dorsiflexors ("foot drop").

Fig. 12.**49**   The block should be performed with the aid of a nerve stimulator.

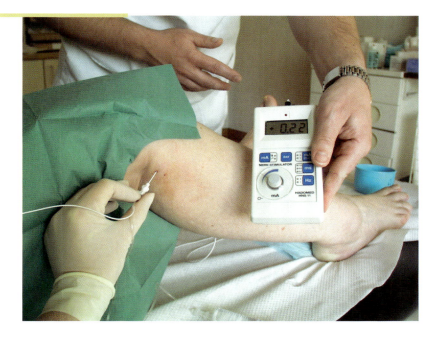

Fig. 12.**50**   A volume of 2–5 ml of local anesthetic is sufficient.

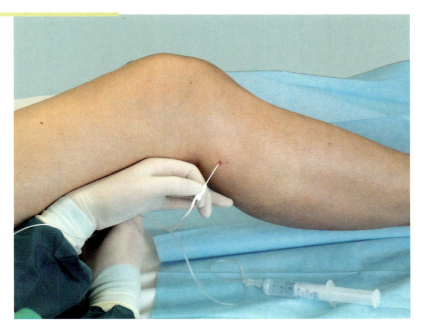

Fig. 12.**51**   The common fibular nerve can also be blocked with the leg extended. Here, too, the nerve is found just distal and posterior to the head of the fibula.

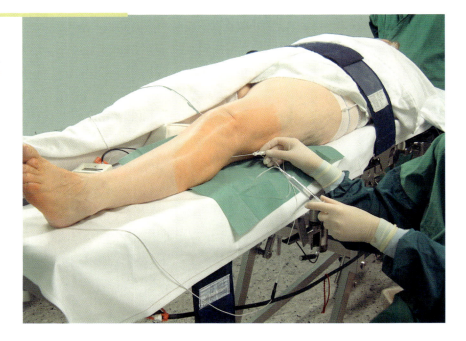

Remarks on the Technique

The fibular nerve can in principle be blocked over its entire course through the popliteal fossa to distal to the head of the fibula. In their anatomical investigations, Snyder et al. (1989) found the nerve constantly 0.5 cm (to 1 cm) medial to the most prominent (posterior) part of the head of the fibula and medial to the tendon of the biceps femoris. A number of variations for blocking the fibular nerve at the knee have been described. An injection of 5-10 ml of LA is adequate for anesthesia. It should be noted that anesthesia of the outside of the lower leg and the dorsum of the foot can be obtained, but the lateral border of the foot is supplied by the sural nerve and this nerve may have to be blocked in addition. The techniques can be subdivided into blocks in the region of the popliteal fossa (see Chapter 11; Adriani 1951; Lecron 1990; Wassef 1989), the head of the fibula (Adriani 1951; Hoerster 1988; Sparks and Higeleo 1989), and distal to the head of the fibula in the fibular extensor compartment (Zinke 1985). The two methods described are easily learned and are regarded as safe (Niesel 1994). Fibular neuritis and fibular paresis have been described as a complication of fibular nerve block (Hoerster 1988). In fibular paresis, pressure injury due to position or a lesion as a result of a tourniquet must be considered (Moore et al. 1994; Stöhr 1996). The most elegant and often the best technique for practical purposes consists in block of the common fibular nerve in the proximal part of the popliteal fossa together with the tibial nerve (see Chapter 11.3).

References

Adriani J. Local and regional anesthesia for minor surgery. Surg Clin North Am. 1951;31:1507.
Auberger HG, Niesel HC. Praktische Lokalanästhesie. 4th ed. Stuttgart: Thieme; 1982:11-127.
Augspurger R, Donohue RE. Prevention of obturator nerve stimulation during transurethral surgery. J Urol. 1980;123:170-1.
Benzon HT, Sharma S, Calimaran A. Comparison of the different approaches to saphenous nerve block. Anesthesiology. 2005;102:633-8
Bergmann RA. Compendium of human anatomic variations. Munich: Urban & Schwarzenberg; 1994:143-7.
Bier A. Über einen neuen Weg Lokalanästhesie an den Gliedmaßen zu erzeugen. Arch Klin Chir. 1908;86:1007.
Bonica JJ. The management of pain. Philadelphia: Lea and Febiger; 1980:1205-9.
Bonica JJ. Local anesthesia and regional blocks. In: Wall PD, Melzack R, eds. Textbook of pain. Edinburgh: Churchill Livingstone; 1984:541-57.
Bonniot A. Anatomie du plexus lombaire chez l'homme [Thesis]. Lyon; 1922/23.
Bouaziz H, Narchi P, Zetlaoui PJ, Paqueron X, Benhamou D. Lateral approach to the sciatic nerve at the popliteal fossa combined with saphenous nerve block. Techniques in Regional Anesthesia and Pain Management. 1999;3:19-22.
Bridenbaugh PhO, Wedel DJ. The lower extremity. In: Cousins MJ, Bridenbaugh PhO. eds. Neural blockade in clinical anesthesia and management of pain. 3rd ed. Philadelphia: Lippincott-Raven; 1998:373-409.
Büttner J, Meier G. Kontinuierliche periphere Techniken zur Regionalanästhesie und Schmerztherapie - Obere und untere Extremität. Bremen: UNI-MED-Verlag; 1999.
Comfort A, Kim V, Lang S, Yip R. Saphenous nerve anesthesia: a nerve stimulator technique. Can J Anaesth. 1996;43:852-7.
Cousins MJ, Bridenbaugh PhO. Neural blockade. In: Cousins MJ, Bridenbaugh PO, eds. Neural blockade in clinical anesthesia and management of pain. 3rd ed. Philadelphia: Lippincott-Raven; 1998:378-88.
Defalque RJ, McDanal JT. Proximal saphenous neuralgia after coronary bypass. Reg Anesth. 1994;(A)19:90.
Ellis H, Feldman S. Anatomy for Anesthetists. 7th ed. Cambridge: Blackwell Science; 1996.
Falsenthal G. Nerve blocks in the lower extremities: Anatomic considerations. Arch Phys Med Rehabil. 1974;55:504-7.
Gasparich JP, Mason JT, Berger RE. Use of nerve stimulator for simple and accurate obturator nerve block before transurethral resection. J Urol. 1984;132:291-3.
Geiger M, Wild M, Bartl A, Völk C, Kunz C, Mehrkens HH. 3-in-1 block—reality or fantasy? Int Monitor Reg Anesth. 2000;(A)12:74.
Hallén J, Rawal N, Harrtvig P. Pharmacokinetic and pharmacodynamic studies of 11C-lidocaine following intravenous regional anesthesia (IVRA) using positron emission tomography. Acta Anaesthesiol Scand. 1991;35:214.
Hoerster W. Blockaden im Bereich des Fußgelenkes. In: Astra Chemicals GmbH, ed. Regionalanästhesie. Stuttgart: Gustav Fischer; 1988:133-9.
Hoffmann P, Meyer O. Der Obturatoriusreflex und seine Ausschaltung durch gezielte Blockade. Reg Anaesth. 1980;3:55-6.
Hong Y, OT, Lopresti D, Carlson C. Diagnostic obturator nerve block for inguinal and back pain: A recovered opinion. Pain. 1996;67:507-9.
Hovelacque A. Anatomie des nerfs craniens et rachidiens du système grand sympathique chez l'homme. Paris: Doin; 1927:534-638.
Jenkner FL. Nervenblockaden. 4th ed. Wien: Springer; 1983:65-75.
Konder H, Moysich F, Mattusch. Akzidentelle motorische Blockade des N. cutaneus femoris lateralis. Reg Anaesth. 1990;13:122-3.
Lecron L. Anesthésie du membre inférieur. In: Lecron L, ed. Anesthésie loco-regionale. 2nd ed. Paris: Arnette; 1990:327-48.
Löfström B. Blockaden der peripheren Nerven des Beines. In: Eriksson E, ed. Atlas der Lokalanästhesie. 2nd ed. Berlin: Springer; 1980:101-15.
Lonsdale M. 3-in-1 block: Confirmation of Winnie's anatomical hypothesis. Anesth Analg. 1988;67:601-2.
Mansour NY. Re-evaluating the sciatic nerve block: Another landmark for consideration. Reg Anesth. 1993;18:322-3.
Meier G. Technik der kontinuierlichen anterioren Ischiadicusblockade (KAI). In: Büttner J, Meier G, eds. Kontinuierliche periphere Techniken zur Regionalanästhesie und Schmerztherapie - Obere und untere Extremität. Bremen: UNI-MED-Verlag; 1999:132-7.
Meier G, Büttner J. Regionalanästhesie - Kompendium der peripheren Blockaden. Munich: Arcis; 2001.
Meier G, Bauereis Ch, Meier Th, Maurer H, Huber Ch. Schmerztherapie mit distalen Ischiadicuskathetern - Anatomische Voraussetzungen. Schmerz. 1999;13(S1):75.
Moore DC, Multoy MF, Thompson GE. Peripheral nerve damage and regional anesthesia [Editorial]. Br J Anaesth. 1994;73:435-6.
Morris GF, Lang SA. Innovations in lower extremity blockade. Techniques in Regional Anesthesia and Pain Management. 1999;3:9-18.
Morris GF, Lang SA, Dust WN, Van der Wal M. The parasacral sciatic nerve block. Reg Anesth. 1997;22:100-4.
Niesel HCh, ed. Regionalanästhesie, Lokalanästhesie, Regionale Schmerztherapie. Stuttgart: Thieme; 1994.
Parks CR, Kennedy WF. Obturator nerve block: a simplified approach. Anesthesiology. 1967;28:775.
Paul W, Wiesner D, Drechsler HJ. Postoperative pain after total knee replacement: Obturator nerve block may be needed additionally to sciatic and high volume femoral nerve block. Int. Monitor Reg Anaesth. 1996;8(3):31-2.
Platzer W. Taschenatlas der Anatomie - Bewegungsapparat. 7th ed. Stuttgart: Thieme; 1999.
Rosenquist RW, Lederhaas G. Femoral and lateral femoral cutaneous nerve block. Techniques in Regional Anesthesia and Pain Management. 1999;3:33-8.
Rybock JD. Diagnostic and therapeutic nerve blocks. In: Tollison CD, ed. Handbook of chronic pain management. Baltimore: Williams and Wilkins. 1989;115-224.
Shannon J, Lang SA, Yip RW. Lateral femoral cutaneous nerve block revisited: A nerve stimulator technique. Reg Anesth. 1995;20:100-4.
Sharrock NE. Inadvertent "3-in-1 block" following injection of the lateral cutaneous nerve of the thigh. Anesth Analg. 1980;59:887-8.
Snyder MD, DeBoard JW, Beger TH, Gibbons JJ. Anatomy of the common peroneal nerve at the knee: A cadaver study. Reg Anesth. 1989;(S)14:38.
Sparks CJ, Higeleo T. Foot surgery in Vanuata: Results of combined tibial common peroneal and saphenous nerve blocks in fifty-six adults. Anesth Intens Care. 1989:17;336-9.
Stöhr M. Iatrogene Nervenläsionen: Injektionen, Operation, Lagerung, Strahlentherapie. 2nd ed. Stuttgart: Thieme:1996.
Sunderland S. Obturator nerve In: Sunderland S (ed.). Nerves and nerve injuries. Edinburgh: Livingstone; 1968:1096-109.
Trainer N, Bowser BL, Dahm L. Obturator nerve block for painful hip in adult cerebral palsy. Arch Phys Med Rehabil. 1986;67:829-30.
Van der Wahl M, Scott AL, Ray WY. Transsartorial approach for saphenous nerve block. Can J Anaesth. 1993;40:542-6.
Vloka JD, Hadzic A. Obturator and genitofemoral nerve blocks. Techniques in Regional Anesthesia and Pain Management. 1999;3:28-32.
Wassef MR The suprapopliteal approach for sciatic nerve block: Effect of needle placement on success rate at sensory nerve distribution. Reg Anesth. 1989;(S)14:88.
Wassef MR. Interadductor approach to obturator nerve blockade for spastic conditions of adductor thigh muscles. Reg Anesth. 1992;18:13-7.
Yazaki T, Ishikawa H, Kanoh S, Koiso K. Accurate obturator nerve block in transurethral surgery. Urology. 1985;26 588.
Zinke R. Die perivasale Anästhetikuminfiltration als einfache Methode zur peripheren Sympathikusblockade bei Schmerzzuständen der Extremitäten. Z Ärztl Fortbild. 1985;79:77.

13   Peripheral Nerve Blocks at the Ankle

13.1   Anatomical Overview

The foot is supplied by five nerves. Four of them are derived from the sciatic nerve (tibial nerve, superficial fibular nerve, deep fibular nerve, and sural nerve). The sural nerve is a joint terminal branch with sensory nerve fibers from the fibular nerve and the tibial nerve. The fifth nerve, the saphenous nerve, is the sensory terminal branch of the femoral nerve from the lumbar plexus. Three of the five nerves run in the subcu-

taneous fat directly above the crural fascia: the saphenous, sural, and superficial fibular nerves. These are anesthetized by subcutaneous infiltration. The remaining two nerves—the tibial nerve and the deep fibular nerve—run below the crural fascia in the ankle region and are anesthetized by selective subfascial injections. (Fig. 13.**1**). Each of these nerves can be blocked separately. The success rate is very high.

Tibial Nerve

The tibial nerve (L4-L5 to S1-S3) is the larger of the two sciatic branches and in the distal segment of the lower leg it becomes superficial medial to the Achilles tendon. It lies behind and lateral to the posterior tibial artery and between the tendons of flexor digitorum longus and tibialis posterior (in front) and the flexor hallucis longus muscles, covered by the flexor retinaculum (Figs.

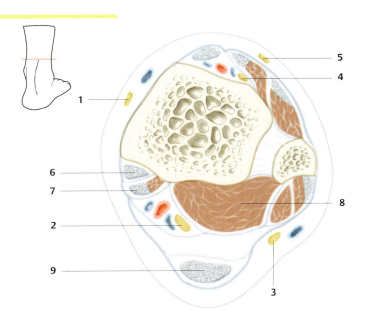

Fig. 13.**1**   Section through the lower leg at the level of the malleoli. Three of the five nerves supplying the foot run in the subcutaneous fat directly over the crural fascia: the saphenous, sural, and superficial fibular nerves. These are anesthetized by subcutaneous infiltration. The remaining two nerves—the tibial and the deep fibular nerves—run under the crural fascia in the ankle region and are anesthetized by direct block. While the former three nerves are essentially responsible for the sensory supply of the skin, the tibial and the deep fibular nerves are important for the sensory (and motor) innervation of more deeply situated structures. (According to Platzer: *Taschenatlas der Anatomie* [*Pocket Atlas of Anatomy*], Vol. 1. Stuttgart: Thieme; 1999.)

1   Saphenous nerve
2   Tibial nerve
3   Sural nerve
4   Deep fibular nerve
5   Superficial fibular nerve
6   Tendon of tibialis posterior
7   Tendon of flexor digitorum longus
8   Flexor hallucis longus
9   Calcaneal tendon (Achilles tendon)

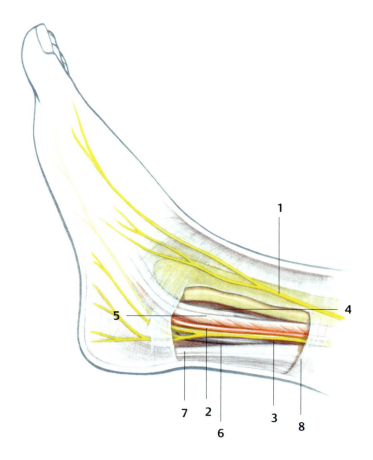

Fig. 13.**2**   Right foot, medial view.

1 Saphenous nerve
2 Tibial artery
3 Tibial nerve
4 Tendon of tibialis posterior
5 Tendon of flexor digitorum longus
6 Tendon of flexor hallucis longus
7 Calcaneal tendon (Achilles tendon)
8 Crural fascia

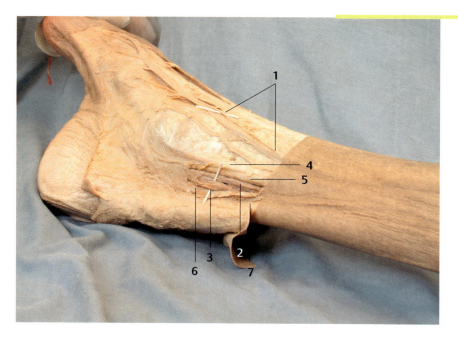

Fig. 13.**3**   Right foot, medial view. The tibial nerve (L4–L5 to S1–S3) reaches the surface in the distal segment of the lower leg medial to the Achilles tendon. It lies behind the posterior tibial artery and between the tendons of flexor digitorum longus and tibialis posterior and flexor hallucis longus, covered by the flexor retinaculum (see Fig. 13.**1**).

1 Saphenous nerve
2 Tibial artery
3 Tibial nerve
4 Tendon of tibialis posterior
5 Tendon of flexor digitorum longus
6 Tendon of flexor hallucis longus
7 Calcaneal tendon (Achilles tendon)

13.**1**-13.**4**). The tibial nerve always runs close to the posterior tibial vessels The tibial nerve gives off medial calcaneal branches on the inside of the heel and then divides behind the medial malleolus into the medial plantar nerve and the lateral plantar nerve. These two nerves run downward toward the sole of the foot, covered by abductor hallucis, and provide the sensory innervation of the sole. The tibial nerve is the motor supply of the flexor muscles (plantar flexion) and the sensory supply of the anterior and medial regions of the sole.

Saphenous Nerve

The saphenous nerve is the sensory terminal branch of the femoral nerve. It passes through the crural fascia in the region of the pes anserinus at the medial knee joint line and runs distally with the long saphenous vein on the medial side of the tibia subcutaneously, reaches the ankle region anterior to the medial malleolus, and continues as far as the great toe, giving off branches on the medial border of the foot (Figs. 13.**1**-13.**3**, 13.**5**). The sensory innervation of the medial region of the heel, the medial malleolus, and the medial border of the foot, sometimes as far as the great toe, is provided by the saphenous nerve.

Sural Nerve

The sural nerve is a cutaneous nerve that is formed by the union of a branch of the tibial nerve (medial sural cutaneous nerve) with a branch of the common fibular nerve (lateral sural cutaneous nerve). The nerves usually unite in the middle third of the leg and there penetrate the fascia. The sural nerve (which is also called the external saphenous nerve) then runs in the subcutaneous layer and passes downward together with the short saphenous vein behind the lateral malleolus to the outer border of the foot (Figs. 13.**6**, 13.**7**). It is the sensory supply of the lateral heel region and lateral malleolus and, as the lateral dorsal cutaneous nerve, it innervates the lateral border of the foot as far as the little toe.

Fig. 13.**4**   Right foot, medial view. Operative exposure of the tibial nerve.

1   Tibial nerve

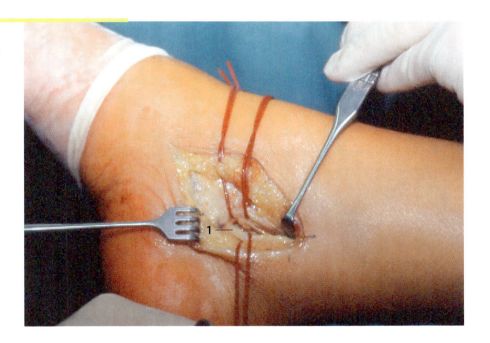

Fig. 13.**5**   Right foot, medial view. The main branch of the saphenous nerve runs together with the long saphenous vein on the inside of the lower leg as far as the ankle; occasionally it can extend as far as the great toe.

1   Saphenous nerve
2   Long saphenous vein

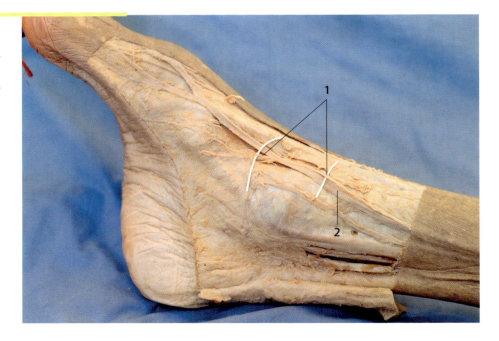

Superficial Fibular Nerve

The superficial fibular nerve (synonym: superficial peroneal nerve) comes from the common fibular nerve and branches off at the head of the fibula. It passes distally lateral to the tibial border, lying subcutaneously directly on the crural fascia, and branches above ankle level in a broad fan shape over the entire dorsum of the foot, to all of which it is the sensory supply (Figs. 13.6-13.9). This superficial branch is also called the musculocutaneous nerve (of the leg) (Bridenbaugh and Wedel 1998)

Deep Fibular Nerve

The deep fibular nerve (synonym: deep peroneal nerve) passes downward on the anterior surface of the interosseous membrane of the leg and lies between tibialis anterior and extensor hallucis longus. It then continues along the dorsum of the foot, covered by the superior and inferior extensor retinaculum. There it innervates the short toe extensors and the skin on the lateral side of the great toe and the medial side of the second toe. During its course in the anterior muscle compartment of the lower leg, the tibial artery is medial to the nerve. However, further distally the nerve crosses beneath

the artery, which then lies lateral to it. At the level of the extensor retinaculum the nerve and artery are crossed by the tendon of extensor hallucis longus coming from the medial side. At the junction with the foot, the anterior tibial artery is therefore lateral to the deep fibular nerve, while the tendon of extensor hallucis longus is medial to the nerve (Figs. 13.6, 13.8, 13.10).

Sensory Innervation of the Foot Region

(Fig. 13.11)

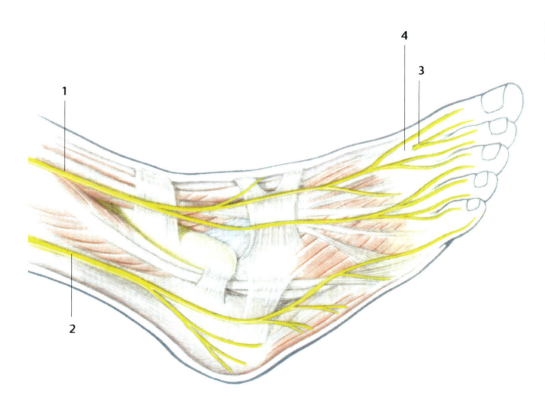

Fig. 13.6   Right foot, lateral view. Note the subfascial position of the deep fibular nerve until its emergence peripherally.

1   Superficial fibular nerve
2   Sural nerve
3   Deep fibular nerve
4   Fascia

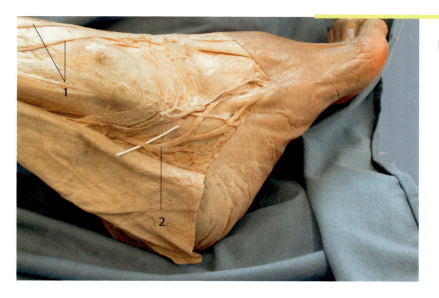

Fig. 13.7   Right foot, lateral view.

1   Superficial fibular nerve
2   Sural nerve

Fig. 13.**8** Right foot, dorsal view. Note the subfascial position of the deep fibular nerve. It continues along the dorsum of the foot covered by the inferior and superior extensor retinaculum. At the junction with the foot, the anterior tibial artery is lateral to the deep fibular nerve, while the tendon of extensor hallucis longus runs medial to the nerve. The sensory terminal branches innervate the skin on the lateral side of the great toe and the medial side of the second toe.

1 Superficial fibular nerve
2 Saphenous nerve
3 Deep fibular nerve
4 Dorsalis pedis artery
5 Tendon of extensor hallucis longus

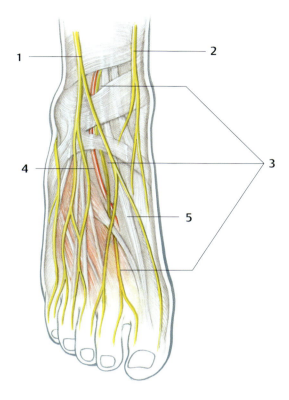

Fig. 13.**9** Right foot, dorsal view.

1 Superficial fibular nerve
2 Saphenous nerve
3 Tendon of extensor hallucis longus

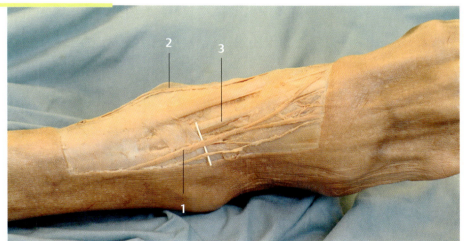

Fig. 13.**10** Sensory terminal branches of the deep fibular nerve.

1 Sensory terminal branches of the deep fibular nerve

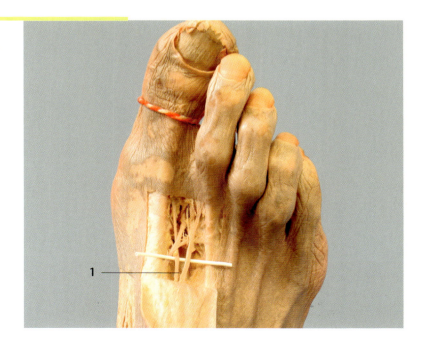

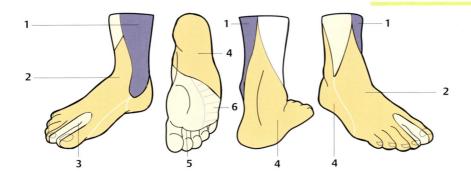

Fig. 13.**11** Sensory supply of the foot. The foot is supplied by five nerves. Four of these originate from the sciatic nerve (tibial nerve, superficial fibular nerve, deep fibular nerve, and sural nerve). The sural nerve is a common terminal branch with sensory nerve fibers from the fibular nerve and the tibial nerve. The fifth nerve, the saphenous nerve, is the sensory terminal branch of the femoral nerve from the lumbar plexus (q.v.).

    1 Saphenous nerve
    2 Superficial fibular nerve
    3 Deep fibular nerve
    4 Sural nerve
    5 Medial plantar nerve
    6 Lateral plantar nerve (tibial nerve)
Blue: Terminal branch of the femoral nerve
        (lumbar plexus)
Yellow: Terminal branches of the sciatic nerve
        (sacral plexus)

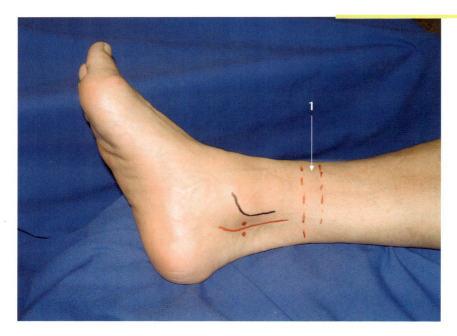

Fig. 13.**12** Right foot, medial view. Saphenous nerve block: starting from the anterior border of the tibia, 10 ml of a medium-acting or long-acting LA is injected subcutaneously four fingers above the medial malleolus as far as the Achilles tendon.

    1 Subcutaneous injection to block
       saphenous nerve

13.2 Saphenous Nerve, Sural Nerve and Superficial Fibular Nerve Block

Position and Landmarks
Anterior border of the tibia, medial and lateral malleolus, Achilles tendon.
The patient lies supine.

Procedure
Following disinfection of the lower leg and foot on the side to be anesthetized, conduction anesthesia is performed with a 6 cm long 24G needle.

Saphenous Nerve Blockade

Landmarks and Procedure
Starting from the anterior border of the tibia, 10 ml of a medium-acting or long-acting local anesthetic (LA) is injected (infiltrated) subcutaneously around the medial lower leg ca. four fingers above the medial malleolus, to the Achilles tendon (Fig. 13.**12**).

Superficial Fibular Nerve Block and Sural Nerve Block

Landmarks and Procedure
Three to four fingers above the lateral malleolus, a subcutaneous skin depot is created with 5-10 ml of LA on the lateral side of the lower leg, and the depot should continue backward as far as the Achilles tendon to block the sural nerve (Figs. 13.**13**, 13.**14**).

Fig. 13.**13**   Superficial fibular nerve and sural nerve block: 5–10 ml of LA is injected to create a subcutaneous skin depot between the anterior border of the tibia about 3–4 fingers above the lateral malleolus. Following the superficial fibular nerve block, injection of LA can be continued further laterally towards the Achilles tendon.

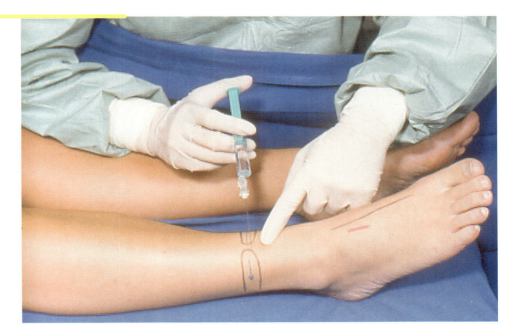

Fig. 13.**14**   Right foot, lateral view. A block of the sural nerve can be performed by laterally continuing the subcutaneous LA injection, as described for common fibular nerve block, as far as the Achilles tendon.

1 Sural nerve
2 Short saphenous vein

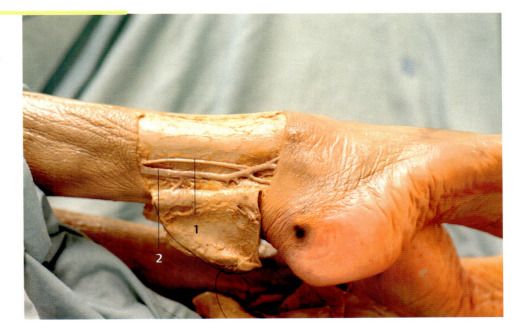

Fig. 13.**15**   Right foot, lateral view. The sural nerve can also be blocked selectively by a subcutaneous injection of ca. 5 ml of LA behind the lateral malleolus.

1 Sural nerve (here exposed surgically)
2 Superficial fibular nerve

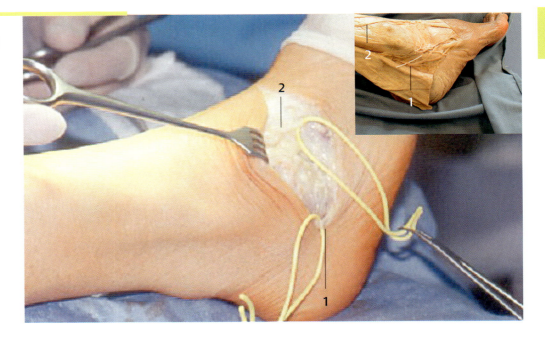

Alternative Method for Selective Block of the Sural Nerve

The sural nerve can also be blocked by subcutaneous infiltration between the Achilles tendon and the lateral malleolus with 5-10 ml of LA (Fig. 13.**15**).

The sural nerve is a purely sensory nerve that innervates the lateral malleolus and the lateral border of the foot.

13.3　Deep Fibular Nerve Block

Landmarks

Tendon of extensor hallucis longus, dorsalis pedis artery.

Procedure

The puncture site is on the dorsum of the foot immediately between the tendon of extensor hallucis longus (medial) and the dorsalis pedis artery (lateral). The needle is advanced between the artery and tendon deep under the fascia, the extensor retinaculum; after negative aspiration, ca. 3 ml of LA is injected (Fig. 13.**16**). The needle is then withdrawn and, after negative aspiration, ca. 3 ml of LA (e.g., mepivacaine 1% [10 mg/ml]or ropivacaine 0.75% [7.5 mg/ml]) is injected again, now lateral to the artery.

- Orientation is sometimes difficult if the pulse is impalpable. Use of a small Doppler probe can be helpful.
- The tendon of extensor hallucis longus is readily palpable on dorsiflexion of the foot. The artery is always lateral to this tendon.
- A selective block is useful only in the case of pain or operations on the medial side of the great toe and/or lateral side of the second toe (e.g., ingrowing toenail).

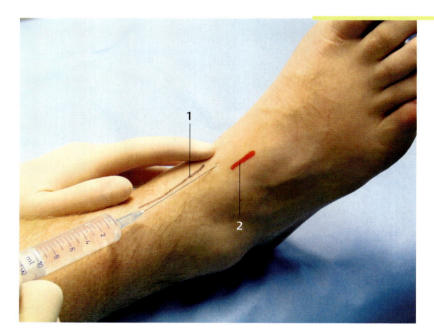

Fig. 13.**16**　The puncture site for the deep fibular nerve block is on the dorsum of the foot immediately between the tendon of extensor hallucis longus (medial) and the dorsalis pedis artery (lateral). The needle is advanced deeply between the artery and tendon under the fascia, the extensor retinaculum, and after negative aspiration, ca. 3 ml of LA is injected. The needle is then withdrawn and, after negative aspiration, ca. 3 ml of LA is also injected lateral to the artery (e.g., mepivacaine 1% [10 mg/ml] or ropivacaine 0.75% [7.5 mg/ml]).

1　Tendon of extensor hallucis longus
2　Dorsalis pedis artery

13.4　Tibial Nerve Block

Landmarks and Position

Medial malleolus, Achilles tendon.

The patient remains supine, and the lower leg is crossed on the tibia of the other leg (Fig. 13.**17**).

Procedure

The nerve is blocked behind the medial malleolus. After disinfection, the skin is infiltrated somewhat lateral to the posterior tibial artery (i.e., between the Achilles tendon and posterior tibial artery) or—if this is not palpable—immediately medial to the Achilles tendon at the level of the cranial section of the medial malleolus. A 5-8 cm long 24G needle is introduced at this point

Fig. 13.**17**   The tibial nerve is blocked behind the medial malleolus. Somewhat lateral to the posterior tibial artery or immediately medial to the Achilles tendon at the level of the cranial segment of the medial malleolus, a 5–8 cm needle is introduced and advanced as far as the posterior border of the tibia (motor response with PNS: plantar flexion of the toes). After reaching the posterior border of the tibia, the needle is withdrawn about 1 cm and 10 ml of a medium-acting or long-acting LA is injected.

  1   Medial malleolus
  2   Posterior tibial artery

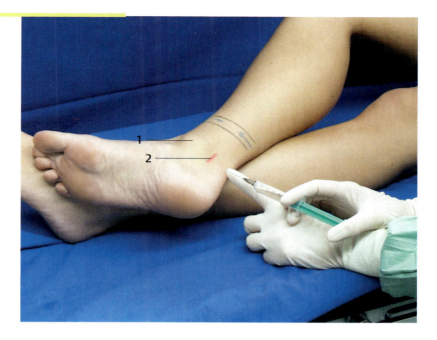

Fig. 13.**18**   Block of the tibial nerve can also be performed with the nerve stimulator. The response consists of plantar flexion of the toes.

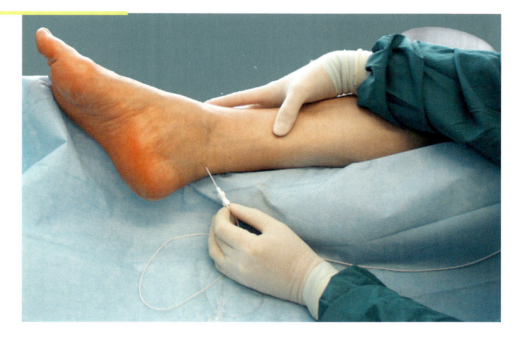

Fig. 13.**19**   When the artery is poorly palpable, it is advisable to enter immediately medial to the Achilles tendon for block of the tibial nerve, aiming for the posterior border of the tibia.

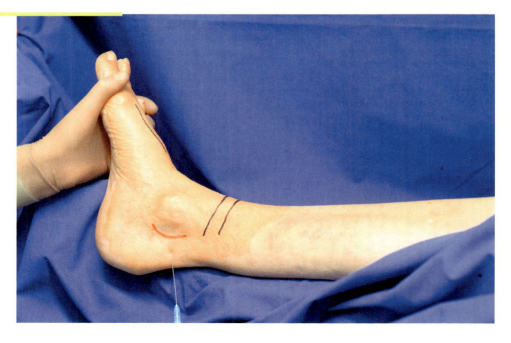

vertically to the skin and is advanced cautiously and with intermittent aspiration as far as the posterior border of the tibia (motor response on PNS: plantar flexion of the toes) (Figs. 13.**17**-13.**19**). Paresthesia is not deliberately sought but is relatively frequent. After reaching the posterior border of the tibia, the needle is withdrawn ca. 1 cm. Following negative aspiration, 10 ml of a medium-acting or long-acting LA is injected. The analgesia extends to the sole of the foot (with the exception of the heel) and the medial border of the foot. Special complications are not to be expected. There have been isolated reports of dysesthesia after this block (Schurmann 1976).

Practical Notes
- Paresthesia should not be sought. However, if paresthesia (plantar) is produced, the patient must be prepared for this unpleasant sensation so that the patient and therapist are not endangered by a sudden withdrawal movement.
- Anesthesia can be performed very well with PNS (response: plantar flexion of the toes) (Frederic and Bouchon 1996).
- An additional injection below the fascia on the contralateral side (medial) of the artery ensures the success of the block even when the course of the tibial nerve is variable relative to the artery, particularly when a nerve stimulator is not used or no paresthesia is produced.

13.5 Ankle Block

Complete block of the foot can be obtained by joint block of all five nerves supplying the foot, the so-called ankle block.

Practical Notes
- The saphenous, superficial fibular and sural nerves can be blocked relatively easily at the upper level of the ankle joint by subcutaneous infiltration anesthesia. If the procedure starts with these subcutaneous blocks, penetration of the skin in the subsequent blocks is pain-free. The order is important for minimizing pain when performing an ankle block.
- A complete circular depot should be avoided so as not to endanger blood perfusion of the foot. Subcutaneous infiltration depots can instead be made at different levels.
- The posterior and anterior tibial (deep fibular) nerves must be sought selectively.
- Epinephrine-free local anesthetics should be used.
- Depending on experience and the anatomical situation, performing an ankle block takes between 5 and 15 minutes; the effect commences after 15 minutes and is complete after 30 minutes. If areas of the foot remain sensitive, these gaps can also be filled by peripheral (subcutaneous) infiltration.
- The pressure of a tourniquet over the subcutaneous infiltration depot is tolerated for up to 2 hours. The actual pain caused by a tourniquet is an ischemic pain and is thus dependent on the ischemic muscle mass that is produced by the tourniquet; for this reason, a tourniquet sited further peripherally (e.g., 2-3 fingers above the malleoli) is always tolerated better.

13.6 Indications, Contraindications, Complications, Side Effects

Indications
- Incomplete lumbosacral plexus anesthesia
- Operations on the foot (e.g., hallux valgus, foot gangrene)
- Pain therapy
- Diagnostic blocks

Contraindications
- General contraindications (see Chapter 15)
- Nerve lesions (relative; previous documentation required)

Complications and Side Effects
There are no reported special complications or side effects.

13.7 Remarks on Ankle Block

Combination of the individual blocks described is traditionally called ankle block and is described in many textbooks. It is an easily performed technique with a low rate of complications and a high rate of success (Kay 1999; Malloy 1999). In operations in the ankle region, it must always be ensured that the block is performed above the ankle region. In these cases it should be considered whether a popliteal block or distal sciatic block (q.v.) is a rational alternative. A complete ankle block—despite its relative safety—is technically rather complex for the beginner as it involves two individual blocks in addition to the superficial ring blocks, namely, block of the posterior tibial nerve and the deep fibular nerve. In view of the variable anastomoses and the large range of anatomical variation, blocking all the nerves requires either a good technique or injection of rather large volumes.

In 100 blocks of the areas of distribution of the sural nerve and saphenous nerve, McCutcheon (1965) reported that only 60% and 84%, respectively, correlated with the information in anatomical textbooks. He obtained a success rate for block of the tibial nerve of only 88%. Others, however, have reported very high success rates of 95% (Kofoed 1982) and 100% (Schurmann 1976). Sharrock and Mineo (1988) found low blood levels of local anesthetic after ankle block, so that it may be assumed that the volumes required for successful anesthesia are well tolerated. The combination of two ankle blocks in one patient is therefore regarded as justifiable (Concepcion 1999). Nevertheless, the maximum dosages of the individual local anesthetics should be respected.

Ankle block can also be performed for operations with a lower leg tourniquet. In a prospective study, Delgado-Martinez et al. (2001) investigated whether block of individual nerves is then adequate. On the basis of their results, they recommend that a complete "ankle block," i.e., anesthesia of all five nerves, can be used. If a tourniquet is required, it can be applied just above the ankle. Different levels of pressure in the cuff are reported (Frederic and Bouchon 1996). A study in volunteers found that pressures of

225 mmHg (± 46 mmHg) with a narrow cuff and 284 mmHg (± 42 mmHg) with a wide cuff can be regarded as safe and effective (Biehl et al. 1993). Other authors regard it as sufficient to measure the individually required pressure with Doppler or a stethoscope (Diamond et al. 1985; Pauers and Carocci 1994). In an electrophysiological study of the use of a tourniquet above the ankle, no increased risk to the nerves was found (Chu et al. 1981). In a retrospective study of 3027 patients who had a tourniquet during operation with a cuff pressure of 325 mmHg, a post-tourniquet syndrome was found in three patients (Derner and Buckholz 1995).

Ankle block is regarded as a safe anesthesia procedure. Complications have been described only rarely. Isolated cases of persistent paresthesia have been reported in a few studies, but these subsided spontaneously after 4-6 weeks (Sharrock and Mineo 1988; Sharrock et al. 1986). In a study of 1295 patients who had an ankle block, four complications were recorded (three vasovagal reactions, one supraventricular tachycardia), while neuritis, hematoma, or infection was not found in any patient (Myerson et al. 1992). In a prospective study of 284 patients, no postanesthetic neuralgia or other complications were found (Kofoed 1982). In other studies, also, no complications were reported (Needoff et al. 1995; Sarrafian et al. 1983; Wassef 1991).

13.8 Summary

So-called ankle block is a low-complication and safe anesthesia procedure for operations on the foot.

The technique is outstandingly suitable for selective block of individual nerves for diagnosis or to complete regional anesthesia. However, it should be ensured that the patient receives as few painful punctures as possible. Remember that complete anesthesia of the foot also can be achieved with a distal sciatic block or popliteal block (see Chapter 11).

13.9 Blocks at the Toes

Anatomical Overview

The sensory nerves supplying the foot are terminal branches of the sciatic nerve. The medial border of the foot is occasionally supplied as far as the great toe by the terminal branch of the femoral nerve, the saphenous nerve. The tibial and deep fibular nerves supply the more deeply located structures (bone, joints, muscles); the tibial nerve also supplies the sole of the foot and the deep fibular nerve supplies the skin on the lateral side of the great toe and the medial side of the second toe. The other nerves run subcutaneously and innervate the skin of the medial (saphenous nerve) and lateral side of the foot (sural nerve) and also the dorsum of the foot and toes (superficial fibular nerve).

Conduction Anesthesia of the Toes (Oberst Conduction Anesthesia)

Digital conduction anesthesia according to Oberst is an easy and reliable method that is employed especially for conduction block in the fingers. However, the method is also employed for conduction anesthesia in the toes.

Landmarks and Position
Dorsal side of the toe, patient in supine position.

Procedure
The toe is punctured bilaterally with a thin needle in the middle of the proximal phalanx from the dorsal side tangentially to the bone, almost reaching the plantar side. By supporting the plantar side of toe with one's own finger, it is possible to check how

Fig. 13.**20**   Conduction anesthesia of the toes with a fine needle. The toes are subcutaneously injected bilaterally at the middle of the proximal phalanx from the dorsum tangentially to the bone, when the plantar side should almost be reached. By plantar support of the toe with one's own finger, the depth of the needle can be felt. 0.5–1 ml of 1 % (10 mg/ml) medium-acting local anesthetic is injected on each side.

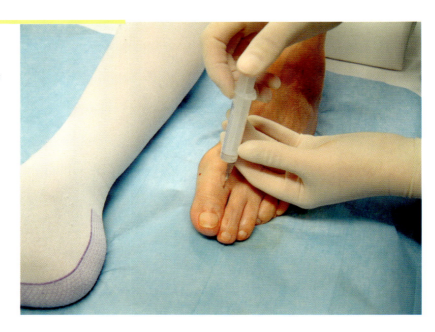

far the needle has reached in the plantar direction. On each side, 0.5-1 ml of a 1 % (10 mg/ml) medium-acting LA is injected (Fig. 13.**20**).

Practical Notes

- The injection should be given slowly as the pressure produced by the injection volume may be perceived as very unpleasant by the patient.
- Oberst conduction anesthesia can be recommended for the great toe but is less suitable for the other toes because of their tough tissue.
- A gentle alternative is interdigital block in the proximal toe region or in the metatarsal region (q.v.).

Remarks on the Technique

In principle there is a risk of block-related gangrene, so only epinephrine-free solutions should be used. No more than 8 ml to a maximum of 10 ml of LA per toe should be infiltrated. These peripheral block techniques are indicated particularly in the outpatient area and in at-risk patients in whom minor operations on the toes or forefoot must be performed (e.g., nail removal, corrective operations for fractures or hammer toe, toe amputations, or other operations in the area of the phalanges).

Because of the risk of gangrene, the digital block techniques are relatively contraindicated in patients with peripheral perfusion disorders including Raynaud syndrome and should only be performed after a thorough consideration of the advantages and disadvantages and alternatives (e.g., distal sciatic, q.v.). In these cases a tourniquet should not be applied for more than 15 minutes, and the maximum dose of local anesthetic per toe is reported to be 8 ml (Adriani 1984).

References

Adriani J. Labat regional anesthesia. Techniques and clinical applications. 4th ed. St. Louis: Green; 1984;373-84.

Biehl WC, Morgan JM, Wagner FW. The safety of the Esmarch tourniquet. Foot Ankle. 1993;14:278-83.

Bridenbaugh PhO, Wedel DJ. The lower extremity. In: Cousins MJ, Bridenbaugh PhO, eds. Neural blockade clinic anesthesia and management of pain. 3rd ed. Philadelphia: Lippincott-Raven; 1998:373-409.

Chu J, Fox I, Jassen M. Pneumatic ankle tourniquet: Clinical and electrophysiologic study. Arch Phys Med Rehabil. 1981;62:570-5.

Concepcion M. Ankle block. Techniques in Regional Anesthesia and Pain Management. 1999;3:241-6.

Delgado-Martinez AD, Marchal JM, Molina M, Palma A. Forefoot surgery with ankle tourniquet: Complete or selective ankle block [Letter]. Reg Anesth. 2001;26:184.

Derner R, Buckholz J. Surgical hemostasis by pneumatic ankle tourniquet during 3027 pediatric operations. J Foot Ankle Surg. 1995;34:236-46.

Diamond EL, Sherman M, Lenet M. A quantitative method of determining the pneumatic ankle tourniquet setting. J Foot Surg. 1985;24:330-4.

Frederic A, Bouchon Y. Analgesia in surgery of the foot. Cah Anesthesiol. 1996;44:115-8.

Kay J. Ankle block. Techniques in Regional Anesthesia and Pain Management. 1999;3:3-8.

Kofoed H. Peripheral nerve blocks at the knee and ankle in operations for common foot disorders. Clin Orthop. 1982;168:97-101.

Malloy RE. Ankle block. In: Benson HT, Malloy RE, Strichartz G, eds. Essentials of pain medicine and regional anesthesia. Philadelphia: Churchill Livingstone; 1999:437.

McCutcheon R. Regional anaesthesia for the foot. Can Anaesth Soc J. 1965;12:465.

Myerson MS, Ruland CM, Allon SM. Regional anesthesia for foot and ankle surgery. Foot Ankle. 1992;13:282-8.

Needoff M, Radford P, Costigan P. Local anesthesia for postoperative pain relief after foot surgery: A prospective clinical trial. Foot Ankle Int. 1995;16:11-3.

Pauers RS, Carocci MA. Low pressure pneumatic tourniquets: Effectiveness at minimum recommended inflation pressures. J Foot Ankle Surg. 1994;33:605-9.

Sarrafian SK, Ibrahim IN, Breihan JH. Ankle-foot peripheral nerve block for mid and forefoot surgery. Foot Ankle. 1983;4:86-90.

Schurmann DJ. Ankle-block anesthesia for foot surgery. Anesthesiology. 1976;44:348-52.

Sharrock NE, Mineo R. Venous lidocaine and bupivacaine levels following midtarsal ankle block. Reg Anesth. 1988;(S)13:75.

Sharrock NE, Waller JF, Fierro LE. Midtarsal block for surgery of the forefoot. Br J Anaesth. 1986;58:37-40.

Wassef MR. Posterior tibial nerve block. A new approach using only landmark of the sustentaculum tali. Anaesthesia. 1991;46:841-4.

General Considerations

14   Special Features of Peripheral Nerve Blocks

14.1   Advantages of Peripheral Nerve Blocks

A reduction in postoperative mortality and morbidity can be assumed from a meta-analysis of central neuraxial blocks (CNB) (Rodgers et al. 2000). There are no comparable studies regarding peripheral nerve blocks. However, it can be assumed that peripheral nerve blocks offer advantages in at-risk patients compared with general anesthesia and also compared with neuraxial blocks. While peripheral blocks are performed quite frequently on the upper limb, they are not yet so frequently used for operations on the lower limb. One reason for this may be that parts of both the lumbar and sacral plexuses always have to be anesthetized for a complete block of the lower limb (two injections). Considerable drops in blood pressure can occur with central neuraxial blocks. The essential advantage of peripheral nerve blocks is therefore the lower interference with circulation. Thus, cardiac arrest was seen significantly less often after peripheral blocks than after spinal anesthesia (Auroy et al. 1997). Furthermore, possible complications (infections, hemorrhage, nerve injury) are less serious than the complications of CNB blocks. While intact coagulation is an absolute requirement for neuraxial blocks, the criteria for peripheral nerve blocks are less strict. A normal coagulation clinically and in the patient's medical records is usually sufficient for performing a peripheral nerve block (see below).

Under certain circumstances, peripheral blocks are the procedure of choice for surgical anesthesia. In the nonfasting patient, regional anesthesia procedures should be preferred; for the upper limb, only peripheral nerve blocks should be considered. Many patients with rheumatic diseases have severely limited mouth opening, often together with extreme deformity of the entire spine. Both general anesthesia and neuraxial blocks are associated with considerable technical difficulties and risks in these patients. Numerous other examples could be cited where peripheral nerve blocks represent the procedure of choice.

Every anesthetist should master the standard techniques of peripheral block of the upper and lower limbs in order to be able to make an individual decision on the best anesthetic procedure in the individual case.

14.2   Problems of Peripheral Nerve Blocks

Incomplete Block

Although small, the possible risk of an incomplete block should be anticipated and prepared for.

The reported incidence of incomplete block varies greatly. Failure rates of up to 30% are reported for axillary plexus anesthesia. Such problems should be explained to the patient and strategies for further procedure must be discussed. The time needed for a complete block to develop may vary with the technique and the local anesthetic employed; some blocks may require up to 40 minutes (or more) to achieve full effect. The performance of peripheral nerve blocks should therefore be well planned logistically. However, with some experience an early prognosis can be made as to whether a completely successful block can be expected. The first evidence of commencement of the block effect is a rise in skin temperature caused by sympathetic block, followed by hypoesthesia and motor weakness. These signs of incipient success of the block should appear within 10–15 minutes; if this is not the case, there is no point in waiting any longer.

The following procedure is recommended in the case of incomplete regional block for *surgery:*

Patients are often irritated by the fact that they still "feel" something but do not actually complain of pain. In this case, mild analgosedation is adequate to solve the problem. The patient should be given an oxygen $_m$ask; monitoring of oxygenation (pulse oximetry) is mandatory, and sometimes monitoring of the patient's ventilation by capnometry is indicated (see p. 226).

If the block is basically inadequate for surgical purposes, no attempts should be made to increase a patient's pain tolerance by higher doses of analgesics and sedatives unless the airway is appropriately secured. If there are no contraindications, general anesthesia (e.g., propofol and a laryngeal mask) is indicated. In most cases, a partial block exists and only a small supplementary amount of an opiate may be sufficient to achieve surgical tolerance (e.g., 10 µg sufentanyl).

If there are contraindications to general anesthesia or reservations on the part of the patient, most peripheral nerve blocks offer the option of selective nerve block supplementation distal to the already performed block. The following are examples.

- *Incomplete interscalene plexus anesthesia for shoulder operation:* supplementation by block of the suprascapular nerve and the supraclavicular nerves.
- *Incomplete supraclavicular or infraclavicular or axillary plexus anesthesia:* supplementation by selective nerve blocks in the upper arm, elbow or wrist region.
- *Incomplete femoral and sciatic nerve block for operations on the ankle or foot:* supplementation by distal *sciatic nerve block*, saphenous nerve block, or foot block.

After a peripheral nerve block has been performed resulting in a partial effect, supplementary blocks should be performed distal to the previous block and only with *"atraumatic" needles with a unipolar tip* (see p. 229) *and with the use of a nerve stimulator.* On no account should blocks be repeated in the area already infiltrated with local anesthetic.

Local Anesthetic Dosages

A greater volume of local anesthetic is required for peripheral blocks.

Peripheral nerve blocks are associated with

seizures significantly more often than are neuraxial blocks (Auroy et al. 1997). In peripheral nerve blocks where larger volumes of local anesthetic are used or when there is a risk of injection into an artery leading to the brain, all safety precautions required for dealing with such an incident must be taken (peripheral venous access, possibility of intubation and ventilation with 100% oxygen, emergency medications). Moreover, it is necessary to ensure patient safety by selecting the least toxic local anesthetic and observing the recommended maximum doses. The injection must always be given slowly while observing the patient.

References

See pp. 244-246.

15 Complications and General Contraindications of Peripheral Blocks

15.1 Complications of Peripheral Nerve Blocks

Besides the specific complications described for the individual techniques, the following complications of peripheral nerve blocks are possible:

- Toxic reactions caused by the local anesthetic
- Neurological injuries (neuropathy)
- Infection

Toxic Reactions Caused by the Local Anesthetic

These can be *due to overdosage* at a correct initial injection site or accidental intravascular injection of a relatively small dose of local anesthetic. After an overdose, the symptoms can be expected to develop at the time of maximum blood levels, depending on the rate of absorption.

However, individual variations in tolerability are large, so there is no fixed definition of "overdose" of local anesthetics (Rosenberg 2004).

In the event of *accidental intravascular injection* of the local anesthetic, small amounts may cause a toxic reaction (see above). For this reason, the maximum doses for many local anesthetics recommended by the manufacturer should be regarded with a degree of skepticism, since much smaller doses can lead to major incidents in the event of

accidental intravascular injection, while much higher doses may be tolerated with correct injection.

Systemic intoxication by local anesthetics is expressed in cerebral and cardiac effects; the cerebral effects usually precede the cardiac effects (Fig. 15.**1**). Early symptoms are a metallic taste on the tongue, tinnitus, dizziness, and acoustic phenomena, followed by muscle twitching, confusion, unconsciousness, seizure, and coma. The cardiac changes occur in parallel with correspondingly higher blood levels; first there is tachycardia and hypertension, followed by bradycardia, hypotension, and arrhythmia possibly progressing to asystole.

When injecting the local anesthetic it is important to watch for early symptoms of intoxication in order to stop administration immediately, e.g., in the case of accidental intravascular injection. To obviate intravascular injection, the local anesthetic must be given slowly, with repeated attempts at aspiration, and with constant verbal communication with the patient ("verbal monitoring") in order to detect early CNS symptoms.

Intoxication symptoms are enhanced by hypoxia and acidosis, so prophylactic oxygen administration is recommended.

In the case of cerebral intoxication, oxygen must be given immediately. In the case of a

seizure, the patient must also be ventilated adequately (if necessary with intubation and mechanical ventilation) and administration of benzodiazepines (midazolam, diazepam) or barbiturates will stop the seizure.

With regard to the cardiac effects, too, the first rule is avoidance of hypoxia and acidosis. Naturally, injection of the local anesthetic must stop immediately and, in addition to administration of positive inotropic and chronotropic medications (atropine, catecholamines) and volume replacement, prolonged mechanical cardiac massage may be required. This may be the case in particular with bupivacaine, as bupivacaine may block the effect of an external electrical pacemaker. More prolonged cardiac massage can sometimes be successful (Fig. 15.**2**).

When selecting the local anesthetic, consideration must be given to its potential toxicity, especially in the event of accidental intravascular injection. Medium-acting local anesthetics are less toxic than the long-acting drugs. Of the currently employed long-acting local anesthetics (racemic) bupivacaine, levobupivacaine [(S)-isomer of bupivacaine], and ropivacaine [(S)-isomer], the least cardiotoxic is ropivacaine. With regard to intracellular energy metabolism also, it has clear advantages compared to levobupivacaine. In contrast to ropivacaine and the medium-acting local anesthetics, levobupivacaine and

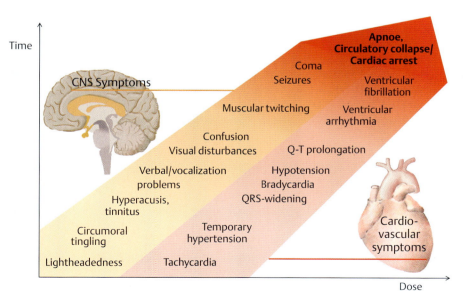

Time

CNS Symptoms

Apnoe,
Circulatory collapse/
Cardiac arrest

Coma
Seizures

Ventricular
fibrillation

Muscular twitching

Ventricular
arrhythmia

Confusion
Visual disturbances

Q-T prolongation

Verbal/vocalization
problems

Hypotension
Bradycardia
QRS-widening

Hyperacusis,
tinnitus

Circumoral
tingling

Temporary
hypertension

Cardio-
vascular
symptoms

Lightheadedness

Tachycardia

Dose

A relatively small dose of local anesthetic, if accidentally injekted intravascularily, may lead directly to seizures with both respiratory and cardiovascular problems, depending on drug and patient condition.

Fig. 15.**1** Cerebral and cardiac symptoms of systemic intoxication by local anesthetics. (From Meier G, Büttner J. *Pocket Compendium of Peripheral Nerve Blocks*, 3rd ed. Munich, Germany. Arcis Publishing Company, 2005.)

bupivacaine may lead to a complete block of ATP synthesis in the myocardium at toxic concentrations (Sztark et al. 1998, 2000). *Allergic reactions* are extremely rare with the use of the amide local anesthetics that are used almost exclusively today.

Neurological Injuries (Neuropathy)

Neurological injuries (Fig. 15.**3**) are reported after peripheral nerve blocks with an incidence between 0.019% (Auroy et al. 1997) and 1.7% (Fanelli et al. 1999). Most post-

operative nerve lesions are not due to a nerve block; other causes such as position-induced injury or injury caused by the operation are common (Cheney et al. 1999; Fanelli et al. 1999). A subfascial hematoma following a femoral nerve block (Jöhr 1987) or axillary plexus anesthesia (Ben-David 1999) can lead to mechanical nerve compression (Jöhr 1987). Occasionally brachial plexus neuropathy or "idiopathic neuritis" or "idiopathic plexitis" occurs in association with an interscalene brachial plexus block (Hebl et al. 2001; Horlocker et al. 2000; Tetzlaff et al. 1997). This is associated with

severe nerve pain, numbness, and motor weakness. An immediate injury due to the puncture has not taken place here; accordingly, the neurological picture cannot be attributed to injury of individual cords or nerves. The syndrome is due to an inflammatory immunological event. Postoperative plexus neuropathy can also occur spontaneously independently of the anesthesia procedure performed. This makes it difficult to make a causal distinction from regional anesthesia (Malamut et al. 1994).
Nerve injuries after peripheral nerve blocks usually have a good prognosis (Fanelli et al.

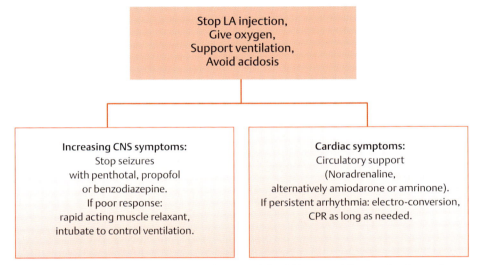

Fig. 15.**2**   Treatment of systemic intoxication by local anesthetics: the first measure is always adequate oxygenation and ventilation (oxygen mask, if necessary intubation, ventilation with 100% O$_2$). (From Meier G, Büttner J. *Pocket Compendium of Peripheral Nerve Blocks*, 3rd ed. Munich, Germany. Arcis Publishing Company, 2005.)

Stop LA injection, Give oxygen, Support ventilation, Avoid acidosis

Increasing CNS symptoms:
Stop seizures
with penthotal, propofol
or benzodiazepine.
If poor response:
rapid acting muscle relaxant,
intubate to control ventilation.

Cardiac symptoms:
Circulatory support
(Noradrenaline,
alternatively amiodarone or amrinone).
If persistent arrhythmia: electro-conversion,
CPR as long as needed.

Allergy for amid local anesthetics is extremely rare and should be treated like any allergic reaction.

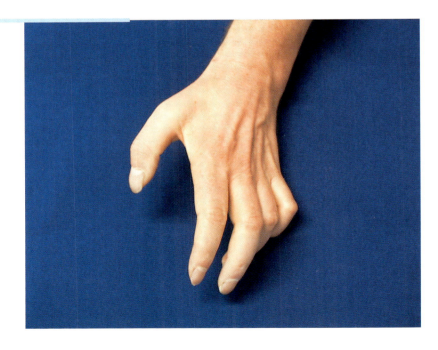

Fig. 15.**3**   Persistent nerve damage due to a traumatic peripheral regional anesthesia (ulnar nerve injury with typical claw hand).

1999; Stan et al. 1995). After weeks to months, complete or extensive resolution of the paresis and pain can be expected (Stöhr et al. 1996). However, depending on the type and degree of nerve injury, residual paresis interfering with function—sometimes associated with causalgiform pain syndromes—can persist in individual cases. Atraumatic needles should be used to reduce the risk of nerve injury, and a deliberate search for paresthesia should be avoided. Continuous axillary plexus anesthesia and distal blocks in the hand and foot can be performed without a nerve stimulator. All other blocks should be performed with the aid of the nerve stimulator. If the patient

reports paresthesia during the injection, the needle position must be changed immediately. Continuous nerve blocks for postoperative pain therapy are sometimes performed under general anesthesia or in an area anesthetized by a central neuraxial block. This should only be done with the aid of a functioning nerve stimulator as the patient cannot give any indication of paresthesia in the event of accidental intraneural injection. Remember that neuromuscular blockade also blocks the response to nerve stimulation.

In general it is preferable to perform peripheral nerve blocks on awake or only lightly sedated patients, particularly when a catheter for pain management is placed (Neal 2001)!

Infection

Local site infections or general infections caused by a single-shot peripheral neural blockade are extremely rate. One case of a fatal streptococcal necrotizing fasciitis as a complication of an axillary brachial plexus block has been published (Nseir 2003). There is a potential risk of infection associated with perineural catheters. Reports enrolling over 900 patients undergoing continuous interscalene analgesia for 2-5 days observed an incidence of catheter site infection of approximately 0.7% (Borgeat 2003). One prospective survey of 211 femoral catheters noted an incidence of infectious complications of 1.4% (Cuvillon 2001).

15.2 General Contraindications to Peripheral Nerve Blocks (Table 15.1)

Infection

Infections in the region of the puncture site constitute an *absolute contraindication* to every kind of regional anesthesia. Infection in the area of innervation to be blocked is not a contraindication as long as the puncture site itself is not affected. Bacteremia is not a contraindication for "single-shot" blocks. However, an indwelling catheter should be avoided, as any foreign body may promote septic colonization (Hempel 1998). For medicolegal reasons, the patient must be informed about the potentially greater infection risk.

Coagulation Disorders

The patient's history and medical examination can provide important information with regard to coagulation-related problems and should be clarified before performing a regional block. Blocks in the neck, head, and trunk regions should not be performed if there is a history and/or clinical confirmation of a coagulation disorder. *Techniques in which vascular puncture is knowingly*

accepted (e.g., transarterial technique), should be avoided.

Taking acetylsalicylic acid (ASA) and low-dose heparinization with unfractionated or low-molecular-weight heparin do not contraindicate use of peripheral nerve blocks as long as there is no evidence of an obvious coagulation disorder. There is little experience regarding the newer antithrombotic agents (fondaparinux, melagatran, ximelagatran) and platelet aggregation inhibitors (ticlopidine, clopidogrel), particularly in association with peripheral blocks. With the exception of the psoas compartment block, few major complications of peripheral nerve blocks have been described in association with medications affecting coagulation, and there have been no reports of persistent nerve injury in this connection. Performing peripheral nerve blocks during medication with antithrombotic medication and/or platelet aggregation inhibitors can therefore be justified after careful analysis of the risks and benefits. Under these circumstances, the block should be performed by an experienced colleague, and following the block qualified monitoring should be ensured for prompt identification of a nerve

compression syndrome as a result of a developing hematoma. Remember that the block itself can delay the appearance of neural symptoms. In this connection, the interscalene block using the Meier technique, the axillary block, and the "mid-humeral approach" in the upper limb, and femoral nerve block and distal sciatic nerve block in the lower limb can be mentioned as safer techniques. Under the conditions listed above and after careful consideration, plexus blocks in the proximity of the clavicle (upper limb) and proximal sciatic nerve blocks (lower limb) can be used. *Because of several serious case reports in association with medications affecting coagulation* (Klein et al. 1997; Weller et al. 2003), *the psoas compartment block should be performed under the same strict conditions as neuraxial blocks* (Gogarten et al. 2003; Horlocker 2003). This also applies to removal of a psoas compartment catheter.

Preoperative coagulation tests should be done in patients on anticoagulation treatment or with history or signs of coagulation disorders. Table 15.2 gives the borderline values recommended by the authors for performing peripheral blocks.

Absolute	Relative
• Infections in the region of the puncture site	• Neurological deficits (prior documentation required)
• Manifest coagulation disorders with blocks in the head, neck, and trunk regions	
• Refusal by the patient	

With regard to specific technical contraindications, see the individual procedures.

Table 15.**1** General contraindications to peripheral nerve blocks

Table 15.2   Borderline coagulation parameters for performing peripheral regional nerve blocks in the head, neck, and trunk regions

	Safe Use	After Careful Consideration
Quick test	> 45 %	45–40 %
Partial thromboplastin time (PTT)	< 45 s	46–50 s (Factor VIII > 25 %)
Platelet count	50 000–500 000	
Bleeding tendency	None	Present

Preexisting Neurological Deficits

Previous neurological disease or peripheral nerve lesions of acute or chronic origin do not per se represent a contraindication to a peripheral regional procedure, but should be well documented before the block is performed.

References

See pp. 244-246.

16   General Principles for Performing Peripheral Blocks

16.1   Hygiene Requirements for Performing Peripheral Nerve Blocks

So-called "single-shot" techniques require the skin to be disinfected three times and puncture should be performed using sterile precautions.

Much higher demands must be made when placing peripheral nerve catheters for continuous administration of local anesthetic (LA). Peripheral regional pain catheters carry a remarkable infection risk.

The strictest hygienic standards are therefore demanded for dealing with continuous regional pain catheters.

The recommendations of the American Centers for Disease Control and Prevention (CDC) on preventing (intravascular) catheter-associated infections can also be applied to regional pain catheters (Meyer and Herrmann 1998). Catheter placement must be performed only after careful hand decontamination. Use of a cap, face mask, and sterile gloves is mandatory, and it is strongly recommended to wear a gown! (Fig. 16.1). The injection site should be disinfected at least three times with an exposure time of 3–10 minutes. Sterile draping of the puncture site must follow promptly. After fixation of the catheter (see below), the puncture site must be covered with a sterile dressing. The time and date of catheter placement must be documented.

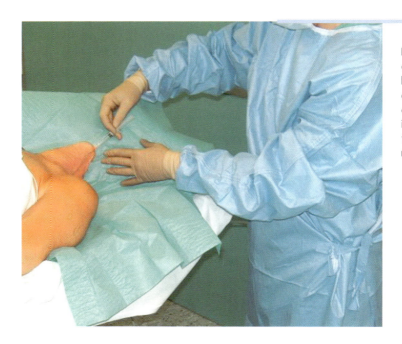

Fig. 16.**1** Particularly when placing continuous peripheral nerve blocks, the strictest hygiene requirements should be followed: cap, sterile gown, facemask, threefold skin disinfection, sterile gloves, and sterile draping. The draping must ensure that a view of the anatomical landmarks and the expected muscle responses is not obscured.

16.2   General Principles of Informed Consent, Positioning and Monitoring

Anesthesia-related mortality has fallen markedly in recent decades and is today estimated at one death per 10 000 anesthesia procedures. Many incidents of complications during both general and regional anesthesia can be avoided. An important requirement is judicious preparation and monitoring and early identification of a problematic situation.

A requirement for every regional anesthesia is the patient's legally effective informed consent. In day surgery or in the outpatient pain clinic, continuous peripheral block tech-

niques can be performed and continued successfully on an outpatient basis (Rawal et al. 1997; Rawal 2000; Ilfeld et al 2002a, b, 2003, 2004). However, the basic conditions (getting home, side effects, etc.) must be carefully discussed and evaluated with the patient and if necessary the relatives or family doctor should also be involved.

Besides the anesthetist's competence, the facilities and equipment are of fundamental importance in regional anesthesia. The treatment room should have a calm atmosphere, be of adequate size, and allow the patient to

be placed in suitable positions. Emergency medications, the possibility of ventilation and intubation, and also a defibrillator must be available. Every patient should have an i. v. line and basic monitoring (ECG, blood pressure monitoring).

In addition to monitoring of the vital parameters, assessment and monitoring of the onset, distribution, and quality of the nerve block is required. The procedure and sequence should be documented.

Patient Informed Consent before Peripheral Nerve Blocks

The procedure of a peripheral nerve block must be explained to the patient. It is important also to mention the possibility of an incomplete block and discuss further procedures in this case. General anesthesia should always be considered, so information must also be provided about this.

A regional block can be planned as a supplement to general anesthesia in major surgery, particularly when continuous peripheral nerve analgesia is planned or for postoperative pain management.

Whether sedation is desired for performance of the block must be discussed.

As well as specific complications of the technique (e.g., Horner syndrome in interscalene block, pneumothorax with blocks close to the clavicle), the patient must be generally informed about toxic reactions caused by the LA and about possible nerve injuries. Hematomas and false aneurysms can also occur after vascular puncture. If continuous peripheral techniques are planned, the risk of infection must be described. It must be pointed out to the patient that some problems can become apparent only after the end of the block (e.g., infection, pneumothorax). The patient should be instructed to report problems of any kind.

Position

The most comfortable position possible should be ensured for the patient. Positioning aids (cushions, pads, etc.) can facilitate the procedure. Position-related injuries in particular must be avoided. Attention must be paid to regions particularly at risk (e.g., ulnar nerve in the ulnar sulcus; fibular nerve at the head of the fibula). Pressure-free positioning of the limb must also be ensured in the postoperative period. This applies especially to continuous techniques. Special pads and splints are available (Fig. 16.2).

Monitoring

Consciousness: Many patients want sedation and this requires special attention and monitoring by the anesthetist. Pulse oximetry should be provided in sedated patients in addition to ECG and blood pressure monitoring.

Circulation: Oscillometric automatic blood pressure measurement has become well established in clinical practice. Wider circulatory monitoring during regional anesthesia is related to the risk classification of the patient and the type of operation.

ECG: There should be continuous ECG monitoring during the performance of a regional anesthesia block and perioperatively. Together with blood pressure monitoring, the ECG is the basis of monitoring patients under regional anesthesia.

Ventilation: Perioperative monitoring of ventilation during regional anesthesia is usually just clinical (visual and acoustic). With indirect measurement of ventilation by means of pulse oximetry, the consequences of reduced alveolar ventilation are identified with a marked delay, particularly when oxygen is being given (hypercapnic normoxia). Additional monitoring of spontaneous respiration (at least as a trend) can be performed by measuring end-expiratory CO_2. To do this, a CO_2 line is placed close to the patient's nose under the oxygen mask (Fig. 16.3).

Oxygenation: The status of pulse oximetry during regional anesthesia is controversial. It has a key position in the monitoring of vital functions, i.e., circulation and ventilation.

Fig. 16.2   Special pads help to prevent nerve injury in the (partially) anesthetized arm.

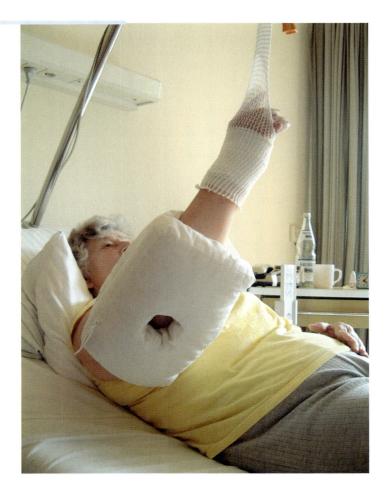

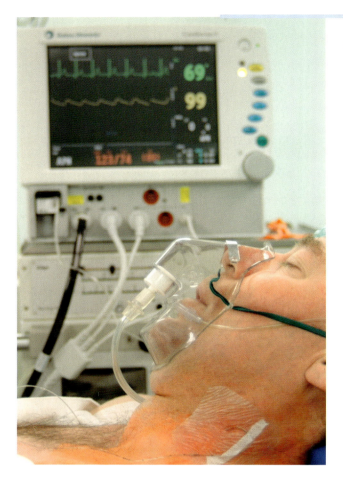

Fig. 16.**3**   Capnography installed under the patient's oxygen mask.

Vasoconstriction is a limiting factor of pulse oximetry.
Temperature: Monitoring of body temperature is indicated particularly in elderly patients, in prolonged operations, and when there is increased blood loss. In regional anesthesia with a marked sympathetic block, heat redistribution occurs and the insulating function of the periphery (vasoconstriction) is eliminated. In addition, the patient finds the cool room temperature (air conditioning) unpleasant. Adequate warming is therefore recommended during all operations. Air warming systems are regarded as particularly suitable.

16.3   Technical Aids for Performing Peripheral Nerve Blocks

Doppler Vascular Ultrasound

Doppler ultrasound is used in regional anesthesia for orientation of the course of blood vessels and to avoid vascular puncture. In difficult anatomical situations, it can be extremely helpful. With different acoustic transducers, the small and very handy devices that are now available can show both superficial (8 MHz) and very deep (4 MHz) veins and arteries (Fig. 16.**4**).

Ultrasound

Ultrasound in regional anesthesia was for a long time used either to diagnose side effects (e.g., phrenic nerve paresis) or to avoid vascular puncture. Use of this technique to show the anatomy and identify peripheral nerves in the region of the brachial plexus and, e.g., the lumbar plexus is a very recent development (Marhofer et al 2005).

This form of diagnostic ultrasound (small parts sonography), which uses high-frequency linear probes (7.5-15 MHz) to diagnose superficial anatomical structures (glands, joints, tendons, and nerves), presents new possibilities for regional anesthesia. Handy high-quality devices enable problem-free use even in the operating theatre (Fig. 16.**5**).
Just like tendons, nerves demonstrate anisotropic behavior in the reflection of ultra-

sound waves because of the layered and bundled structure of the tissue. The angle and the intensity of the reflection depend on the angle of emission of the ultrasound waves in relation to the long axis of the nerve. The best pictures are obtained when the signal is emitted at a right angle to the long axis of the nerve. This means that a sector scanner is unsuitable for use in this area as it exhibits suitable reflection conditions only in the central field but not in the marginal areas. Linear multifrequency digital 7.5-10 MHz acoustic transducers are regarded as optimal; they employ device

software dedicated to the purpose of small parts sonography. Ultrasound enables the spatial distribution of the LA to be visualized and allows one to observe how nerves are encompassed by the LA. The LA acts like a contrast agent on ultrasound because of its watery consistency. It is thus possible to predict the block of nerves and the spread (e.g., in divisions of a plexus) with certainty. Ultrasound-guided block of peripheral nerves is very suitable for the brachial plexus area and for femoral nerve block ("3-in-1 technique," see Chapter 9). As the pleura is imaged during a supraclavicular

block technique, a pneumothorax can be avoided (Otaki et al. 2000).

Use of the technique requires some practice and a high-quality device. Under these conditions, ultrasound may be of considerable importance in the future in regional anesthesia procedures and also in monitoring the position of catheters. Brown (1998) has attributed to this procedure the potential to revolutionize the procedure of brachial plexus anesthesia.

Figures 16.**6**-16.**12** show examples of scans of peripheral nerves using the ultrasound technique.

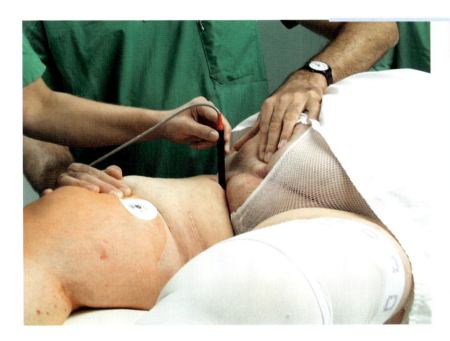

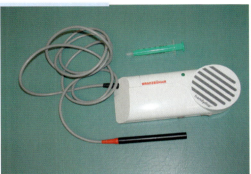

Fig. 16.**4**   Vascular Doppler for tracing the course of blood vessels, especially useful in difficult anatomical situations.

Fig. 16.**5**   Ultrasound device for orientation in peripheral nerve blocks.

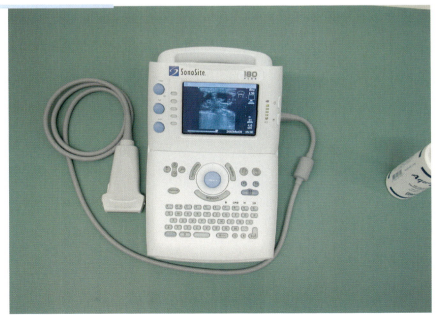

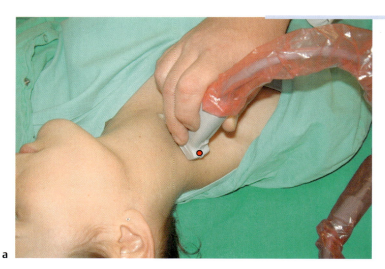

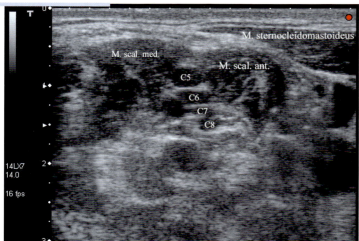

Fig. 16.**6 a**   Ultrasound guidance for interscalene approach to the brachial plexus. The red dot indicates the position of the ultrasound transducer.

Fig. 16.**6 b**   The ultrasound transducer is moved laterally until the lateral border of the sternocleidomastoid can be distinguished. The scalenus anterior and scalenus medius muscles can be identified beneath it. The plexus can be identified as a chain of round to oval structures representing the cross sections of the roots (C5–C8, T1) (Photographs: Kapral/Marhofer, Toshiba Apilo, 14–10 MHz probe, linear.)

Fig. 16.**6 c**   Spread of 15 ml of local anesthetic.

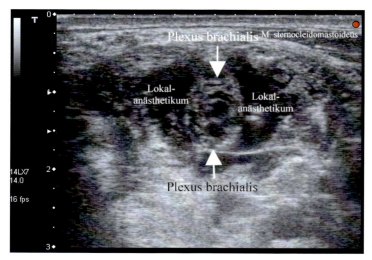

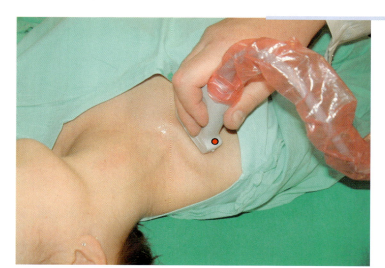

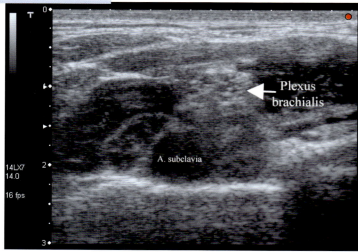

Fig. 16.**7 a**   Ultrasound guidance for supraclavicular approach to the brachial plexus. The red dot indicates the position of the ultrasound transducer.

Fig. 16.**7 b**   Ultrasound monitoring in the supraclavicular and infraclavicular regions can minimize the risk of pleural injury when a brachial plexus block is performed in this area (Photograph: Kapral/Marhofer, Toshiba Apilo, 14–10 MHz probe, linear.)

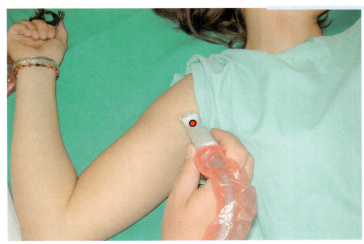

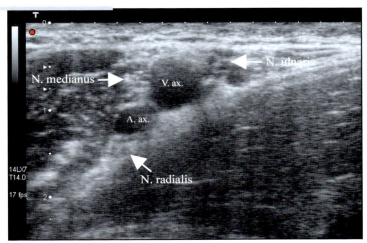

Fig. 16.**8 a**　Ultrasound guidance for axillary approach to the brachial plexus. The red dot indicates the position of the ultrasound transducer.

Fig. 16.**8 b**　This site appears the most suitable for beginners using the ultrasound method as the anatomy is familiar and the structures can readily be distinguished ultrasonographically. (Photograph: Kapral/Marhofer, Toshiba Apilo, 14–10 MHz probe, linear.)

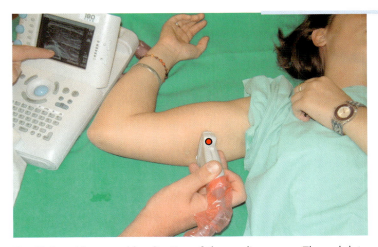

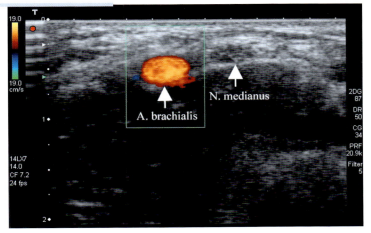

Fig. 16.**9 a**　Ultrasound localization of the median nerve. The red dot indicates the position of the ultrasound transducer.

Fig. 16.**9 b**　The peripheral nerves, e.g., in the distal upper arm or elbow, can be shown well ultrasonically. An essential requirement is detailed knowledge of the planes and anatomy and ultrasound images of the peripheral nerves. (Photograph: Kapral/Marhofer, Toshiba Apilo, 14–10 MHz probe, linear.)

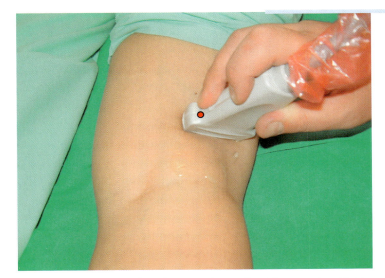

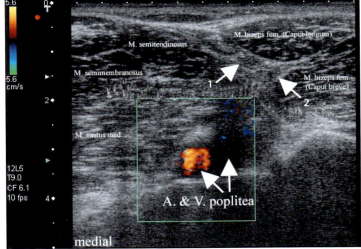

Fig. 16.**10 a**　Ultrasound guidance in the popliteal fossa region (right leg). The red dot indicates the position of the ultrasound transducer.

1　Tibial nerve
2　Common fibular nerve

Fig. 16.**10 b**　Ultrasonography of the popliteal fossa shows the popliteal vessels well. The sciatic nerve, which has already divided into the fibular and tibial nerves, can easily be identified. (Photograph: Kapral/Marhofer, Toshiba Apilo, 14–10 MHz probe, linear.)

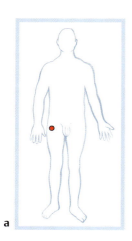

a

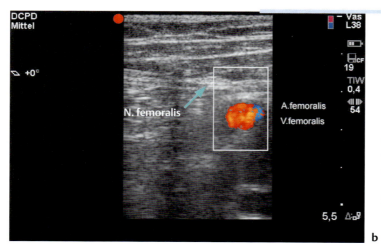

b

Fig. 16.**11 a**   Ultrasound imaging of the
femoral nerve (right leg). The red dot indicates the position of the ultrasound transducer.

Fig. 16.**11 b**   Because of its relatively superficial position, the femoral nerve is highly suitable for ultrasound-guided nerve block distal to the inguinal ligament with the femoral
artery as another close landmark. (Photograph: G. Meier/Steffgen, SonoSite Titan, 10–
5 MHz probe, linear.)

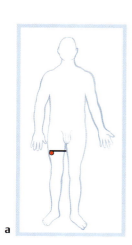

a

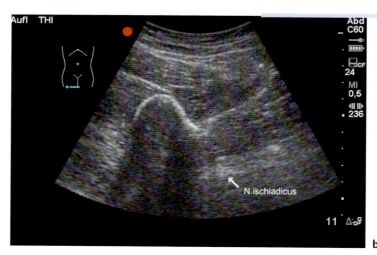

b

Fig. 16.**12 a**   Ultrasound imaging of the sciatic nerve (right thigh, anterior). The red dot
indicates the position of the ultrasound
transducer.

Fig. 16.**12 b**   The digital high-frequency
linear probe can penetrate only a few centimeters, but the linear probe is unsuitable
for ultrasound-guided block of ventral sciatic
blocks. The digital low-frequency curved-
array probe (2–4 MHz) enables an excellent
deep view deep, but with the disadvantage
of poorer resolution. However, it is well
suited for orientation and determination of
the skin–nerve distance (here 11 cm). (Photograph: G. Meier/Steffgen, SonoSite Titan,
Curved Array, 5–2 MHz.)

Surface Thermometer

Depending on the proportion of sympathetic
fibers, block of peripheral nerves leads to
regional sympathetic block. The proportion
of sympathetic fibers is very high, for
instance, in the brachial plexus and the sciatic nerve. The effects of the block can be
checked very well by monitoring the skin
temperature. As the C-fibers (postganglionic
sympathetic fibers) are blocked first, a rise
in skin temperature distal to the site of the
block is an early indication of the onset of
the block. The rise in skin temperature is 2-8
Celsius degrees depending on the baseline
and can be measured quickly and easily with
a surface thermometer.
A suitable thermometer (adjustable to surface temperature) is, for example, First Temp
Genius (Sherwood Medical) (Fig. 16.**13**).

Peripheral Nerve Stimulation (PNS)

The need for peripheral nerve stimulation in
performing conduction anesthesia continues
to be controversial (Schwarz et al. 1998).
Regional anesthesia can also be performed
successfully without nerve stimulation. This
applies particularly for techniques that for
anatomical reasons (common fascial sheath
around the nerves) allow a loss-of-resistance
technique (e.g., axillary plexus anesthesia).
PNS can then be used for additional orientation. However, use of a nerve stimulator
should be mandatory in difficult anatomical
situations and in nerve blocks involving a
large skin-nerve distance (e.g., sciatic nerve).
PNS is particularly indicated for nerves with
predominantly motor fibers (e.g., femoral
nerve) as paresthesia cannot always be produced because of lack of sensory fibers,
which means an increased risk of injuries to
the nerve. In purely motor neurons, an over-

proportionate incidence of intraneural injection can be expected (Graf and Martin 2001;
Urmey 1997).
PNS cannot be regarded as a substitute for
anatomical knowledge but it is a valuable
aid to precise localization of the nerve. In
clinical practice, peripheral nerve stimula-
tion enables verification of correct needle
position and thus usually helps to avoid
nerve damage.
The following are the *minimum requirements
for a nerve stimulator* nowadays (Kaiser
2003) (Fig. 16.**14**).
Electrical design:
- Adjustable constant current
- Monophasic rectangular output pulse
- Adjustable pulse duration (0.1-1.0 ms)
- Adjustable current intensity (0-5.0 mA)
- Exact adjustability
- Digital display of actual current value
- Stimulating frequency 1-2 Hz

Fig. 16.**13** Suitable surface thermometer for objective confirmation of the success of the block.

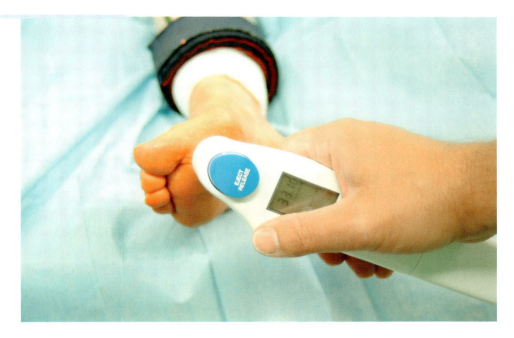

Fig. 16.**14** Nerve stimulators for performing peripheral nerve blocks.

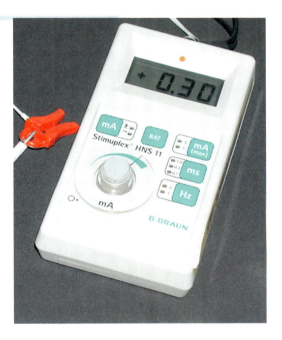
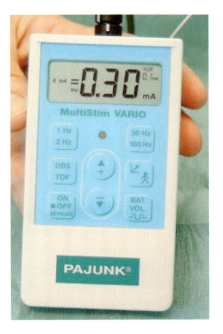

Device safety:
- Alarm when circuit is interrupted
- Alarm when impedance is too high
- Alarm on internal device error
- Outputs clearly assigned
- Reliable instructions for use stating tolerated deviations

Advantages of Peripheral Nerve Stimulation
- Cooperation with the patient is not necessary, so regional anesthesia can also take place under light sedation and in patients who are unable to cooperate (e.g., children, "confused" patients).
- Peripheral blocks can be performed in regions that are already partially or completely anesthetized by more proximal blocks (e.g., plexus or neuraxial blocks).

- The risk of nerve injury is reduced to the minimum as direct contact of the needle with the nerve is deliberately avoided.

The distance between the exploring needle and the nerve can be estimated from the strength of the current required. If a very small current (0.2 mA) produces an adequate muscle contraction, the needle is in immediate proximity to the nerve. Too close proximity of the needle tip (current < 0.3 mA/ 0.1 ms) should be avoided for considerations of safety, particularly in a sedated patient (Choyce et al. 2001). In regional blocks in patients without polyneuropathy, successful, effective, and safe blocks can be achieved with minimal currents of 0.3 mA and a pulse duration of 0.1 ms (Neuburger et al. 2001). Currents over 0.5 mA lead to more failures and incomplete anesthesia.

Stimulation of purely sensory nerves (e.g., saphenous nerve) is also possible, but the use of a longer pulse (1.0 ms) is recommended (Comfort et al. 1996).

Practical Notes
- The pulse duration is given as "ms" for millisecond. Note: In the Anglo-American language area the pulse duration is sometimes given as μsec (0.1 ms = 100 μsec).
- When the nerve stimulator is operated after perforation of the skin, it should first be ensured using a low amplitude that the needle tip is not already in the vicinity of the nerve, as uncontrolled muscle contractions might occur otherwise. The subsequent search for the nerve begins at a current amplitude of 1.0 mA

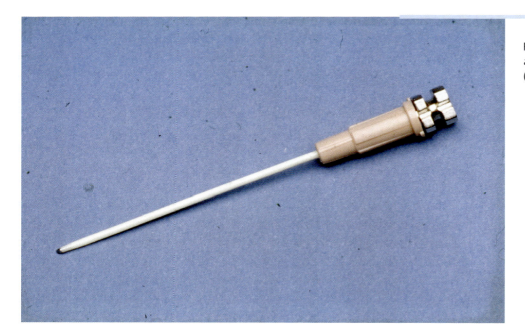

Fig. 16.**15** Combination needle–cannula for axillary plexus anesthesia (18G, 51 mm) (Pajunk, Geisingen).

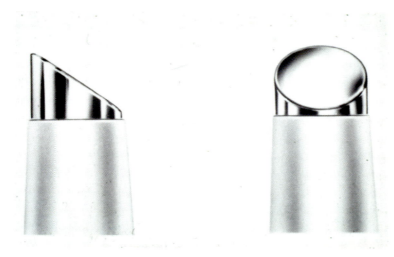

and a pulse width of 0.1 ms with decreasing current.

- In sedated patients or in blocks that are difficult for anatomical reasons, the selection of a longer pulse (1.0 ms) initially in order to obtain a response promptly is appropriate. As soon as contractions in the key muscle are produced, the nerve stimulator is switched to the shorter pulse (0.1 ms).
- Injection at a response below 0.3 mA and a pulse width of 0.1 ms should be avoided, because this indicates a very close proximity of the needle tip to the nerve, with a probably higher risk of nerve damage but resulting in no better success of the peripheral nerve block.
- Practical clinical experience has shown that a response at 0.2-0.3 mA/1.0 ms often corresponds to a response of 1 mA/0.1 ms (Neuburger et al. 2001). In order to avoid anesthesia failures, at least 0.5 mA/0.1 ms should be looked for when stimulating a mixed nerve.

- In patients with polyneuropathy (e.g., diabetes mellitus), selection of a longer pulse (1.0 ms) is rational.
- A minimum distance between the electrode and stimulation needle has not been established. The site of placement of the cutaneous electrode appears to be unimportant during nerve localization for peripheral nerve blocks (Hadzic 2004), when constant-current nerve stimulators are used.
- Contrary to the statements of the manufacturers, PNS can also be used in patients with implanted cardiac pacemakers/defibrillators (Kaiser 2003). However, it should be ensured that the pacemaker aggregate, the cardiac electrodes, and the heart are not on the line connecting the skin electrode to the stimulation needle.

Stimulation Needles and Catheters

Needles insulated on the shaft and conductive at the tip (monopolar or unipolar) are used as stimulation needles. Which type of insulated needle should be used depends crucially on the anatomical requirements and the (catheter) technique to be performed. If a technique can be performed successfully with "loss of resistance" (e.g., axillary plexus anesthesia), a needle with a 45° bevel ("short" bevel) is appropriate. In conductive anesthesia, where resistance-free sliding of the needle is of advantage (e.g., sciatic block), a needle with a pencil-point tip or a 30° bevel is better. Needles with a so-called sharp or long bevel (15°) slide best through the tissue, but the risk of injuring the nerve is greater (Hirasawa et al. 1990; Selander 1993; Selander et al. 1977).

However, the direction of the needle is also important in nerve injuries. Where anatomically possible, it should be at an acute angle and parallel to the course of the nerve (Hempel and Baur 1982). For needles with a 15° bevel, combination with a nerve stimulator is recommended in every case (Hirasawa et al. 1990).

Noninsulated needles are also employed in combination with a nerve stimulator, but this combination is not recommended.

Needles for the Catheter Technique

Insulated needles should be also used for nerve stimulation when catheter techniques are employed. There are two techniques, which differ in both material and procedure:
- Needles with a surrounding plastic cannula
- Insulated needles (with catheter-through-needle technique)

Needles with Surrounding Plastic Cannula
The advantage of the 45°, short-bevel needle is the possibility of using it for "loss-of-resistance" techniques, as an obvious perforation click is felt when the neurovascular sheath is penetrated. Compared to a hollow needle, the advantage of a solid steel stylet is said to be the avoidance of "punch injuries" of the nerve.

After successful stimulation and after the stylet is removed and the LA is injected, the indwelling cannula can initially be left in place for further injection or top-ups, or the catheter is advanced through the needle, e.g., for longer operations or for pain therapy (continuous technique).

- "Combination" needle for axillary plexus anesthesia (18G, 51 mm; for infants or school children use 20G) (also suitable for femoral nerve block) with solid steel stylet, plastic cannula and 45° bevel with rounded edges (in a set with 20G catheter with side opening). (Pajunk, Geisingen [Fig. 16.**15**].)
- "Combination" needle for high axillary plexus anesthesia (or 3-in-1 technique) 16G, 83 mm, with solid steel stylet and 45° bevel with rounded edges (in a set with 19G catheter with side opening). (Pajunk, Geisingen.)
- "Contiplex" D needle, unipolar needle with 15° or 30° bevel with plastic cannula. (B Braun [Fig. 16.**16**].)
- Insulated needle with surrounding plastic cannula and catheter, pencil-point, facet, or Tuohy tip. (Pajunk, Geisingen.)

Insulated Needles (with Catheter-through-Needle Technique)
After successful identification of the nerve and injection of the LA, the catheter can be advanced through the needle. The insulated needles have a 30° bevel or a pencil-point tip with a side opening. The catheter can be advanced in the desired direction through the side opening. The diameter of the needles should be kept as small as possible in consideration of tissue trauma. Nevertheless, it must be ensured that the needle is sufficiently stable, e.g., for deep blocks, and that a catheter of adequate diameter (20G) can be introduced.
- Plexolong catheter set; insulated needle with pencil-point tip and side opening

(19.5G, 60 mm) for brachial plexus anesthesia (interscalene, infraclavicular) and distal sciatic nerve block, 20G catheter with central end-orifice. (Pajunk, Geisingen [Fig. 16.**17**].)
- Plexolong catheter set; insulated needle with pencil-point tip or Tuohy tip (19.5G, 120 mm) for psoas compartment block, 20G catheter with central end-orifice. (Pajunk, Geisingen.)
- Plexolong catheter set; insulated needle with facet tip or Tuohy tip (19.5G, 100 mm) for proximal or distal sciatic nerve block, 20G catheter. (Pajunk, Geisingen.)
- Plexolong catheter set; insulated needle with facet tip (19.5G, 150 mm) for anesthesia of the sciatic nerve and psoas compartment block, 20G catheter with central end-orifice. (Pajunk, Geisingen.)

Stimulating Catheters

Special catheters are available that have a stimulation tip for checking their position. These catheters can be employed for precise placement of the catheter, for instance, in difficult anatomical situations (Pham-Dang 2003). A stimulating catheter is also suitable for the differential diagnosis of dislocation/tachyphylaxis (e.g., Stimulong Plus, Pajunk, Geisingen; StimuCath, Arrow International) (Fig. 16.**18**). Adequate stimulation response before new administration of LA indicates that there is no catheter dislocation. If it is inadequate, an attempt can be made to correct the catheter position by withdrawing it.

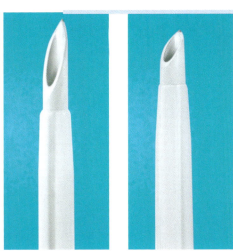

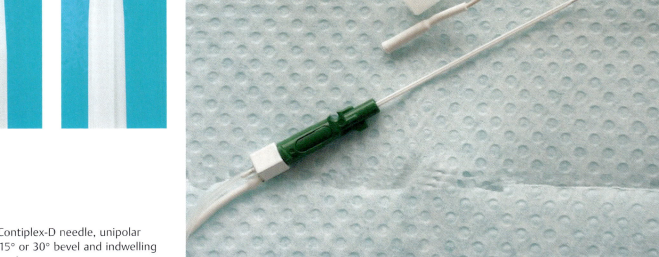

Fig. 16.**16**   Contiplex-D needle, unipolar needle with 15° or 30° bevel and indwelling needle (B Braun).

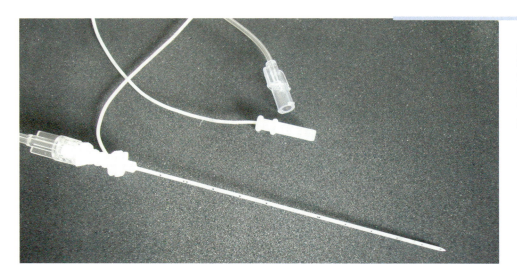

Fig. 16.**17** Insulated needles for catheter-through-needle technique; Plexolong catheter set, Pajunk, Geisingen. The needle is available in different lengths (5–15 cm) and with different tips (faceted bevel tip, pencil-point tip with lateral opening and Tuohy tip).

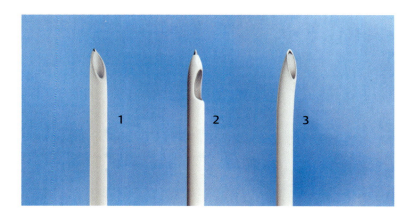

1 Faceted bevel needle
2 Special pencil-point needle (Sprotte)
3 Tuohy needle

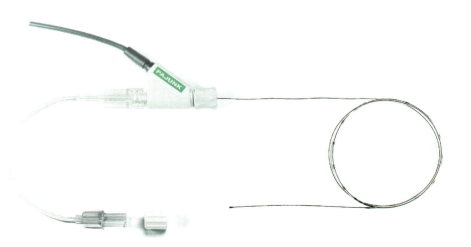

Fig. 16.**18** A stimulation catheter enables the position of the catheter tip to be checked by electrostimulation with a nerve stimulator.

16.4   General Principles for Performance of Regional Anesthesia

- The puncture site and its surrounding area are disinfected and draped with sterile fenestrated drapes.
- Infiltration anesthesia with a 26G needle: too deep injection has to be avoided, as it carries the risk of premature block of the target nerve or plexus.
- A skin puncture can then be made with a lancet or sharp needle. This is recommended when using a short-bevel needle in order to advance it through the tissue with minimal force. At the same time, this prevents punched-out material from being carried inward (Fig. 16.**19**).
- The needle is advanced subcutaneously with slight rotation of the needle tip (if necessary slightly "shaking" the needle tip to loosen it from the surrounding tissue).
- In the *loss-of-resistance technique*, advance the needle until there is a "fascial click."
- The nerve stimulator is then attached.
- A longer pulse (1.0 ms) should be selected when stimulating sensory nerves.

- The distance of the skin electrode from the site of stimulation is not important, but the distance must be adequate to ensure sterility.
- Maximal muscle contractions should be avoided as the patient can find these unpleasant.
- The stimulation needle is advanced carefully. Whenever possible, perform intermittent aspirations to detect an intravascular position.
- Continuous aspiration should not be performed as the catheter lumen can become occluded by tissue.
- If the patient reports pain during the puncture, a further infiltrating injection of LA can be given provided a response has not yet occurred in the key muscle.
- When there is a motor response, the current is reduced gradually until key muscle contractions are still just visible at a pulse amplitude of 0.3 mA to a maximum of 0.5 mA and 0.1 ms pulse width. The LA is then injected.

- Placement of a catheter should usually be done after injection of the LA as experience has shown that the catheter can then be advanced more easily. If a stimulation catheter is used, neither LA nor saline solution should be given before the catheter is placed, as both impair stimulating response.
- The catheter is usually advanced 3-5 cm beyond the distal end of the needle. If the catheter ends in an incorrect position, it should be withdrawn to the original stimulation position.
- The catheter can be fixed by suturing or by use of a sterile adhesive dressing (Fig. 16.**20**).
- A sterile dressing should include an absorbent dressing for the first 25 hours. This can then be replaced by a transparent dressing.
- Document the depth of puncture and the skin level of the catheter in the patient's record.

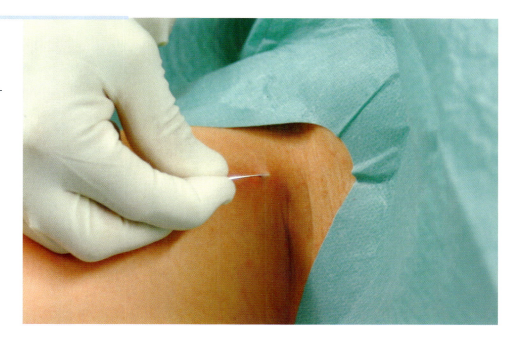

Fig. 16.**19**   An incision with a lancet is required to enable passage through the skin, particularly when using short-bevel or blunt pencil-point "atraumatic" needles; it also prevents introduction of possibly contaminated skin particles.

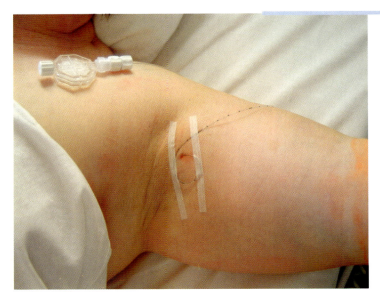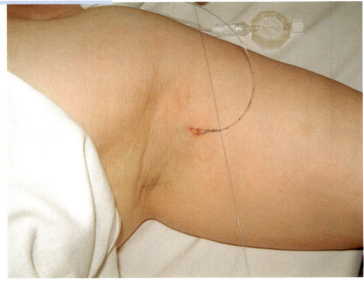

Fig. 16.**20**   The catheter can be fixed temporarily with sterile adhesive strips, or for longer use with a suture.

16.5   Analgesia/Sedation for Regional Anesthesia/Peripheral Nerve Block

For Peripheral Nerve Blocks

Regional blocks for postoperative pain therapy can be performed in the anesthetized patient or under spinal anesthesia if they are placed with correct use of a nerve stimulator and employing atraumatic insulated needles. However, the awake, cooperative patient is the best guarantee for avoiding nerve injury, particularly when pain catheters are placed. Under sedation with midazolam or propofol, patients are often restless and difficult to control.

The following *recommendations for analgosedation* enable performance of a regional peripheral nerve block in a sedated and cooperative patient (Table 16.**1**):
Sufentanyl 5 μg + midazolam 1 mg i. v. (Gentili et al. 1999).

Alternatively: remifentanil 0.05 μg/kg body weight (b.w.)/min, if necessary after a "loading dose" of 0.3 μg/kg.
This dose of remifentanil provides ideal conditions for placement of a nerve block but requires monitoring of ventilation. It is advisable to give oxygen through a mask during placement of the block. After a successful block, a patient on a remifentanil infusion must be adequately monitored!

Concomitant Medication during Surgery under Regional Anesthesia

Remifentanil has also proved effective at the above dosage for analgosedation during surgery (Lauwers et al. 1999).

Intraoperative Sedation with Remifentanil under Regional Anesthesia
Remifentanil 0.05 μg/kg b.w./min (Graf and Martin 2001).
Taking the desired effect and the side effects into account, Holas et al. (1999) recommend the combination of propofol and remifentanil at the following dosage:
Remifentanil 0.03 μg/kg b.w./min + propofol 0.7 mg/kg b.w./h (Ford et al. 1984).
Target-controlled infusion with propofol is recommended for sedation during regional blocks (Janzen et al. 2000; Sutcliffe 2000). This can also be patient-controlled (Irwin et al. 1997).

Variant 1	Sufentanyl 5 μg + midazolam 1 mg
Variant 2	"Loading Dose": remifentanil 0.3 μg/kg Followed by: remifentanil 0.05 μg/kg/min

Table 16.**1**   Intravenous analgosedation for setting up a nerve block (normal-weight adult)

16.6 General Principles for Administration of Local Anesthetics in Peripheral Nerve Block

Local Anesthetics

Medium-acting and long-acting amide LAs are most frequently used in regional anesthesia today (Table 16.**2**).

The choice of LA for a peripheral block is influenced by the following considerations: An LA with a *rapid onset* is desirable. Because of their chemical structure, medium-acting LAs have advantages in this respect. However, the latency time obtained in a combined femoral-sciatic nerve block with 0.75% (7.5 mg/ml) ropivacaine was similar to 2% (20 mg/ml) mepivacaine (Casati et al. 1999).

When the "single-shot" technique is used, a long-acting LA is often required depending on the *anticipated duration of surgery*; moreover, the long-acting LA may provide correspondingly long-lasting *postoperative analgesia*. With ropivacaine, an average duration of analgesia of 12-14 hours can be expected (Casati et al. 1999; Wank et al. 2002), and in individual cases the effect may last up to 20 hours. A partial motor block can be observed for almost the same period. Patients must be informed about the probable duration of the block, so that they do not worry unnecessarily.

Relatively high doses of LA are administered in peripheral blocks. Many peripheral techniques include the risk of accidental intravascular injection. For this reason, the *local anesthetic with the lowest toxicity should be preferred*. Medium-acting LAs are less toxic than long-acting ones. Among the long-acting LAs, ropivacaine is less toxic than bupivacaine. While it is argued that ropivacaine is of lower potency for central blocks compared to bupivacaine (D'Angelo and James 1999), numerous studies confirm the equipotency of ropivacaine to bupivacaine in peripheral blocks (Altintas 2005; Casati et al. 2000a, 2001; Eroglu et al 2004; Greengrass et al. 1998; Hickey et al. 1992; Hilgier 1985; Klein et al. 1998). Being less lipophilic than bupivacaine, ropivacaine provides a better differential block at lower concentrations than bupivacaine (Borgeat et al. 2001).

Pulmonary function as a consequence of ipsilateral hemidiaphragmatic paresis decreased more after interscalene brachial plexus blocks with 0.33% (3.3 mg/ml) bupivacaine than with 0.33% (3.3 mg/ml) ropivacaine in patients with chronic renal failure. Block quality was similar in both groups (Altintas et al 2005).

Mixtures of a long-acting LA with a medium-acting one are occasionally used. This combines the relatively short onset of the medium-acting LA with the long duration of the long acting one. It must be remembered that the toxicity of local anesthetics is additive.

Dosage

Depending on age and physical constitution a volume of *30-50 ml of a 1% (1 mg/ml) solution of a medium-acting LA can be recommended* for all peripheral nerve blocks close to the trunk (Table 16.**3**).

A medium-acting LA (e.g., mepivacaine or lidocaine) will be used primarily. The recommended maximum dose of mepivacaine is 500 mg. Dosages of up to 750 mg in adults of normal weight are tolerated without problems (Cockings et al. 1987; Simon et al. 1990). After an initial dose of 400 mg of mepivacaine, repeat doses of up to 400 mg can be given up to three times at two-hour intervals for axillary continuous plexus anesthesia without fear of toxic blood levels or clinical signs of overdose (Büttner et al. 1989 b). As a long-acting LA, ropivacaine has proved to be less toxic than bupivacaine and to have similar potency in peripheral nerve blocks (see above). For axillary plexus block, a dose of up to *300 mg of ropivacaine 0.75% (7.5 mg/ml)* has proved to be effective without side effects (Wank et al. 2002).

In *combined femoral-sciatic nerve block*, the established maximum doses will have to be exceeded to achieve an adequate effect for the two techniques. Normally the toxicity of the LAs presents no clinically relevant problem in such cases because of the delayed absorption of LA in lower-limb nerve blocks

Table 16.**2** Overview of commonly used local anesthetics. The distribution coefficient gives information about the lipid solubility of the individual local anesthetics

Substance	Potency in vitro (Procaine = 1)	Molecular Weight	pK_a (25°C)	Distribution Coefficient	Protein Binding	Duration of Action (hours)
Mepivacaine	4	246	7.6	0.8	77%	1.5–3
Bupivacaine	16	288	8.16	27.5	96%	1.5–8
Ropivacaine	14–16	276	8.05	6.7	95%	3–6
Lidocaine	4	234	7.9	2.9	65%	2–4

Table 16.**3** Dosage of local anesthetics in peripheral blocks close to the trunk (normal-weight adult)

Local Anesthetic	Volume ("Single Shot")
Medium-acting (30–50 ml)	Lidocaine 1% (10 mg/ml) Alternatively, mepivacaine 1% (10 mg/ml)
Long-acting (30–40 ml)	Ropivacaine 0.5% (5 mg/ml)/0.75% (7.5 mg/ml) Alternatively, bupivacaine 0.5% (5 mg/ml)

Alkalinization of the local anesthetic:
1 ml NaHCO$_3$ 8.4% to 10 ml mepivacaine/lidocaine 1% (10 mg/ml)

Clonidine 0.5-1.0 μ/kg added to the local anesthetic leads to prolongation of the block; in chronic pain states, an intensification of the block can occasionally be noted.

Table 16.**4** Additions to the local anesthetic in peripheral nerve blocks

(Magistris et al. 2000), provided accidental intravascular injection does not occur. When continuous techniques are performed, the two blocks can be initiated with a medium-acting LA. If a continuous technique is not used and longer-lasting analgesia is desired, a combination of a medium-acting LA (lidocaine or mepivacaine) with ropivacaine can be given. The total dose in this case should not be more than 150 mg of ropivacaine and 300-400 mg of mepivacaine.
Addition of epinephrine can generally be omitted in peripheral blocks.

Measures to Shorten the Latency Time

A problem of peripheral nerve blocks is their relatively long onset time, and numerous attempts have been made to shorten it. There are essentially three approaches:
- Carbonization of the LA
- Alkalinization of the LA
- Warming of the LA

Carbonization of the Local Anesthetic
The anticipated advantage of using a LA in the carbonic acid salt formulation instead of the HCl preparation (e.g., mepivacaine-CO$_2$ vs. mepivacaine-HCl) has not been confirmed (Dreesen et al. 1986; Krebs and Hempel 1985). Shorter onset times were not found with peripheral blocks, although high blood levels did indicate a faster absorption of the CO$_2$-containing formulation.

Alkalinization of the Local Anesthetic
Numerous randomized, mostly double-blind, studies were able to show a faster onset of peripheral nerve blocks as a result of alkalinization of the LA solution (Büttner and Klose

1991; Capogna et al. 1995; Coventry and Todd 1989; DiOrio and Ellis 1988; Gormley et al. 1996; Hilgier 1985; Quinlan et al. 1992; Tetzlaff et al. 1990; 1995). Moreover, better tolerance of the blood-free field tourniquet (Tetzlaff et al. 1993), more profound motor block (Tetzlaff et al. 1995), and a better overall block effect (Quinlan et al. 1992) were observed. Only a few studies showed no beneficial effect of alkalinization on the onset time (Auroy et al. 1997; Candido et al. 1995; Chow et al. 1998), probably as a result of too great an increase in the pH (Auroy et al. 1997; Candido et al. 1995), which may have resulted in precipitation of the local anesthetics.
The optimal proportions of LA and added sodium bicarbonate are influenced by the LA used and its concentration. The following proportions are well tested and recommended (Table 16.**4**):
Mepivacaine 1% (10 mg/ml)(or 1.5% [15 mg/ml]) 10 ml + NaHCO$_3$ 8.4% 1 ml.
Alkalinization of ropivacaine is theoretically possible (e.g., 0.1 ml bicarbonate/20 ml ropivacaine) (Fulling and Peterfreund 2000) but is not recommended for routine clinical use because of the risk of precipitation (Milner et al. 2000).

Warming the Local Anesthetic
Warming the LA to body temperature leads to a significantly faster onset of effect (Heath et al. 1990). The mechanism is unclear. Overheating must be excluded.

Adjuvants

Attempts to improve the quality of the block and prolong the duration of action by adding various adjuvants have been reported.

Clonidine
When added to different LAs, clonidine leads to a significant prolongation of postoperative analgesia (Büttner et al. 1992; Casati et al. 2000b; El Saied et al. 2000). However, no effect could be demonstrated in conjunction with 0.75% (7.5 mg/ml) ropivacaine for axillary plexus block (Erlacher et al. 2000). The optimal dosage appears to be 0.5-1 μg clonidine/kg b.w. added to the LA solution (Bernard and Macaire 1997; Singelyn et al. 1996). Higher dosages are accompanied by systemic side effects such as sedation and hypotension (Büttner et al. 1992). In intravenous regional anesthesia there was better toleration of a tourniquet with the addition of 150 μg of clonidine (Gentili et al. 1999). Infected tissues under peripheral neural block are normally more resistant than healthy areas to anesthesia; clonidine added to mepivacaine seems to enhance both anesthesia during surgery and postoperative analgesia (Iohom 2005). Addition of clonidine (1-2 μg/ml) to a continuous perineural ropivacaine infusion showed no clinically relevant benefits (Ilfeld 2003a; Ilfeld 2005).

Opioids
Any anticipated benefit of adding opioids to local anesthetics for peripheral nerve block has not been confirmed (Bouaziz et al. 2000; Magistris et al. 2000; Murphy et al. 2000; Nishikawa et al. 2000).

Neostigmine
Neostigmine appears to have some beneficial effects on postoperative analgesia but does not lead to a faster block (Bone et al. 1999).

References

See pp. 244-246.

17 Continuous Peripheral Nerve Blocks

Advantages

The superiority of peripheral nerve blocks for postoperative analgesia after major shoulder and knee surgery compared to systemic intravenous PCA (patient controlled analgesia) with opioids has been demonstrated clearly (Borgeat et al. 1997; Capdevila et al. 1999; Singelyn et al. 1998). For postoperative analgesia after extensive knee surgery, continuous epidural analgesia and a continuous femoral nerve block via catheter were assessed as equally effective; because of the lower risk, the peripheral block should be preferred (see below). However, apart from the superiority with regard to the analgesic effect, a significant benefit on the duration of rehabilitation and on the quality of the rehabilitation is also achieved (Capdevila et al. 1999).

With the aid of a continuous peripheral nerve block, possible major complications in association with neuraxial blocks can be avoided.

Selective nerve block of the affected lower limb enables early mobilization as only one limb is affected. However, it must be borne in mind that motor weakness is present in the affected limb.

In contrast to epidural block, prolonged urinary diversion is not required.

The contraindications with regard to neuraxial techniques are much wider than for peripheral blocks, so that a peripheral nerve catheter for continuous pain management can be placed in cases where a neuraxial procedure is contraindicated or not technically feasible.

Indications

- Severe postoperative pain
- Posttraumatic pain states
- Physiotherapy treatment
- Sympathetic block
- Prevention and treatment of amputation stump and phantom pain

Local Anesthetics: Administration, Dosage

Different types of administration can be distinguished:

- Intermittent administration of a bolus
- Continuous administration
- Patient-controlled bolus delivery with or without basic continuous infusion

Which of the listed methods will be used depends, among other things, on organizational factors. Numerous variants of local anesthetic administration for postoperative pain therapy through continuous peripheral nerve catheters have been studied (Meyer and Hermann 1998; Mezzatesta et al. 1997; Singelyn and Gouverneur 2000; Singelyn et al. 1999).

The following dosage recommendations can be given for the long-term use of local anesthetics (Table 17.1):

Ropivacaine 0.2%-0.375% (2-3.75 mg/ml), 6-10 ml/h.

Alternatively: bupivacaine 0.125%-0.375% (1.25-3.75 mg/ml), 5-10 ml/h, max. 30 mg/h. Ropivacaine should be preferred because of the lower toxicity and the lower motor impairment by ropivacaine in the low concentration ranges (Borgeat et al. 2001). In the first 24 hours postoperatively, 0.2% (2 mg/ml) ropivacaine at a dosage of

0.25 mg/kg b.w./h proved insufficiently effective (Salonen et al. 2000). Therefore, 0.33-0.375% (3.3-3.75 mg/ml) ropivacaine is often used in this situation.

It should be kept in mind that the clearance of local anesthetic from the body is reduced by high age, renal dysfunction, hepatic dysfunction, and cardiac dysfunction. In these circumstances, doses need to be reduced according to age- and disease-related influences on the pharmacodynamics and pharmacokinetics (Rosenberg 2004).

The use of *infusion or syringe pumps* has proved useful for techniques of continuous analgesia. Continuous delivery can be provided through perfusor syringes, which are usually limited to a volume of 50 ml. A consequent disadvantage is the requirement for frequent change of syringe with relatively high infusion rates (6-10 ml/h). However, syringe pumps with a freely selectable volume per bolus have been available for some years, and are suitable for greater volumes (60-100 ml).

Devices that enable both continuous and patient-controlled intermittent delivery (PCA) are well tried and tested. A commercially available plastic bag (Polybag) containing 200 ml of ropivacaine can be attached to these pumps. If a higher concentration of ropivacaine is desired, 240 ml of a 0.33% (3.3 mg/ml) solution can be made by adding 40 ml of 1% (10 mg/ml) ropivacaine (Table 17.2). As well as the advantage of less frequent change of bags, which is important from the hygiene aspect, these devices provide the patient with greater mobility. The use of large-volume infusion units leads to considerably improved organizational possibilities.

Table 17.**1**   Recommended dosages for long-term use of local anesthetics

Ropivacaine 0.2–0.375% (2–3.75 mg/ml), 6–10 ml/h (max. 37.5 mg/h)
(Alternatively: bupivacaine 0.125–0.375% (1.25–3.75 mg/ml), 5–10 ml/h (max. 30 mg/h)

Table 17.**2**   Suggestions for increasing the concentration of Naropin 2 mg/ml in the "Polybag"

Ropivacaine (Naropin Polybag 200 ml/ actual volume 210 ml)	Standard	420 mg Ropivacaine	210 ml Volume	2 mg/ml Ropivacaine
	ml Additional Volume	Total mg	Total Volume	Concentration mg/ml
Increase in concentration by addition of Naropin 10 mg/ml	10	520	220	2.4
	20	620	230	2.7
	40	820	250	3.3
	60	1020	270	3.8

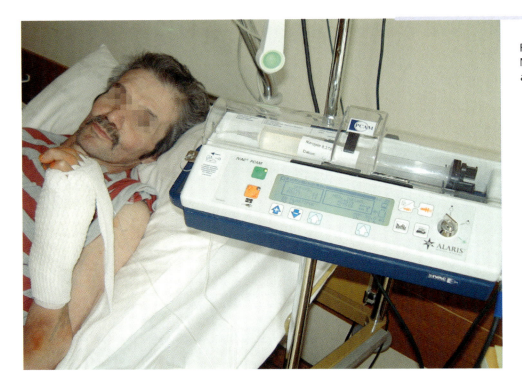

Fig. 17.**1**   Syringe pump PCAM P5000 (Alaris Medical Systems) for continuous infusion and/or bolus delivery of local anesthetic.

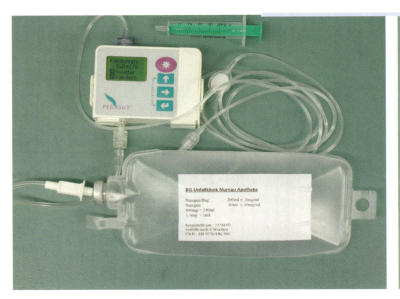
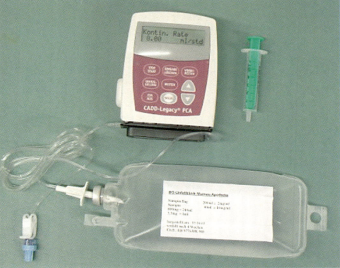

Fig. 17.**2**   Pump systems for continuous delivery of local anesthetics in peripheral nerve blocks; bolus delivery is also possible. Pegasus Vario-PCA (LogoMed); Deltec CADD Legacy PCA (SIMS Deltec).

Elastomer pumps are also gaining increasing interest; these are filled with a certain volume of local anesthetic (usually 250 ml) and infuse the local anesthetic solution at a fixed delivery rate (e.g., 5 or 10 ml/h). These systems work very reliably, but a bolus delivery by the patient is not possible with most of the currently available systems.

Syringe Pumps/Infusion Pumps

The following are proven examples.
Syringe pumps
- PCAM P5000 (Alaris Medical Systems)
- Perfusor syringes 60-100 ml (BD)
  (Fig.17.**1**)

Infusion pumps (Figs. 17.**2**, 17.**3**)
- Deltec CADD Legacy PCA (SIMS Deltec)
- Rythmic PCAP (Alaris Medical Systems)
- Multifuse PCA (B Braun)
- Pegasus Vario-PCA (LogoMed)
- Graseby 9300 PCA (Graseby)
- I-Pump-System (Baxter)
- Microject Pump (Arrow)

Most of these pump systems can be used in conjunction with the Polybag 200 ml Naropin 0.2 % (2 mg/ml) (Astra Zeneca).
Mechanical elastomer pumps (disposable) (Fig.17.**4**)
- Baxter
- Accufusor
- B Braun

Care of Peripheral Pain Catheters in a General Ward

The requirements for care of catheters for peripheral continuous nerve blocks are fundamentally the same as for neuraxial catheters. However, special features differing from neuraxial blockades must be taken into account.

Changes of the syringes or local anesthetic bags and tubing or filters can in principle be delegated to nonmedical staff, provided this staff has sufficient knowledge and experience with regard to possible complications, side effects, and first measures in case of incidents (Van Aken et al. 2001). Accordingly, approved training as a specialist nurse

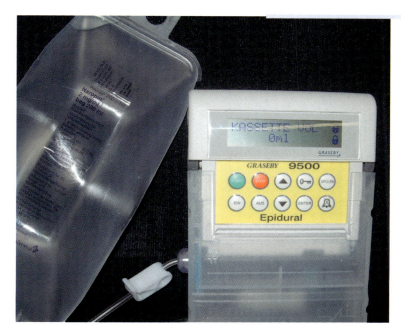
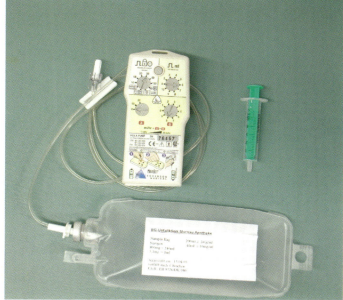

Fig. 17.**3** Pump systems for continuous delivery of local anesthetics in peripheral nerve blocks; bolus delivery is also possible. Graseby 9300 PCA (Graseby); Microject Pump (Arrow).

Fig. 17.**4** Mechanical elastomer pumps (disposable items) for continuous delivery of local anesthetic in peripheral nerve blocks. The pumps are filled with the desired substance (e.g., ropivacaine 0.2–0.33 % [2–3 mg/ ml]; filling volume up to 250 ml), and then release the LA at a defined rate (e.g., 10 ml/h).

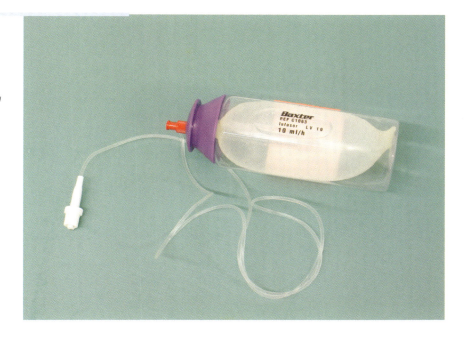

in anesthesia/intensive care is not required, but it is necessary to check qualifications before delegating tasks and to ensure the availability of a specialist doctor at short notice during all procedures. Which doctor is responsible for instruction and checking qualifications depends on the organization of pain therapy in the individual hospital. A clear agreement between the specialist departments and nursing services management on competence and areas of responsibility is strongly recommended.

If analgesia is inadequate, the following causes should be considered:
- A surgical complication
- Catheter dislocation
- Ineffective dose of local anesthetic

Surgical complication: Experience has shown that even with normally effective pain catheters, complications such as compartment syndrome or infection may lead to an above-average requirement for local anesthetic or additional analgesics. Uncritical augmentation of the block can be dangerous in this situation. Instead, the surgeon should be informed in order to assess the situation. *Catheter dislocation:* The original stimulation depth of the needle and the length of catheter inserted should be noted to facilitate detection of dislocation. However, advancement of the catheter too far can also be the cause of inadequate analgesia. Thus, an interscalene plexus catheter that has been advanced too far can cause a complete

motor and sensory block in the hand, but with persistent pain in the region of the operated shoulder. A successful block can be achieved by retracting the catheter ca. 3 cm (from an original depth of ca. 9 cm). Occasionally, a catheter that has been advanced too far beyond the tip of the needle may move away from the target nerves. In this case, too, withdrawal to about the depth at which the nerve was originally stimulated with the needle can lead to successful analgesia. If there are doubts about the correct position of a regional pain catheter, a single effective dose of local anesthetic can be given to check whether a successful block occurs. If this is not the case, the catheter should be removed.

Peripheral Nerve Catheters for Outpatient Regional Pain Management

Operations associated with considerable postoperative pain are more frequently performed on an outpatient basis. A precondition for this is, of course, adequate postoperative pain therapy (Ghosh and Sallam 1994; Wedderburn et al. 1996). In addition to their high degree of effectiveness, the advantages of peripheral nerve catheters, particularly for outpatient postoperative pain therapy, include the lack of respiratory depression and significantly less nausea and vomiting (versus opioids).

These two factors often make early discharge impossible in the outpatient area; this is often the case when regional pain therapy is lacking (Candido et al. 2001; Grant et al. 2001; Ilfeld and Enneking 2002; Ilfeld et al. 2002a; Klein 2002; Klein et al. 2001; Krone et al. 2001; Mulroy et al. 2001; Rawal 2001; Rawal et al. 2002). Significant superiority was shown for postoperative pain therapy by continuous peripheral nerve block in the outpatient area compared to conventional pain therapy (Illfeld et al. 2002a, 2002b; Rawal et al. 2002). These advantages were

- Less pain
- Less sleep disturbance
- Less need for analgesics
- Fewer side effects (nausea, gastrointestinal symptoms, etc.)
- Greater general satisfaction (of patients and medical staff)

In these studies, no local anesthetic- or catheter-related complications were observed.

A precondition for continuous peripheral regional analgesia in the outpatient area is a properly informed and cooperative patient. A competent contact person must be available around the clock and the distance to the responsible clinic should be reasonably short, so that the patient can easily go there in the event of problems that cannot be resolved by telephone. For the ambulant area, disposable elastomer pumps are available that allow continuous administration with a fixed basic rate (Infuser LV5/10, capacity 250 ml, Baxter; Easy pump C-block RA, capacity 400 ml, B Braun). The advantage of these disposable infusion pumps is their low occurrence of malfunction (Capdevila #et al. 2003); a disadvantage is that some of them do not allow a change in administration pattern, e.g., to bolus.

The patient must be given adequate detailed information, both verbal and written, about risks and problems that can arise

It is important to always select a concentration of local anesthetic that enables the patient to preserve some residual sensation and maintains motor function optimally.

This appears to be the case with 0.2% (2 mg/ml) ropivacaine. The limb must nevertheless be well padded to prevent any position-related nerve damage (ulnar nerve injury, fibular nerve injury). In using blocks of the lower limb it is assumed that patients are capable of completely relieving the affected limb from loading using crutches since there is a risk of falling when sensation and/or motor function are limited.

Telephone contact should be made with the patient at least once a day. The patient must be informed about possible changes at the puncture site that might indicate developing infection. In this case patients must be informed that they should make contact with the responsible doctor promptly. Removal of the catheter should be performed by a competent person who can make a correct assessment.

Complications of Peripheral Nerve Catheters for Pain Management

Infection

All continuous peripheral nerve catheters are at risk for infection. Superficial erythema of the puncture site is observed with an incidence of 5–10% (Meier et al. 1997). Major infections occur in < 1% of cases (Fig.17.**5**). The following preventive measures should be observed:

- Absolute asepsis when placing the catheter
- Daily inspection of the puncture site

Crucial evidence is not so much erythema but rather pain in the region of the puncture site and secretions draining from the puncture site (not to be confused with local anesthetic, which occasionally flows backward through the puncture site). Pain in the region of the puncture site should be given particular consideration as this is the most sensitive indicator of early infection. In case of doubt, the catheter should be removed as soon as possible, and antibiotic therapy should be considered. Usually the infection is caused by *Staphylococcus aureus* and/or *Staphylococcus epidermidis*, which have high sensitivity to antibiotics. The patient should be continuously monitored in the following days as an abscess can develop even after removal of the catheter. If an abscess is present, surgical intervention may be required.

Nerve Injury due to Peripheral Catheters

There is no information reported on the incidence of nerve injury due to peripheral nerve catheters for continuous pain treatment. A question as yet unresolved is how long a patient should be observed in order to check whether there is a nerve injury due to the puncture or the catheter. Occasionally, the surgeon wants to perform a postopera-

tive neurological assessment. In this case it is advisable to perform the block with a medium-acting local anesthetic, and then, after neurological examination, start continuous infusion of the local anesthetic (after giving an adequate bolus). In such cases, ropivacaine, with its better sensory-motor separation, is recommended.

Catheter Tear, Looping

Rupture or accidental shearing of peripheral nerve catheters has been described (Lee and Goucke 2002). These complications can occur during catheter placement, particularly when the catheter with guide wire is withdrawn before removal of the needle through which the catheter was introduced. Accordingly, the needle must always be withdrawn before the guide wire is removed. When catheters have been secured with a skin suture, it is essential to ensure that the catheter is not ruptured at removal. It is a matter of discussion whether accidental catheter rupture or tearing during removal should be approached surgically. Removal can sometimes be extremely difficult, and a preoperative CT scan can occasionally be very helpful in locating the catheter. In any case, the operation should be performed in the operating theater under the general conditions of an operation, and with adequate anesthesia.

When it is threaded too far, knots and looping of the catheter are possible (Krebs and Hempel 1984). If persistent resistance occurs during removal of the catheter, the procedure should be stopped and a radiograph with contrast performed. In this case the catheter may have to be removed surgically.

Duration In Situ of Peripheral Nerve Catheters for Pain Management

The time for which peripheral pain catheters are left in situ should be kept as short as possible because of the risk of infection. The average duration is generally reported as 4–6 days (Büttner et al. 1989a; Meier et al. 1997). The necessity of the pain catheter must be reevaluated daily. If in doubt, a "cessation trial" can clarify the question of further need for the catheter. For chronic pain therapy, average maintenance of 37.4 days with a maximum of 240 days has been reported (Schreiber et al. 1997). In these cases, subcutaneous tunneling of the catheter is recommended. Subcutaneous implantation of a port system for axillary block for long-term analgesia in patients with CRPS I and II has also been described (Aguilar et al. 1995, 1998). The longest duration was 16 months.

Meier and colleagues have presented the results of 3683 peripheral nerve catheters taking into account the duration in situ and complications. These are summarized in Table 17.**3**.

Fig. 17.**5**   Abscess after continuous peripheral nerve block; pain is often the first early
sign of local inflammation and must be carefully investigated.

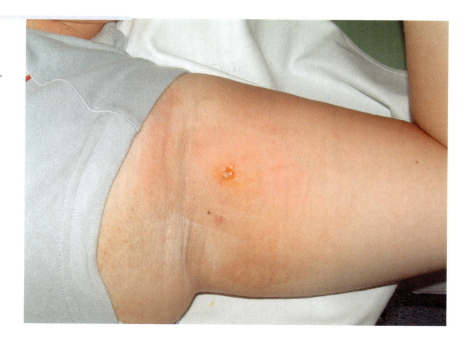

Table 17.**3**   Results of 3683 peripheral nerve
catheters

Technique	Number	Age (years) (mean)	Chronic Polyar-thritis	Days in situ (average)	Incorrect Position	Successful Correction
Interscalene plexus	206	56 (max. 82)	88%	5.6 (max. 20)	11 (5.3%)	6 (55%)
Axillary plexus	2769	52 (max. 83)	89%	4.4 (max. 23)	110 (3.9%)	65 (63%)
"3 in 1"	405	43 (max. 80)	83%	5.1 (max. 23)	10 (2.5%)	6 (60%)
Sciatic (distal)	303	56 (max. 82)	81%	4.5 (max. 21)	26 (8.5%)	21 (81%)
Total	3683	52	85%	5.0	157 (5.0%)	98 (65%)

Technique	Dislocation	Local Inflamma-tion	Abscess	Systemic Infection	Patient Satisfac-tion
Interscalene plexus	8 (4%)	6 (3%)	0	0	96%
Axillary plexus	120 (4%)	120 (4%)	2	0	95%
"3 in 1"	18 (4%)	20 (5%)	0	0	96%
Sciatic (distal)	9 (3%)	15 (5%)	0	0	94%
Total	4%	4%	0.05%	0	95%

Documentation

Full recording and documentation of all
regional pain catheters is essential. A central
record of all catheters currently in action is
required (e.g., recovery room, computer-
assisted record). This enables daily monitoring of all patients and thus documentation
of all problems and complications. To prevent any gaps arising in the information,
each patient should receive a special form
for documentation of dosages and special
features (Fig. 17.**6**).

Trauma Center Murnau
Department of Anesthesia
Pain Service

Name:_____   Regional anesthesia:_____

Date of birth:_____   Date inserted:_____

Ward:_____Room no.:_   Skin–nerve space:_____

Indication:_____   Distance catheter tip–skin(cm):_____

Date	Time	Anesthetic agent mg/ml	ml/h	Insertion site	Patient condition	VAS at rest	VAS with motion	Sig.

Catheter removed (date):   Bacteria test: yes O, no O
                                  Results   pos O   neg O

Comments:_____

                                  Signature:

VAS (Visual analog scale): 0 = no pain; 10 = maximum imaginable pain

Fig. 17.**6**   Example of a documentation sheet for recording control of patient with a peripheral pain catheter.

References, Chapters 14–17

Aguilar JL, Domingo V, Samper D. Long term brachial plexus anesthesia using a subcutaneous implantable injection system. Reg Anesth. 1995:20:242-5.

Aguilar JL, Mendiola MA, Valdivia J. Long-term continuous axillary brachial plexus blockade using an implanted port In: Urmey WF, ed. Techniques in regional anesthesia and pain management. Philadelphia: Saunders; 1998:74-8.

Altintas F, Gumus F, Kaya G et al. Interscalene brachial plexus block with bupivacaine and ropivacaine in patients with chronic renal failure: Diaphragmatic excursion and pulmonary function changes. Anesth Analg. 2005;100:1166-71

Auroy Y, Narchi P, Messiah A. Serious complications related to regional anesthesia. Anesthesiology. 1997;87:479-86.

Ben-David B, Stahl S. Axillary block complicated by hematoma and radial nerve injury. Reg Anesth Pain Med. 1999;24:264-6

Bernard JM, Macair P. Dose-range effects of clonidine added to lidocaine for brachial plexus block. Anesthesiology. 1997;87:277-84.

Bone HG, Van Aken H, Brooke M. Enhancement of axillary brachial plexus block anesthesia by coadministration of neostigmine. Reg Anesth Pain Med. 1999;24:405-10.

Borgeat A, Schäppi B, Biasca N. Patient-controlled analgesia after major shoulder surgery. Anesthesiology. 1997;87:1343-7.

Borgeat A, Kalberer F, Jacob H. Patient-controlled interscalene analgesia with ropivacaine 0.2% versus bupivacaine 0.15% after major open shoulder surgery: The effects on hand motor function. Anesth Analg. 2001;92:218-23.

Borgeat A, Dullenkopf A, Ekatodramis G, Nagy L. Evaluation of the lateral modified approach for continuous interscalene block after shoulder surgery. Anesthesiology. 2003;99:436-42

Bouaziz H, Kinirons BP, Macalou D, et al. Sufentanil does not prolong the duration of analgesia in a mepivacaine brachial plexus block: A dose response study. Anesth Analg. 2000;90:383-7.

Brown DL. Anatomic imaging: Seeing into the future. Reg Anesth. 1998;23:529-30.

Büttner J, Klose R. Alkalinisierung von Mepivacain zur axillären Katheterplexusanaesthesie. Reg Anaesth. 1991;14:17-24.

Büttner J, Klose R, Hammer. Die kontinuierliche axilläre Plexusanästhesie - eine Methode zur postoperativen Analgesie und Sympathikolyse nach handchirurgischen Eingriffen. Handchir Mikrochir Plast Chir. 1989a;21:29-32.

Büttner J, Klose R, Hoppe. Serum levels of mepivacaine-HCl during continuous axillary brachial plexus block. Reg Anesth. 1989b;14:124-7.

Büttner J, Ott B, Klose R. Der Einfluss von Clonidinzusatz zu Mepivacain: Axilläre Plexus-brachialis-Blockade. Anaesthesist. 1992;41:548-54.

Candido KD, Winnie AP, Covino BG. Addition of bicarbonate to plain bupivacaine does not significantly alter the onset or duration of plexus anesthesia. Reg Anesth. 1995;20:133-8.

Candido KD, Franco CD, Khan MA, et al. Buprenorphine added to the local anesthetic for brachial plexus block to provide postoperative analgesia in outpatients. Reg Anesth Pain Med. 2001;26:352-6.

Capdevila X, Barthelet Y, Biboulet P. Effects of perioperative analgesic technique on the surgical outcome and duration of rehabilitation after major knee surgery. Anesthesiology. 1999;91:8-15.

Capdevila X, Macaire Ph, Aknin PH. Patient controlled perineural analgesia after ambulatory orthopedic surgery: a comparison of electronic versus elastomeric pumps. Anesth Analg. 2003;96:414-7.

Capogna G, Celleno D, Laudano D. Alkalization of local anesthetics. Which block, which local anesthetic? Reg Anesth. 1995;20:369-77.

Casati A, Fanelli G, Borghi B. Ropivacaine or 2% mepivacaine for lower limb peripheral nerve blocks. Anesthesiology. 1999;90:1047-52.

Casati A, Fanelli G, Albertin A, et al. Interscalene brachial plexus anesthesia with either 0.5% ropivacaine or 0.5% bupivacaine. Minerva Anesthesiol. 2000a;66:39-44.

Casati A, Magistris L, Fanelli G, et al. Small-dose clonidine prolongs postoperative analgesia after sciatic-femoral nerve block with 0.75% ropivacaine for foot surgery. Anesth Analg. 2000b;91:388-92.

Casati A, Fanelli G, Magistris L. Minimum local anesthetic volume blocking the femoral nerve in 50% of cases: a double-blinded comparison between 0.5% ropivacaine and 0.5% bupivacaine. Anesth Analg. 2001;92:205-8.

Cheney FW, Domino KB, Caplan RA. Nerve injury associated with anesthesia. Anesthesiology. 1999;90:1062-9.

Chow MY, Sia ATH, Koay CK. Alkalinization of lidocaine does not hasten the onset of axillary brachial plexus block. Anesth Analg. 1998;86:566-8.

Choyce A, Cahan VWS, Middleton WJ, Knight PR, McCartney CJL. What is the relationship between paresthesia and nerve stimulation for axillary brachial plexus block? Reg Anesth Pain Med. 2001;26:100-4.

Cockings E, Moore PL, Lewis RC. Transarterial brachial plexus blockade using high doses of 1.5% mepivacaine. Reg Anesth. 1987;12:159-64.

Comfort VK, Lang SA, Yip RW. Saphenous nerve anesthesia—a nerve stimulator technique. Can J Anaesth. 1996;43:852-7.

Coventry DM, Todd JG. Alkalinization of bupivacaine for sciatic nerve blockade. Anaesthesia. 1989;44:467-70.

Cuvillon P, Ripart J, LaLourcey L et al. The continuous femoral nerve block catheter for postoperative analgesia: bacterial colonization, infectious rate and adverse effects. Anesth Analg. 2001;93:1045-9

D'Angelo R, James RL. Is ropivacaine less toxic than bupivacaine? [Editorial]. Anesthesiology. 1999;90:941-3.

DiOrio S, Ellis R. Comparison of pH-adjusted and plain solutions of mepivacaine for brachial plexus anaesthesia [Abstract]. Reg Anesth. 1988;13:1S-3.

Dreesen H, Büttner J, Klose R. Wirkungsvergleich und Serumspiegel von Mepivacain-HCl und Mepivacain-CO$_2$ bei axillärer Plexus-brachialis-Anaesthesie. Reg Anaesth. 1986;9:42-5.

El Saied AH, Steyn MP, Ansermino JM. Clonidine prolongs the effect of ropivacaine for axillary brachial plexus blockade. Can J Anaesth. 2000;47:962-7.

Erlacher W, Schuschnig C, Orlicek F. The effects of clonidine on ropivacaine 0.75% in axillary perivascular brachial plexus block. Acta Anaesthesiol Scand. 2000;44:53-7.

Eroglu A, Uzunlar H, Sener M, Akinturk Y, Erciyes N. A clinical comparison of equal concentration and volume of ropivacaine and bupivacaine for interscalene brachial plexus anesthesia and analgesia in shoulder surgery. Reg Anesth Pain Med 2004; 29:539-43.

Fanelli G, Casati A, Garancini P. Nerve stimulator and multiple injection technique for upper and lower limb blockade: Failure rate, patient acceptance, and neurologic complications. Anesth Analg. 1999;88:847-52.

Ford DJ, Pither CE, Raj P. Comparison of insulated and uninsulated needles for locating peripheral nerve stimulator. Anesth Analg. 1984; 63:925-8.

Fulling PD, Peterfreund RA. Alkalinization and precipitation characteristics of 0.2% ropivacaine. Reg Anesth Pain Med. 2000;25:518-21.

Gentili M, Bernard JM, Bonnet F. Adding clonidine to lidocaine for intravenous regional anesthesia prevents tourniquet pain. Anesth Analg. 1999;88:1327-30.

Ghosh S, Sallam S. Patient satisfaction and postoperative demands on hospital admission and community services after day surgery. Br J Surg. 1994;81:1635-8.

Gogarten W, Van Aken H, Büttner J. Rückenmarksnahe Regionalanästhesie und Thromboembolieprophylaxe/antithrombotische Medikation. Anasthesiol Intensivmed. 2003;44:218-30.

Gormley WP, Hill DA, Murray JM. The effect of alkalinisation of lignocaine on axillary brachial plexus anaesthesia. Anaesthesia. 1996;51:185-8.

Graf BM, Martin E. Periphere Nervenblockaden - Eine Übersicht über neue Entwicklungen einer alten Technik. Anaesthesist. 2001;50:312-22.

Grant S, Nielsen KC, Greengrass RA, et al. Continuous peripheral nerve block for ambulatory surgery. Reg Anesth Pain Med. 2001;26:209-14.

Greengrass RA, Klein SM, D'Ercole JF. Lumbar plexus and sciatic nerve block for knee arthroplasty: comparison of ropivacaine and bupivacaine. Can J Anaesth. 1998;45:1094-6.

Hadzic A, Vloka JD, Claudio RE, Hadzic N, Thys DM, Santos AC. Electrical nerve localization. Effects of cutaneous placement and duration of the stimulus on motor response. Anesthesiology. 2004;100:1526-30

Heath PJ, Brownlie GS, Herrick MJ. Latency of brachial plexus block, the effect on onset time of warming local anaesthetic solutions. Anaesthesia. 1990;45:297-301.

Hebl JR, Horlocker TT, Pritchard DJ. Diffuse brachial plexopathy after interscalene blockade in a patient receiving cisplatin chemotherapy: The pharmacologic double crush syndrome. Anesth Analg. 2001;92:249-51.

Hempel V, Baur KF. Regionalanästhesie für Schulter, Arm und Hand. München: Urban & Schwarzenberg; 1982.

Hempel V. Interscalenusblock bei Infektionen der Schulter. Anaesthesist. 1998;47:940.

Hickey R, Rowley CL, Candido KD. A comparative study of 0.25% ropivacaine and 0.25% bupivacaine for brachial plexus block. Anesth Analg. 1992;75:602-6.

Hilgier M. Alkalinization of bupivacaine for brachial plexus block. Reg Anesth. 1985;8:59-61.

Hirasawa Y, Katsuni Y, Küsswetter W, Sprotte G. Experimentelle Untersuchungen zu peripheren Nervenverletzungen durch Injektionsnadeln. Reg Anaesth. 1990;13:11-5.

Holas A, Krafft P, Marcovic M. Remifentanil, propofol or both for conscious sedation during eye surgery under regional anaesthesia. Eur J Anaesth. 1999;16:741-8.

Horlocker T, O'Driscoll SW, Dinapoli RP. Recurring brachial plexus neuropathy in a diabetic patient after shoulder surgery and continuous interscalene block. Anesth Analg. 2000;91:688-90.

Horlocker TT. Regional anesthesia in the anticoagulated patient. Defining the risks. (The second ASRA consensus conference on neuraxial anesthesia and anticoagulation.) Reg Anesth Pain Med. 2003;28:172-97.

Ilfeld BM, Enneking FK. A portable mechanical pump providing over four days of patient-controlled analgesia by perineural infusion at home. Reg Anesth Pain Med. 2002;27:100-4.

Ilfeld BM, Moery T, Enneking F. Continuous infraclavicular brachial plexus block for postoperative pain control at home. Anesthesiology. 2002a;96:1297-304.

Ilfeld BM, Morey T, Wang RD. Continuous popliteal sciatic nerve block for postoperative pain control at home. Anesthesiology. 2002b;97:959-65.

Ilfeld BM, Timothy E, Wright TW, Chidgey LK, Enneking FK. Continuous interscalene brachial plexus block for postoperative pain control at home: A randomized, double-blinded, placebo-controlled study. Anesth Analg 2003;96:1089-95.

Ilfeld BM, Morey TE, Enneking FK. Continuous infraclavicular perineural infusion with clonidine and ropivacaine compared with ropivacaine alone: a randomized, double-blinded, controlled study. Anesth Analg. 2003;97:706-12.

Ilfeld BM, Timothy E, Wright TW, Chidgey LK, Enneking FK. Interscalene perineural ropivacaine infusion: A comparison of two dosing regimens for postoperative analgesia. Reg Anesth Pain Med 2004;29:9-16.

Ilfeld BM, More TY, Thanikkary LJ, Wright TW, Enneking FK. Clonidine added to a continuous interscalene ropivacaine perineural infusion to improve postoperative analgesia: A randomized, double-blind, controlled study. Anesth Analg. 2005;100:1172-8.

Iohom G, Machmachi A, Diarra DP et al. The effects of clonidine added to mepivacaine for paronychia surgery under axillary brachial plexus block. Anesth Analg. 2005;100:1179-83.

Irwin MG, Thompson N, Kenny GNC. Patient-maintained propofol sedation. Assessment of a target-controlled infusion system. Anaesthesia. 1997;52:525-30.

Janzen PRM, Hall WJ, Hopkins PM. Setting targets for sedation with a target-controlled propofol infusion. Anaesthesia. 2000;55:666-9.

Jöhr M. Späte Komplikation der kontinuierlichen Blockade des N. femoralis. Reg Anaesth. 1987;10:37-8.

Kaiser H. Periphere elektrische Nervenstimulation. In: Niesel HC, Van Aken H, eds. Lokalanästhesie, Regionalanästhesie, Regionale Schmerztherapie, 2 nd ed. Stuttgart: Thieme; 2003:140-59.

Klein SM. Beyond the hospital: continuous peripheral nerve blocks at home [Editorial]. Anesthesiology. 2002;96:1283-4.

Klein SM, D'Ercole F, Greengrass RA. Enoxaparin associated with psoas hematoma and lumbar plexopathy after lumbar plexus block. Anesthesiology. 1997;87:1576-9.

Klein SM, Greengrass RA, Steele SM, et al. A comparison of 0.5% bupivacaine, 0.5% ropivacaine, and 0.75% ropivacaine for interscalene brachial plexus block. Anesth Analg. 1998;87:1316-9.

Klein SM, Nielsen KC, Martin A, et al. Interscalene brachial plexus block with continuous intraarticular infusion of ropivacaine. Anesth Analg. 2001;93:601-5.

Krebs P, Hempel V. Eine neue Kombinationsnadel für die hohe axilläre Plexus-brachialis-Anästhesie. Anasthesiol Intensivmed. 1984;25:219.

Krebs P, Hempel V. Mepivacain zur axillären Plexusanästhesie. Reg Anaesth. 1985;8:33-5.

Krone SC, Chan VW, Regan J, et al. Analgesic effects of low-dose ropivacaine for interscalene brachial plexus block for outpatient shoulder surgery: a dose finding study. Reg Anesth Pain Med. 2001;26:439-43.

Lauwers M, Camu F, Breivik H, et al. The safety and effectiveness of remifentanil as an adjunct sedative for regional anesthesia. Anesth Analg. 1999;88:134-40.

Lee BH, Goucke CR. Shearing of a peripheral nerve catheter. Anesth Analg. 2002;95:760-1.

Magistris L, Casati A, Albertin A, et al. Combined sciatic-femoral nerve block with 0.75% ropivacaine: effects of adding a systemically inactive dose of fentanyl. Eur J Anaesth. 2000;17:348-53.

Malamut RI, Marques W, Engl JD. Postsurgical idiopathic brachial neuritis. Muscle Nerve. 1994;17:320-4.

Marhofer P, Greher M, Kapral S. Ultrasound guidance in regional anaesthesia. Br J Anaesth 2005;94:1-3.

Meier G, Bauereis C, Heinrich C. Der interscalenäre Plexuskatheter zur Anästhesie und postoperativen Schmerztherapie. Anaesthesist. 1997;46:715-9.

Meyer J, Herrmann M. Prävention katheteras-soziierter Infektionen. Anaesthesist. 1998;47:136-42.

Mezzatesta JP, Scott DA, Schweitzer SA. Continuous axillary brachial plexus block for postoperative pain relief—intermittent bolus versus continuous infusion. Reg Anesth. 1997;22:357-62.

Milner QJ, Guard BC, Allen JG. Alkalinizaton of amide local anesthetics by addition of 1% sodium bicarbonate solution. Eur J Anaesthesiol. 2000;17:38-42.

Mulroy MF, Larkin KL, Batra MS, et al. Femoral nerve block with 0.25 or 0.5% bupivacaine improves postoperative analgesia following outpatient arthroscopic anterior cruciate ligament repair. Reg Anesth Pain Med. 2001;26:24-9.

Murphy DB, McCartney CJ, Chan VW. Novel analgesic adjuncts for brachial plexus block: A systematic review. Anesth Analg. 2000;90:1122-8.

Neal JM. How close is close enough? Defining the "paresthesia chad" [Editorial]. Reg Anesth Pain Med. 2001;26:97-9.

Neuburger M, Rotzinger M, Kaiser H. Elektrische Nervenstimulation in Abhängigkeit von der benutzten Impulsbreite. Anaesthesist. 2001;50:181-6.

Nishikawa K, Kanaya N, Nakayama M. Fentanyl improves analgesia but prolongs the onset of axillary brachial plexus block by peripheral mechanism. Anesth Analg. 2000;91:384-7.

Nseir S, Pronnier P, Soubrier S et al. Fatal streptococcal necrotizing fasciitis as a complication of axillary brachial plexus block. Br J Anesth. 2004;92:427-9.

Otaki C, Hayashi H, Amano M. Ultrasound-guided infraclavicular brachial plexus block: an alternative technique to anatomical landmark-guided approaches. Reg Anesth Pain Med. 2000;25:600-4.

Pham-Dang C, Kick O, Collet T et al. Continuous peripheral nerve blocks with stimulating catheters. Reg Anesth Pain Med. 2003;28:83-8.

Quinlan JJ, Oleksey K, Murphy FL. Alkalinization of mepivacaine for axillary block. Anesth Analg. 1992;74:371-4.

Rawal N. Patient-controlled regional analgesia at home. Techniques in Regional Anesthesia and Pain Management. 2000;62-6.

Rawal N. Analgesia for day-case surgery. Br J Anaesth. 2001;87:73-87.

Rawal N, Hylander J, Nydahl PA. Survey of postoperative analgesia following ambulatory surgery. Acta Anaesthesiol Scand. 1997;41:1017-22.

Rawal N, Alvin R, Axelsson K, et al. Patient-controlled regional analgesia (PCRA) at home. Anesthesiology. 2002;96:1290-6.

Rodgers A, Walker N, Schug S, et al. Reduction of postoperative mortality and morbidity with epidural or spinal anaesthesia: results from overview of randomized trials. BMJ. 2000;321:1-12.

Rosenberg PH, Veering B Th, Urmey WF. Maximum recommended doses of local anesthetics: a multifactorial concept. Reg Anesth Pain Med. 2004;29:564-75.

Salonen MH, Haasio J, Bachmann M. Evaluation of efficacy and plasma concentrations of ropivacaine in continuous axillary brachial plexus block: High dose for surgical anesthesia and low dose for postoperative analgesia. Reg Anesth Pain Med. 2000;25:47-51.

Schreiber T, Meissner W, Ullrich K. Continuous vertical infraclavicular brachial plexus block: an alternative to the axillary plexus catheter? [Abstract]. Int Monitor Reg Anaesth. 1997;9(3):49.

Schwarz U, Zenz M, Strumpf M, Junger S. Braucht man wirklich einen Nervenstimulator für regionale Blockaden? Anästhesiol Intensivmed. 1998;12:609-15.

Selander D, Dhuner KG, Lundborg G. Peripheral nerve injury due to injection needles used for regional anesthesia. Acta Anaesthesiol Scand. 1977;21:182-8.

Selander D. Peripheral nerve injury caused by injection needles. B J Anaesth. 1993;71:323.

Simon MA, Gielen MJ, Lagerwerf AJ. Plasma concentrations after high doses of mepivacaine with epinephrine in combined psoas compartment/sciatic nerve block. Reg Anesth. 1990;15:256-60.

Singelyn FJ, Gouverneur JM. Extended "three-in-one" block after total knee arthroplasty: continuous versus patient-controlled techniques. Anesth Analg. 2000;91:176-80.

Singelyn FJ, Gouverneur JM, Robert A. A minimum dose of clonidine added to mepivacaine prolongs the duration of anaesthesia and analgesia after axillary brachial plexus block. Anesth Analg. 1996;83:1046-50.

Singelyn FJ, Deyaert M, Joris D. Effects of intravenous patient-controlled analgesia with morphine, continuous epidural analgesia, and continuous three-in-one block on postoperative pain and knee rehabilitation after unilateral knee arthroplasty. Anesth Analg. 1998;87:88-92.

Singelyn FJ, Seguy S, Gouverneur JM. Interscalene brachial plexus analgesia after open shoulder surgery: Continuous versus patient-controlled infusion. Anesth Analg. 1999;89:1216-20.

Stan TC, Krantz MA, Solomon DL. The incidence of neurovascular complications following axillary brachial plexus block using a transarterial approach. Reg Anesth. 1995;20:486-92.

Stöhr M. Iatrogene Nervenläsionen. 2nd ed. Stuttgart: Thieme; 1996.

Sutcliffe N. Sedation during loco-regional anaesthesia. Acta Anaesth Belg. 2000;51:153-6.

Sztark F, Malgat M, Dabadie P. Comparison of the effects of bupivacaine and ropivacaine on heart cell mitochondrial bioenergetics. Anesthesiology. 1998;88:1340-9.

Sztark F, Nouette-Gaulain K, Dabadie P. Absence of stereospecific effects of bupivacaine isomers on heart mitochondrial bioenergetics. Anesthesiology. 2000;93:456-62.

Tetzlaff JE, Yoon HJ, Brems J, et al. Alkalinization of mepivacaine accelerates onset of interscalene block for shoulder surgery. Reg Anesth. 1990;15:242-4.

Tetzlaff JE, Yoon HJ, Brems J, et al. Alkalinization of mepivacaine improves the quality of interscalene brachial plexus block for shoulder surgery [Abstract]. Anesth Analg. 1993;76:S432.

Tetzlaff JE, Yoon HJ, Brems J, et al. Alkalinization of mepivacaine improves the quality of motor block associated with interscalene brachial plexus anesthesia for shoulder surgery. Reg Anesth. 1995;20:128-32.

Tetzlaff JE, Dilger J, Yap E. Idiopathic brachial plexitis after total shoulder replacement with interscalene brachial plexus block. Anesth Analg. 1997;85:644-6.

Urmey FW. Femoral nerve block for the management of postoperative pain. In: Urmey FW, eds. Techniques in Regional Anesthesia and Pain Management. 1997;2:88-92.

Van Aken H, Klose R, Wulf H. Zum täglichen Wechsel von Spritzenpumpe, Leitung und Filtern bei liegendem Periduralkatheter, Stellungnahme des wissenschaftlichen Arbeitskreises Regionalanästhesie der DGAI. Anasth Intensivmed. 2001;42:973-4.

Wank W, Büttner J, Rissler Maier K. Pharmacokinetics and efficacy of 40 ml ropivacaine 7.5 mg/ml (300 mg), for axillary brachial plexus block—an open pilot study. Eur J Drug Metab Pharmacokinet. 2002;27:53-9.

Wedderburn AW, Morris GE, Dodds SR. A survey of postoperative care after day case surgery. Ann R Coll Surg Engl. 1996;78(2 Suppl):70-1.

Weller RS, Gerancher JC, Crews JC. Extensive retroperitoneal hematoma without neurological deficit in two patients who underwent lumbar plexus block and were later anticoagulated. Anesthesiology. 2003;98:581-5.

Index